Asthma – A Link Between Environment, Immunology, and the Airways

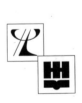

Asthma – A Link Between Environment, Immunology, and the Airways

Proceedings of the XVIth World Congress of Asthma, Buenos Aires, October 17–20, 1999

Edited by
Hugo E. Neffen, Carlos E. Baena-Cagnani, Leonardo Fabbri,
Steven Holgate, Paul O'Byrne

Hogrefe & Huber Publishers
Seattle · Toronto · Bern · Göttingen

Library of Congress Cataloging-in-Publication Data

is available via the Library of Congress Marc Database under the
LC Catalog Card Number 99-65053.

Canadian Cataloguing in Publication Data

World Congress of Asthmology (16th : 1999 : Buenos Aires, Argentina)
    Asthma – a link between environment, immunology, and the airways

Includes index.
ISBN 0-88937-220-9

1. Asthma – Congresses. I. Neffen, Hugo. II. Title.

RC591.W67   1999   616.2'38   C99-931929-9

© Copyright 1999 by Hogrefe & Huber Publishers

USA: P.O. Box 2487, Kirkland, WA 98083-2487
                  Phone (425) 820-1500, Fax (425) 823-8324
CANADA: 12 Bruce Park Avenue, Toronto, Ontario M4P 2S3
                  Phone (416) 482-6339
SWITZERLAND: Länggass-Strasse 76, CH-3000 Bern 9
                  Phone (031) 300-4500, Fax (031) 300-4590
GERMANY: Rohnsweg 25, D-37085 Göttingen
                  Phone (0551) 49609-0, Fax (0551) 49609-88

Printed and bound in Argentina
by Indugraf S.A. - Loria 2251, Buenos Aires.

ISBN 0-88937-220-9

Contents

v

New Technology – Research vs. Clinical Diagnosis

Preface

We are delighted to present this book entitled *Asthma: A Link Between Environment, Immunology, and the Airways*, which represents the proceedings of the XVI World Congress of Asthma organized by INTERASMA, the International Association of Asthmology, in Argentina.

Asthma is a world-wide public health problem. The number of admissions to hospitals, consultations, and prescriptions for asthma drugs are increasing, and asthma mortality rates have risen in various parts of the world. In addition, asthma has an enormous impact on the quality of life of patients and is also a considerable burden from a socio-economic point of view. Therefore, the Scientific Program of the XVI World Congress of Asthma was designed in order to discuss the current evidence-based knowledge on asthma as well as other allergic immunologic, and respiratory-related problems.

The most important advances in the field of asthma, linking the environment, immunology, and the airways, have been included, and the most distinguished basic and clinical researchers have contributed to this book.

The concept of asthma inflammation and the role of the various components driving this inflammation, for instance, the bronchial mucosa, the airway smooth muscle, and neurogenic factors, have been clarified in recent decades. Despite the fact that many questions have not yet been answered, a considerable understanding of the pathophysiology of asthma has been gained. The allergic basis of its pathogenesis, including the role of Th2 lymphocytes, eosinophils, cytokines, adhesion molecules, transcription factors, and chemokines, is currently better understood. Nevertheless, certain types of asthma with neutrophilic inflammation still have to be clarified; these are also discussed in this book.

Environmental factors, indoor and outdoor pollutants, allergens, and smoking all play important roles in asthma, as has been shown in various experimental and epidemiological studies. The interface between environmental factors, the immune system, and airways is the key to understanding the expression of the asthma phenotype in susceptible individuals.

There is also very important news concerning the epidemiology of asthma. The ISAAC study and the European Community Respiratory Health Survey (ECRHS) have provided reliable information on the prevalence and severity of asthma. Other elegant cohort and cross-sectional studies are helping us to understand the magnitude of the "asthma epidemic," its geographical variability, likely causal factors, and the natural history of the disease.

The diagnosis and treatment of asthma is, of course, a very sensitive issue. New developments are helping us to learn what is happening in the airways of asthma patients, while different "markers of asthma" are being extensively studied. New drugs, such as leukotriene receptor antagonists, the clinical usefulness of combination therapy, such as inhaled corticosteroids with long-acting β_2 agonists, and new developments like humanized anti-IgE monoclonal antibodies and anti-IL-5, or allergen peptides for allergic vaccines are providing promising perspectives for the treatment of asthma.

This book deals with all these and many other fascinating topics as we approach the close of a century that has been full of success and discoveries in the field of asthma. However, many doubts about etiology and pathogenesis that remain to be understood will go through to the next millennium. Our wish is that this book may contribute to encouraging new questions and new research – to looking for a better understanding and more answers about asthma in the new millennium.

Hugo E. Neffen
President of the Congress

Carlos E. Baena-Cagnani
President, Scientific Committee

Asthma: A Challenge for the Next Millennium

Stephen Holgate*

Introduction

In his classical treatise on *Asthma: Its Pathology and Treatment*, first published in 1859, Dr. Henry Hyde Salter described asthma as an episodic disorder of the airways causing intermittent breathlessness, with healthy breathing between attacks [1]. This concept of asthma became widely accepted with the disease being considered a disorder of airways smooth muscle which contracted too much and too easily. From a therapeutic standpoint, drugs were identified that relaxed the constricted airways (bronchodilators) such as ephedrine, theophylline and adrenaline. The discovery of α and β adrenoceptors by Ahlquist in 1948 [2] led to a further refinement with the synthesis of isoprenaline (isopreterenol) which was produced as an inhaled formulation and found wide popularity in the 1960s. However, between 1963 and 1966 links of excess isoprenaline to increased asthma mortality [3] drove further drug discovery and the identification by Lands in 1967 [4] of subtypes of the β receptor (β_1 and β_2) and the subsequent development of both short and long acting β_2 agonists for inhalation. Undoubtedly these drugs have provided asthmatic patients with highly effective medications for relieving asthma symptoms, but a salutary lesson was learnt, again in the early 1980s, when excess mortality in New Zealand was again linked to over prescribing of an inhaled β_2 agonist [5]. It seems unlikely that this drug class will be improved upon much further although, as with all inhaled drugs, there is still room for better methods for delivering drugs to the airways and, therefore, optimizing drug effect.

The Era of Drugs to Prevent or Control Asthma

In 1967 Howell and Altounyan reported the first clinical trial on the efficacy of sodium cromoglycate (a derivative of Khellin) in preventing episodes of asthma. At about the same time, Pepys described the early and late asthmatic response to allergen challenge and the ability of cromoglycate to inhibit both responses [7]. Although there continues to be an ongoing debate regarding the cellular target for cromoglycate's efficacy, there is general agreement that the mast cell is at least one target [8]. However, sodium cromoglycate and related drugs (e. g., nedocromil sodium) are relatively weak inhibitors of human mast cell function. With the knowledge that there are pivotal biochemical mechanisms that can uncouple IgE-high affinity receptor signalling in mast cells (e. g., SHP-1, SHP-2, SHIP-1) [9], there is still ample opportunity to create more effective mast cell stabilizing drugs for asthma and related disorders.

Throughout the last two decades, inhaled corticosteroids have provided the bedrock for modern asthma management with their capacity to reduce airway inflammation and improve asthma control through "anti-inflammatory pathways," probably involving inhibition of cytokine-mediated transcription factor activation (e. g., NF-κB, AP-1). Topical corticosteroids have been progressively improved both in potency and efficacy, but concerns are still raised over adverse systemic effects, especially in those with mild disease. While it is possible that structure activity studies will further improve the therapeutic index of this drug class, a more promising approach is the separation of transrepression from transcription functions, the anti-inflammatory effects being mediated via transrepression (i. e., binding of the corticosteroid/corticosteroid receptor complex to proinflammatory transcription factors – AP-1, NF-κB), while the metabolic and endocrine effects are mediated via direct gene activation through binding of the steroid-receptor complex to the promoter region of endocrine. and metabolism controlling genes [10]. A variety of other methods are also being explored to inactivate pro-inflammatory transcription factor activation including gene therapy and the use of "decoys."

---

* Southampton General Hospital, Southamptom, UK

The Rising Trends of Asthma and Allergic Diseases

Most allergic diseases are linked to atopy, the predisposition to generate immunoglobulin (Ig)E to common environmental agents. Because IgE is able to sensitize mast cells anywhere in the body, atopic individuals frequently express disease in more than one organ, e. g., coexistent asthma, rhinitis, eczema, and food allergy.

Population-based studies reveal large geographical differences in the prevalence of allergic disease with countries such as the UK, Australia, and New Zealand having figures 10–15-fold higher than Central and Eastern Europe and Asia. Although atopic disorders show strong heritability, it is differences in the environments that are likely to account for geographical variations. Also of particular concern is the rising trend in all allergic disorders, both in the developed and developing world. The increase has been especially noticeable in the last two decades, predominantly affects the young, and seems to be linked to a Western-type lifestyle [11].

Treatment options for allergic diseases are currently based on allergen avoidance and use of corticosteroids to prevent or control inflammation and antihistamines and sympathomimetics for treating symptoms. Allergen immunotherapy is undoubtedly effective in some allergic disorders (e. g., pollenosis, insect allergy), but not in others (e. g., eczema, food allergy). Central to an understanding of how genetically susceptible (atopic) individuals develop IgE against certain environmental factors is a knowledge of how the immune system recognizes and responds to the offending agents. This involves uptake and processing of allergens by professional antigen presenting cells (APCs – especially dendritic cells), the presentation of small allergen peptides to the T cell receptor and parallel engagement of costimulatory molecules [12]. In those destined to develop an allergic response, naïve T-lymphocytes (Th0) differentiate to a subtype (Th2) that secretes a group of cytokines responsible for switching B lymphocytes to produce IgE and the selective recruitment and activation of mast cells, basophils and eosinophils. In contrast, Th1 responses drive cell-mediated immunity and inhibit Th2 to responses through the release of interferon-γ (IFN-γ).

Inhibiting Allergen Sensitization

Since most atopic disorders are acquired early in life, there is great interest in identifying those environmental factors that lead to Th2 polarization and the emergence of allergic disease with a view to primary prevention by enhancing IFN-γ production. In children who later develop allergic disease there is impaired production of IFN-γ by T cells at birth, possibly through reduced IL-12 production that leads to persistence of the fetal Th2 response into the post-natal period [13]. One explanation for the protective effects of bacteria including *Mycobacteria* in allergic sensitization in early life is their action in increasing IL-12 production [14]. This concept has given rise to the "hygiene hypothesis," in which alterations to infant diets, early use of antibiotics, and reduced exposure to bacteria and their products contributes to persistence of the Th2 response after birth [15]. The co-administration of IL-12 with allergen vaccines has proven to be a powerful, although transient, adjuvant for IFN-γ production [16]. Unfortunately, when administered to humans, IL-12 produces a wide range of side effects that preclude its use as a therapeutic. Another approach has been to take advantage of the capacity of *Mycobacteria* to evoke a strong local cell mediated reaction and stimulate IL-12 and IFN-γ production. Of particular interest is the use of the soil saprophyte, *Mycobacterium vaccae* to achieve this since it is not a pathogen in animals [17]. Clinical trials of this "vaccine" for rhinitis and asthma are in progress, with early results showing some efficacy [18].

The immune system of vertebrates has evolved a defence mechanism that detects bacterial DNA because of their excess of unmethylated cytosine/guanosine dinucleotide repeats (CpG) and offers a possible explanation for the protective action of bacteria on Th2 responses [19]. Synthetic DNA oligonucleotides containing CpG motifs activate dendritic cells to increase their expression of co-stimulatory molecules and promote the generation of Th1-like immune responses via IL-12 [19]. Recent murine studies show that CpG DNA can be used alone or with antigen to induce antigen-specific Th1-like responses even in the presence of pre-existing Th2 responses [20]. Human studies in allergic asthma are being initiated.

Inhibiting IgE Responses

FcεR1 comprises an α chain which binds with strong affinity to the Fc portion of IgE, two γ chains responsible for cell signalling and a β chain which regulates receptor signalling. Although there is still debate about the precise molecular interaction between IgE and FcεR1α, mouse monoclonal antibodies (Mabs) have been produced that inhibit IgE binding to both to FcεR1α and the low affinity IgE receptor (FcεR2 or CD23) but are unable to cross-link IgE bound to mast cells or basophils and, therefore, fail to initiate mast cell activation [21]. When administered to atopic individuals, intravenous chaemeric (CGP 51901) and humanized (E25) anti-IgE Mabs reduce circulating IgE to almost undetectable levels. In patients with allergic asthma, nine weekly injections of E-25 almost abolished the early (mast cell-mediated) and late (leukocyte-mediated) bronchoconstrictor responses to inhaled allergen. The Mab E-25 is also effective in allergic asthma, reducing exacerbations and oral corticosteroid requirement by 50% as well as improving baseline lung function and bronchodilator use [21]. Anti-IgE therapy has also proven to be efficacious in allergic rhinitis [22].

In 1990, a decapeptide within the CH4 domain of IgE was shown to elicit antibodies that blocked anaphylactic histamine release in rabbits [23]. This "vaccine" has since been shown to be efficacious against food allergy in humans [24]. Other peptide sequences from the FcεR1 binding regions of IgE offer great promise as anti-allergic vaccines [25], and while some concern has been expressed that removal of IgE will reduce protection against parasites, animal studies have so far failed to show this.

Inhibiting Mediator Effects

The clear involvement of inflammatory mediators such as histamine, prostaglandins and leukotrienes which interact in allergic responses, has stimulated the development of drugs which either inhibit their formation or block their effects. An alternative approach is to neutralize mediators once they have been released similar to the binding of cytokines by soluble receptors. Nature may provide such molecules in order to minimize tissue reactions, hard ticks have evolved proteins in their saliva that do just this. *Rhipicephalus appendiculatus* is a tick that produces three histamine-binding proteins (Ra-HBPs) in its saliva. FS-HBP2 has two internal histamine binding pockets and a folding pattern not dissimilar to lipocalin [26]. Ra-HBP1, Ra-HBP2, and Ra-HBP3 have been cloned and the recombinant proteins expressed. *In vitro* they have been shown to inhibit the allergen-induced contraction

of sensitized tissues and one such molecule is currently in clinical trial. It is highly likely that other selective mediator inhibitors are awaiting discovery in tick saliva whose activity could be harnessed to create novel therapeutics [26].

The recent discovery that many allergens possess enzymatic activities raises the issue as to whether these biological properties create some advantage for molecules in becoming sensitizing agents. The cysteine protease of the dust mite allergen *Der P₁* can cleave the human low affinity IgE receptor (FcεR2 CD23), IL-2 receptor and occludin (a key protein in epithelial tight junctions), which in turn could increase IgE synthesis, Th2 polarization, and allergen penetration into mucosal tissues, respectively [27]. The importance of proteolytic enzymes in enhancing sensitization is now being realized as is the potential benefit from blocking this activity as a therapeutic target.

Targeting Proallergic Cytokines

Interleukin-4 and its homologue IL-13 are pivotal in regulating the allergic phenotype and operate through the signal transducer and activator of transcription (STAT)-6 [28]. IL-4 (but not its homologue IL-13) is obligatory for maintaining the Th2 T-cell phenotype, although for other functions either cytokine is effective. If the genes for IL-4 or STAT-6 are deleted in mice, IgE production and antigen-induced airway inflammation are inhibited. While humanized blocking Mabs against IL-4 have been developed, the preparation of a recombinant soluble form of human IL-4r α-chain without its transmembrane and cytoplasmic regions (sIL-4r) has shown efficacy both in a mouse model of ovalbumin-induced immediate hypersensitivity [29] and more recently in atopic asthma [30]. Although the IL-4 homologue, IL-13 binds to one type of IL-4r (IL-4α/IL-13α), it will not be recognized by soluble IL-4r. IL-13 is produced in large amounts by asthmatic airways and has been incriminated as an important cytokine in mouse models of asthma [31, 32]. One approach to inhibit IL-4 and IL-13 has been to use a double mutant of IL-4 (Arg-121-Asp and Tyr-124-Asp, BAY 16–9996), which binds as an antagonist to both IL-4 and IL-13 receptor [33]. In a murine model, an antagonistic IL-4 mutant protein was shown to completely prevent the allergic antibody response to a sensitizing antigen as well as cutaneous and anaphylactic hypersensitivity upon challenge [34]. Within IL-4 or IL-13 responsive cells, STAT-6 itself is also a selective target, inhibition of which will prevent signalling by both IL-4 and IL-13 [28].

Interleukin-5, IL-3, and granulocyte macrophage colony stimulating factor (GM-CSF) are essential for the development and recruitment of eosinophils, IL-5 being eosinophil-specific. In animal models, administration of an anti-IL-5 blocking Mab inhibits eosinophil recruitment from the bone marrow into tissues resulting in ablation of the late phase response to inhaled antigen and accompanying bronchial hyperresponsiveness [35]. Recently, a humanized anti-IL-5 Mab (SB-240563), when administered to atopic asthmatic subjects as a single intravenous dose of 10 mg/kg, has been shown to reduce both blood and sputum eosinophils, but in contrast to findings in animal models, it failed to inhibit either allergen provoked late-phase bronchoconstriction or hyperresponsiveness [36]. This somewhat surprising result questions the association between IL-5 secretion and induced eosinophil recruitment as being obligatory for the human late phase allergic response, but does not reduce interest in this approach for treating chronic eosinophil-mediated disorders which rely on IL-5 [37].

The recent discovery that RANTES, MCP-2, MCP-3, MCP-4, and eotaxin – members of the CC chemokine family – are powerful chemoattractants for eosinophils in allergic responses (through utilization of a common CCR-3 receptor) opens up another important target for intervening in allergic disease [37]. A Mab directed toward CCR-3 blocks eosinophil migration [38]. Human Mabs against eotaxin itself are being developed but on account of chemokine redundancy, this will probably have a less effective strategy than inhibiting CCR-3 receptors. Using either bacteriophage expression libraries or combinatorial chemistry, highly selective peptide and nonpeptide CCR-3 receptor antagonists have been discovered. Recent research indicates that CCR-3 and IL-5r agonists work cooperatively in recruiting eosinophils into target tissues [37].

The discovery that IL-10 from activated T cells, monocytes, and B cells mediates at least part of the tolerance observed with allergen immunotherapy [39] has provided the basis for a novel therapeutic approach. Human recombinant IL-10 is currently being assessed as an immunotherapeutic in respiratory allergy.

Immunotherapy

The aim of immunotherapy is through vaccination with allergen or its derivatives to produce selective inhibition of allergen specific responses. While undoubtedly efficacious in a number of serious allergic disorders (e. g., insect or penicillin anaphylaxis), considerable care has to be exercised in order not to provoke local and systemic anaphylactic reactions. Indeed, such adverse reactions have limited the uptake of immunotherapy in some countries. In an attempt to circumvent this, many allergens have now been cloned and mutated to reduce interactions with IgE without changing the epitopes responsible for the development of T-cell tolerance. Strategies are also in place to develop peptides that will induce T-cell tolerance but, unlike the native allergen, fail to trigger IgE-dependent mast-cell activation. Since immunotherapy is thought to be protective, at least in part, by inducing a Th1 IFN-γ response [39], attempts to enhance the efficacy of allergen immunotherapy by generating allergen peptides in *Mycobacterium vaccae* are being pursued.

A further breakthrough has been the use of antigen-selective DNA vaccines, which induce allergen synthesis in the host to stimulate a powerful protective immune response. For example, Leong and coworkers have cloned a major peanut allergen into a synthetic vector in which the DNA is protected from digestion by chitosan, a naturally occurring polysaccharide used for the controlled intestinal delivery of many pharmaceutical agents [40]. After ingestion, the nanoparticles of polysaccharide adhere to the intestinal epithelial cells facilitating uptake of the peanut-specific DNA. When administered orally to mice, this "vaccine" protects against sensitization and subsequent anaphylaxis upon peanut challenge. However, a critical question is whether DNA vaccines can produce tolerance if given to an already sensitized subject. It is encouraging that at least one controlled study has shown that sublingual administration of a grass pollen extract is beneficial in established seasonal allergic rhinitis [41].

Concluding Comments

Elucidating the cause for the rising trends of asthma and allergic disease represent a real challenge for scientists. An understanding of how genetic influences contribute to the asthma and allergic phenotype is of great importance if we are to define how the altered environment leads to new disease. In the case of asthma, polarization of the T-cell responses to a Th2 pattern is of paramount importance, but this alone is unlikely to account fully for the occurrence of asthma, with so many environmental factors playing a role (e. g., pollution, diet, viruses, allergens). The concept that an additional component is needed is driven by the discovery of an abnormal epithelial-mesenchymal trophic unit in this disease, as evidenced by epithelial activation damage and subepithelial collagen deposition. Since the trophic unit is pivotal to the growth and branching of the airways in foetal development, attention might focus on lung specific morphogenic genes to discover novel ways to interfere with this disease at a more fundamental level rather than suppressing inflammation alone.

In addition, the clear recognition that some patients respond to one drug (e. g., leukotriene receptor antagonist) and some to another (e. g., sodium cromoglycate) has led to the important concept of subtypes of disease and pharmacogenetics. Polymorphisms involving receptors and mediator pathways both in respect of disease pathogenesis and drug effects are likely to be of considerable importance in shaping the agenda for asthma management in the future. If this is realized, then tailoring patients' treatments to their individual needs will fulfil the primary objective of a practicing physician rather than the current policy of trying to use one type of therapy to treat everyone irrespective of heterogeneity of disease or their response to treatment.

Taking all these developments into account, we must not forget that over the last 100 years enormous progress has been made in asthma diagnosis and treatment. However, with the current continued increase in disease trends, there remains a large unmet clinical need that only high-quality and disease-orientated research will resolve.

Address for correspondence:

Prof. Stephen Holgate
University Medicine
Level D, Centre Block
Southampton General Hospital
Southampton SO16 6YD
UK
Tel. +44 1703 796-960
Fax +44 1703 701-771
E-mail wmc1 @soton.ac.uk

References

1. Salter HH. On asthma: Its pathology and treatment (pp. 24–60). London: Churchill 1859.

2. Ahlquist RP. A study of adrenotropic receptors. Am J Physiol 1948; 153:586–600.

3. Inman WHW, Adelstein AM. Rise and fall of asthma mortality in England and Wales in relation to use of pressurised aerosols. Lancet 1969; ii:279–285.

4. Lands AM, Arnold A, McAuliff JP, Luduena FP, Brown TG. Different ratio of receptor systems activated by sympathetic amines. Nature 1967; 214:597–598.

5. Crane J, Pearce N, Flatt A, Burgess C, Jackson R, Kwong T, Ball M, Beasley R. Prescribed fenoterol and death from asthma in New Zealand 1981–83: Case control study. Lancet 1989; i:918–922.

6. Howell JBL, Altounyan REC. Double-blind trial of disodium cromoglycate in the treatment of allergic bronchial asthma. Lancet 1967; ii:539–542.

7. Pepys J, Hargreave FE, Chan M, McCarthy DS. Inhibitory effects of disodium cromoglycate on allergen inhalation tests. Lancet 1968; ii:134–137.

8. Djukanovic R, Holgate ST. Lessons to be learned from sodium cromoglycate and related drugs. In MA Kaliner, DD Metcalfe (Eds), The mast cell in health and disease. Series: Lung Biology in Health and Disease (Exec. Ed. C. Lenfant), Vol. 62, 1993 pp. 467–482.

9. Daëron M. ITIM-bearing negative co-receptors. Immunologist 1997; 5:79–85.

10. Barnes PJ. Glucocorticosteroids. In Kay AB (Ed), Allergy and allergic diseases (pp. 619–641). Oxford: Blackwell 1997.

11. Peat JK, Li J. Reversing the trend: reducing the prevalence of asthma. J Allergy Clin Immunol 1999; 103: 1–10.

12. Palmer EM, van Seventer GA. Human T helper cell differentiation is regulated by the combined action of cytokines and accessory cell-dependent co-stimulatory signals. J Immunol 1997; 158:2654–2662.

13. Jung T, Moessner R, Kieckhoff K, Heidrich S, Neumann C. Mechanisms of deficient interferon-γ production in atopic diseases. Clin Exp Allergy 1999; 29: 912–919.

14. Shirikawa T, Enomoto T, Shimazu SI, Hopkin JM. The inverse association between tuberculin response and atopic disorder. Science 1997; 275:77–79.

15. Strachan DP, Harkins LS, Johnston IDA, Anderson HR. Childhood antecedents of allergic sensitisation in young British adults. J Allergy Clin Immunol 1997; 99:6–12.

16. Rampel JD, Wang MD, Hayglass KT. *In vivo* IL-12 administration induces profound, but transient, com-

mitment to T-helper cell type I associated patterns of cytokine and antibody production. J Immunol 1997; 159:1490–1496.

17. Wang C-C, Rook AW. Inhibition of an established allergic response to ovalbumin in BALB/c mice by killed *Mycobacterium vaccae*. Immunology 1998; 93:307–313.

18. Hopkin JM, Shaldan S, Ferry B, Coull P, Antrobus P, Enomoto T, Yamashita T, Furimoto F, Stanford J, Shirikawa T, Rook G. Mycobacterial immunisation in grass pollen immunisation and rhinitis. Thorax 1998; 53(Suppl 4):A16.

19. Krieg AM. An innate immune defence mechanisms based on the recognition of CpG motifs in microbial DNA. J Lab Clin Med 1996; 128:128–133.

20. Chu RS, Targoni OS, Krieg AM, Lehmann PV, Harding CV. CpG oligodeoxynucleotides act as adjuvants that switch on T-helper 1 (Th1) immunity. J Exp Med 1997; 186:1623–1628.

21. Patalano F. Injection of anti-IgE antibodies will suppress IgE and allergic symptoms. Allergy 1999; 54: 103–110.

22. Casale T, Bernstein IL, Busse WW et al. Use of an anti-IgE humanised monoclonal antibody in ragweed-induced allergic rhinitis. J Allergy Clin Immunol 1997; 100:110–121.

23. Stanworth DR, Jones VM, Lavin IV, Naggar S. Allergy treatment with a peptide vaccine. Lancet 1990; 336:1279–1281.

24. Romanski B, Bartuzi Z, Stanworth DR. Assessment of a novel anti-allergy vaccine in subjects with severe food allergy and at risk of anaphylaxis to food. Int Rev Allergol Clin Immunol 1998; 4:164–173.

25. Rudolf MP, Vogel M, Kricek F, Ruf C, Zürcher AW, Reuschel R, Auer M, Meischer S, Stadler BM. Epitope specific antibody response to IgE by mimotope immunisation. J Immunol 1998; 160:3315–21.

26. Paesen GC, Adams PL, Harlos K, Nuttall PA, Stuart DI. Tick histamine-binding proteins: isolation, cloning and three-dimensional structure. Mol Cell 1999; 3:861–71.

27. Sharma S, Lewis SA, Oakley IG, Tiley RS, Curran CC, Fung DCK, Lamont AG, Garland LG. Airway hyperreactivity and inflammation induced by intratracheal exposure to house dust mite extract in rats. Am J Respir Crit Care Med 1999; 159(3):A231.

28. Foster PS. STAT-6: an intracellular target for the inhibition of allergic disease. Clin Exp Allergy 1999; 29:12–15.

29. Renz H, Bradley K, Enssel K, Loader JE, Larsen GL, Gelfand EW. Prevention of the development of immediate hypersensitivity and airway hyperresponsiveness *in vivo* with soluble IL-4 receptors. Int Arch Allergy Immunol 1996; 106:167.

30. Borish LC, Nelson HS, Lanz M et al. Phase I/II study of interleukin-4 receptor (IL04r) in moderate asthma. J Allergy Clin Immunol 1998; 101:S8–9.

31. Grunig G, Warnock M, Wakil AE, Venkayya R, Brombacher F, Rennick DM, Sheppard D, Mohrs M, Donaldson DD, Locksley RM, Corry DB. Requirement for IL-13 independently of IL-4 in experimental asthma. Science 1998; 282:2261–2163.

32. Zhu Z, Homer RJ, Wang Z, Chen Q, Geba GP, Wang J, Zhang Y, Elias JA. Pulmonary expression of interleukin-13 causes inflammation, mucus hypersecretion, subepithelial fibrosis, physiologic abnormalities, and eotaxin production. J Clin Invest 1999; 103: 779–788.

33. Tony H-P, Shen B-J, Reusch P, Sebald W. Design of human interleukin-4 antagonists to inhibiting interleukin-4-dependent and interleukin-13-dependent responses in T cells and B cells with high efficiency. Eur J Biochem 1994; 225:659.

34. Grunewald SM, Werthemann A, Schnarr B, Klein CE, Bröcker EB, Mohrs M, Brombacker F, Sebald W, Duschl A. J Immunol 1998; 160:4004–4009.

35. Danzig M, Cuss F. Inhibition of interleukin-5 with a monoclonal antibody attenuates allergic inflammation. Allergy 1997; 52:787–794.

36. Leckie MJ, ten Brinke A, Lordan J. SB 240563, a humanised anti-IL-5 monoclonal antibody: initial single, dose safety and activity in patients with asthma. Am J Respir Crit Care Med 1999; 159(3):A624.

37. Teran L. Chemokines and IL-5: Major players of eosinophil recruitment in asthma. Clin Exp Allergy 1999; 29:287–290.

38. Heath H, Qin S, Rao P et al. The importance of CCR-3 demonstrated using an antagonistic monoclonal antibody. J Clin Invest 1997; 99:178–84.

39. Durham S, Till SJ. Immunologic changes associated with allergen immunotherapy. J Allergy Clin Immunol 1998; 102:157–164.

40. Roy K, Mao HQ, Haeng SK, Leong KW. Oral gene delivery with chitosan-DNA nanoparticles generate immunological protection in a murine model of peanut allergy. Nature Med 1999; 5:387–391.

41. Clavel R, Bousquet J, André C. Clinical efficacy of sublingual-swallowed immunotherapy. A double blind placebo-controlled trial of a standardised five grass pollen extract in rhinitis. Allergy 1998; 53:493–498.

International Time Trends in Asthma Mortality

Richard Beasley, Julian Crane, Neil Pearce*

Keywords: Asthma, mortality, time trends, epidemiology

Until recently epidemiological studies of asthma mortality have focused on investigating the causes of asthma mortality epidemics identified from the time trend data. With the identification of the role of isoprenaline forte and fenoterol as the primary causes of the asthma mortality epidemics, and with the resolution of the epidemics following regulatory action restricting their availability, attention has now shifted to the causes of the more gradual variations in mortality that have been observed in other countries at different times over the last 40 years. Although the role of different management and nonmanagement factors in these time trends is less certain, an increasingly coherent understanding of their relative contribution is being obtained, as well as the requirements for further epidemiological studies.

Introduction

Examination of international patterns of asthma mortality over the last 40 years reveals two apparently distinct patterns (Figure 1). One pattern is that of epidemics of asthma mortality which occurred in a number of countries in the 1960s and again in New Zealand in the 1970s/1980s. The other pattern is that of more gradual variations in asthma mortality in many countries, including gradual increases in mortality until the mid-1980s and a gradual reduction in some, but not all, countries during the last decade. Whereas the major causes for the epidemics of asthma mortality have been identified, the relative contributions of different factors to the more gradual changes in asthma mortality are less clear. This review focuses primarily on these gradual variations in asthma mortality and the issues which need to be addressed in future research.

Epidemics in the 1960s

Following the relatively stable asthma death rates during the first half of this century, asthma mortality increased dramatically in at least six western countries in the 1960s: England and Wales, Scotland, Ireland, New Zealand, Australia, and Norway (Figure 1) [1]. In these countries, the mortality rates increased two- to ten-fold within a two- to five-year period. Other countries such as the United States, Denmark, Canada, and Germany did not experience epidemics, although in some countries such as Japan, significant increases in asthma mortality were noted within more narrowly defined age groups [2].

The most likely explanation for the epidemics was that they were related to the use of the high dose β-agonist aerosol isoprenaline forte [1, 3]. Epidemics occurred only in countries where the high dose preparation of isoprenaline was available, there was a close association between the sales of isoprenaline forte and asthma mortality, and case series identified that many of the patients who died from asthma had used excessive amounts of this drug in the situation of severe asthma [4]. The mortality rates in countries experiencing epidemics declined following warnings from regulatory bodies, a marked reduction in the sales of isoprenaline forte, and other changes in medical practice, such as increases in hospital admissions and the introduction of inhaled corticosteroids.

The Second New Zealand Epidemic

In the mid-1970s, a second asthma mortality epidemic began in New Zealand, but not in other countries (Figure 1). Similar to the earlier epidemic, the

---

* Department of Medicine, Wellington School of Medicine, Wellington, New Zealand

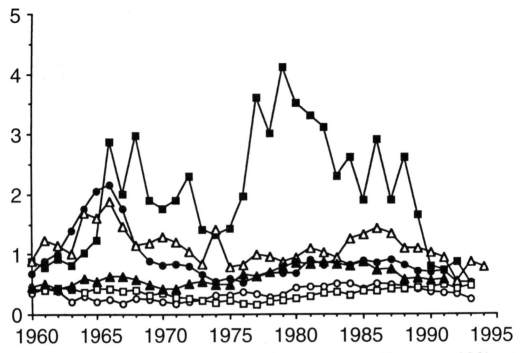

Figure 1. International patterns of asthma mortality (deaths per 100,000 persons) in persons aged 5–34 years, 1960–1994, showing the different trends. ■ = New Zealand, ● = England and Wales, Δ = Australia, ▲ = West Germany, ○ = Canada, □ = United States.

Table 1. Prescribed inhaled β-agonist and the relative risk of dying from asthma[a]: Results from published case-control studies when analyzed in an identical manner.

Specific β-agonist[b]	1st NZ Study	2nd NZ Study	3rd NZ Study	Saskatchewan Study
Salbutamol	0.7	0.7	0.6	0.9
Fenoterol	1.6	2.0	2.1	5.3

[a] Relative risk of death, unadjusted odds ratios. [b] During the period of these studies salbutamol and fenoterol were available in preparations dispensing 100 μg/puff and 200 μg/puff, respectively.

overuse of the high dose β-agonist fenoterol (which shares similar pharmacological properties to iso-prenaline [5]) was identified as the major, but prob-ably not the only cause of the epidemic. This evi-dence was derived primarily from a series of case-control studies in which an increased risk of asthma death was found in patients prescribed fenoterol but not other asthma medications (Table 1) [6–8]. Fur-ther studies indicated that the association between fenoterol and asthma mortality could not be attrib-uted to confounding by severity [9–11].

A subsequent case-control study from Saskatch-ewan, Canada undertaken specifically to address the "fenoterol hypothesis" also found that the pre-scription of the high dose preparation of fenoterol was associated with an increased risk of death when compared with the more commonly prescribed β-agonist, salbutamol (Table 1) [12]. Although the au-thors raised the possibility of a general β-agonist class effect, their subsequent analyses indicated that the general class effect was largely confounded by severity [11, 13].

Similar to the experience with isoprenaline forte, the withdrawal of fenoterol in New Zealand led to a greater than 50% reduction in asthma mortality within a 12 month period [14]. Consistent with the case control studies, time trend data did not suggest a class effect of inhaled β-agonist drugs in the epidemic. Similarly, the time trend data were also inconsistent with the hypothesis that the epidemic may have occurred because of under-prescribing of inhaled corticosteroids or socio-economic factors such as unemployment [14].

Gradual Increase in Asthma Mortality

Although no other countries have apparently experienced epidemics, a more gradual increase in asthma deaths has occurred in many countries during the 1970s and 1980s. This background increase has occurred not only in countries which experienced the first epidemic of deaths in the 1960s, but also in other countries unaffected by previous increases in mortality. It has been difficult to determine the causes of this trend, as death from asthma is a complex phenomenon and many factors relevant to the causation of asthma mortality have changed to differing degrees in different countries during this period. Despite this complexity, a number of observations can be made.

Magnitude

In a number of countries the magnitude of this "gradual" increase has been substantial. For example, between the mid-1970s and mid-1980s, the mortality rate increased by more than 40% in many countries (Table 2) [15–17]. In many of these countries, the marked increases in mortality occurred after a period of previously stable mortality rates. This suggests that the traditional distinction between epidemic and nonepidemic increases in mortality may be inappropriate. In particular, it may be misleading in terms of not acknowledging the magnitude of the increases in mortality in certain countries, thereby leading to a lack of recognition of the importance of the trends and the requirement for research into the causative factors.

Variation

There is both a wide variation in the reported asthma mortality rates in some countries with similar lifestyles and comparable approaches to the man-

Table 2. Asthma mortality (deaths per 100,000 persons) in 10 countries between the mid-1970s and mid-1980s in persons aged 5 to 34 years.

Country	1975–1977	1985–1987	% Increase
Australia	0.86	1.42	65
Canada	0.33	0.47	42
England & Wales	0.57	0.90	58
France	0.24	0.51	113
Japan	0.44	0.59	34
Singapore	0.75	0.88	17
Sweden	0.37	0.54	46
Switzerland	0.31	0.45	45
USA	0.19	0.40	111
West Germany	0.59	0.78	32

agement of asthma (e. g., Australia, England, and Canada), and conversely, similar asthma mortality rates in other countries with different lifestyles and approaches to the management of asthma (e. g., Japan, Sweden, and the United States) (Table 2) [15–17]. There appears to be no unifying hypothesis that explains these international variations. However, it is likely that with the better understanding of the causes of these variations, will come a better understanding of the relative importance of the risk factors for asthma mortality internationally.

Prevalence

The gradual increase in mortality rates has occurred during the same period in which the prevalence of asthma symptoms has increased. This increase in the prevalence of asthma symptoms has been observed in a wide range of countries with differing lifestyles and in some countries has been of considerable magnitude [18]. One interpretation of these observations is that the increase in mortality can be at least partly explained by the increases in prevalence, and that changes in case fatality rates are more informative than consideration of either prevalence or mortality rates in isolation of each other.

Case Fatality Rates

It is evident from these considerations that when making international comparisons of asthma mortality, it is necessary to also consider differences in the asthma prevalence rates of the countries being compared. This is now possible with the standardized international asthma prevalence data published from the European Community Respiratory Health Survey (ECHRS) [19] and the International Study of Asthma and Allergies in Childhood (ISAAC) [20]. These data have allowed an assessment of national case fatality rates which provides a different perspective of the international differences in asthma mortality rates (Table 3). This specific analysis based on the ISAAC data [21] indicates that amongst Western countries, at least a five-fold difference may exist in the case fatality rates, defined by the ratio of the asthma mortality rates to the prevalence rates of severe asthma within each country. This suggests that while the prevalence of severe asthma is one determinant of asthma mortality rates, other factors unrelated to the occurrence of severe disease may also play a major role.

Population Groups

Analysis of trends in asthma mortality rates within countries often reveals differences between specific population groups [22–25]. This is illustrated by studies from the USA, in which the asthma mortality rates are greater in disadvantaged populations such as the Blacks and Hispanics, those who are poorly educated, live in large cities, or are poor [22, 23, 26, 27]. It is likely that through the investigation of such high risk populations, our understanding of the risk factors that contribute to asthma mortality will be improved.

Environmental Exposures

One feature which is not evident from national mortality data is the occurrence of epidemics in discrete locations, associated with environmental exposures. Probably the best studied example is that of the epidemics of life-threatening attacks of asthma (and fatal asthma) in Barcelona in the 1980s, associated with environmental exposure to airborne soybean dust [28, 29]. These and other studies suggest that repeated environmental exposure to a single sensitizing agent can lead to recurrent episodes of life-threatening attacks of asthma in a community whenever exposure reaches a sufficient level [30, 31]. They also illustrate the difficulties that exist in identifying and determining the relative contribution of different environmental (and other) risk factors for asthma mortality.

Seasonal Trends

Seasonal trends in asthma mortality have been observed in a number of countries including the United Kingdom [32], France [33], and the USA [34]. In each of these countries, asthma mortality in the 5- to 34-year age group is highest in the summer months, in contrast to the older age groups, in which the peak occurs in the winter. It is likely that this trend in the younger age group relates to reduced access to or availability of medical care during the summer holidays, in view of the associated reduction in hospital admissions during this period. In contrast, the reverse trend in the older group with an increase in hospital admissions in winter, is most

Table 3. Comparison of asthma mortality rates with prevalence rates of severe asthma in 12 countries.

	Asthma Mortality Rate*	Prevalence of Severe Asthma**	Ratio
Australia	0.86	8.3	0.10
Canada	0.25	8.0	0.03
England & Wales	0.52	8.7	0.06
Finland	0.21	3.1	0.07
France	0.40	2.8	0.14
Italy	0.23	2.0	0.12
Japan	0.73	2.1	0.35
New Zealand	0.50	8.0	0.06
Sweden	0.12	2.0	0.06
USA	0.47	10.0	0.05
West Germany	0.44	5.7	0.08

* Asthma mortality rate (per 100,000) in persons aged 5–34 years in 1993. ** Asthma prevalence rates defined as self-reported episodes of wheezing sufficient to limit speech in previous 12 months, in 13–14 year old children, 1993–1995 (adapted from [21]).
NB: Mortality and prevalence data are not available in the same age group.

likely to be due to a greater frequency of respiratory tract infections.

Role of β-Agonist Therapy

The possible relationship between β-agonist therapy and this gradual trend of increasing asthma mortality needs to be considered. Although it has been noted in several countries that a close association exists between increasing mortality and sales of β-agonist drugs, it is uncertain whether this represents a causal relationship, a response to changes in the prevalence of severe asthma, or merely reflects changes in the approach to asthma management. The two major issues which need to be considered are (1) the extent to which fenoterol may have contributed to the more gradual increases in mortality observed in countries in which its use has been less widespread than in New Zealand; and (2) the contribution of the more selective β-agonist drugs which have been marketed in lower dose preparations and that have not been incriminated in asthma mortality epidemics.

These issues have been addressed in Japan, in which the death rate doubled in the 10 years following the mid-1980s. Initial studies have reported a relationship between asthma deaths and over-reliance or excessive dependence on β-agonists, and a five-fold increased risk of death with the use of fenoterol compared with other β-agonist drugs [35, 36]. In view of the parallel between asthma mortality since the mid-1980s and both the increase in the sales of fenoterol (since its introduction in 1985) and total β-agonist sales, these findings suggest that the trend of increasing asthma mortality in Japan may well be due, at least in part, to the use of fenoterol [37]. Similar epidemiological studies investigating the role in asthma mortality of specific β-agonists and β-agonists as a class in other countries are now urgently required.

Most Recent Trends

There has been a gradual fall in asthma mortality since the late 1980s in some but not all countries in which accurate mortality statistics are kept (Figure 1). Countries in which such reductions have been observed include Australia, Canada, Denmark, West Germany, Sweden, England, and Wales. It is possible that this reduction may relate to changes in management, in particular the greater use of inhaled corticosteroid therapy. In support of this view are the studies which have shown improved clinical outcome with inhaled corticosteroid therapy [38], and their protective effects against mortality [39]. However, the time trend evidence is not conclusive in this regard, particularly as some countries such as the United States and Japan have experienced increases in mortality during this period, despite similar marked increases in the use of inhaled corticosteroid therapy. It is likely that other (unknown) factors may well account for a significant component of the recent mortality decline in those countries in which this trend has been observed.

Acknowledgments

The Wellington Asthma Research Group is supported by program grants from the Health Research Council of New Zealand and the Guardian Trust. We thank Ms Denise Fabian for her expert secretarial assistance.

Address for correspondence:

Prof. Richard Beasley
Department of Medicine
Wellington School of Medicine
PO Box 7343
Wellington
New Zealand
Tel. +64 4 385-5589
Fax +64 4 389-5427
E-mail Beasley@wnmeds.ac.nz

References

1. Stolley PD. Why the United States was spared an epidemic of deaths due to asthma. Am Rev Respir Dis 1972; 105:883–890.

2. Mitsui S. Death from bronchial asthma in Japan. Sino-Jpn J Allergol Immunol, Soshiran 1986; 3:249–257.

3. Stolley PD, Schinnar R. Association between asthma mortality and isoproterenol aerosols: A review. Prev Med 1978; 7:319–338.

4. Fraser PM, Speizer FE, Waters SD, Doll R, Mann NM. The circumstances preceding death from asthma in young people in 1968 to 1969. Br J Dis Chest 1971; 65:71–84.

5. Crane J, Burgess C, Beasley R. Cardiovascular and hypokalaemic effects of inhaled salbutamol, fenoterol and isoprenaline. Thorax 1989; 44:136–140.

6. Crane J, Pearce N, Flatt A, Burgess C, Jackson R, Kwong T, Ball M, Beasley R. Prescribed fenoterol and death from asthma in New Zealand, 1981–83: Case-control study. Lancet 1989; 1:917–922.

7. Pearce N, Grainger J, Atkinson M, Crane J, Burgess C, Culling C, Windom H, Beasley R. Case-control study of prescribed fenoterol and death from asthma in New Zealand, 1977–1981. Thorax 1990; 45:170–175.

8. Grainger J, Woodman K, Pearce N, Crane J, Burgess C, Keane A, Beasley R. Prescribed fenoterol and death from asthma in New Zealand, 1981–1987: A further case-control study. Thorax 1991; 46:105–111.

9. Sackett DL, Shannon HS, Browman GW. Fenoterol and fatal asthma. Lancet 1990; i:46 (letter).

10. Beasley R, Burgess C, Pearce N, Grainger J, Crane J. Confounding by severity does not explain the association between fenoterol and asthma death. Clin Exp Allergy 1994; 24:660–668.

11. Pearce N, Hensley MJ. Epidemiologic studies of β-agonists and asthma deaths. Epidemiol Rev 1998; 20:173–186.

12. Spitzer WD, Suissa S, Ernst P, Horwitz RI, Habbick B, Cockcroft D, Bovin JF, McNutt M, Buist AS, Rebuck A. The use of β-agonists and the risk of death and near death from asthma. N Engl J Med 1992; 326:501–506.

13. Suissa S. The case-time-control design. Epidemiology 1995; 6:248–253.

14. Pearce N, Beasley R, Crane J, Burgess C, Jackson R. End of the New Zealand asthma mortality epidemic. Lancet 1995; 345:41–44.

15. Jackson R, Sears MR, Beaglehole R, Rea HH. International trends in asthma mortality: 1970 to 1985. Chest 1988; 94:914–918.

16. Sears MR, Taylor DR. The b2-agonist controversy: observations, explanations and relationship to epidemiology. Drug Safety 1994; 11(4):259–283.

17. Sears MR. Worldwide trends in asthma mortality. Bull Int Union Tuberc Lung Dis 1991; 66:79–83.

18. National Institutes of Health, National Heart, Lung and Blood Institute and World Health Organisation Workshop Report (1995). Chapter 2, Epidemiology. In Global Initiative for Asthma: Global strategy for asthma management and prevention, pp. 10–24.

19. Burney PGJ, Luczynska C, Chinn S, Jarvis D. The European Community Respiratory Health Survey. Eur Respir J 1994; 7:954–960.

20. Asher MI, Keil U, Anderson HR, Beasley R, Crane J, Martinez F, Mitchell EA, Pearce N, Sibbald B, Stewart AW et al. International Study of Asthma and Allergies in Childhood (ISAAC): Rationale and methods. Eur Respir J 1995; 8:483–491.

21. Asher MI, Anderson HR, Stewart AW, Crane J, Ait-Khaled N, Anabwani G, Beasley R, Björkstén B, Burr M, Clayton TO, Ellwood PE, Keil U, Lai CKW, Mallol J, Martinez F, Mitchell EA, Montefort S, Pearce N, Robertson CF, Shah JR, Sibbald B, Strachan D, von Mutius E, Weiland SK, Williams HC. Worldwide variations in the prevalence of asthma symptoms: ISAAC. Eur Respir J 1998; 12:315–335.

22. Weiss KB, Wagener DK. Changing patterns of asthma mortality: Identifying populations at high risk. JAMA 1990; 264:1683–1687.

23. Sly MR. Mortality from asthma, 1979–1984. J Allergy Clin Immunol 1988; 82:705–717.

24. Ehrlich RI, Bourne DE. Asthma deaths among coloured and white South Africans: 1962 to 1988. Resp Med 1994; 88:195–202.

25. Sears MR, Rea HH, Beaglehole R, Gillies AJD, Holst PE, O'Donnell TV, Rothwell RPG, Sutherland DC. Asthma mortality in New Zealand: A two year national study. NZ Med J 1985; 98:271–275.

26. Weiss KB, Gergen PJ, Wagener DK. Breathing better or wheezing worse? The changing epidemiology of asthma morbidity and mortality. Annu Rev Pub Health 1993; 14:491–513.

27. McFadden ER Jr, Warren EL. Observations on asthma mortality. Ann Int Med 1997; 127:142–147.

28. Anto JM, Sunyer J. Asthma Collaborative Group of Barcelona. A point source asthma outbreak. Lancet 1986; i:900–903.

29. Anto JM, Sunyer J, Rodriguez-Roisin R, Suarez-Cervera M, Vazquez L. Toxicoepidemiological Committee. Community outbreaks of asthma associated with inhalation of soybean dust. N Engl J Med 1989; 320:1097–1102.

30. Packe GE, Ayres JG. Aeroallergen skin sensitivity in patients with severe asthma during a thunderstorm. Lancet 1986; 1: 850–851.

31. Suphioglu C, Singh MB, Taylor P, Bellomo R, Holmes P, Puy R, Knox RB. Mechanism of grass pollen-induced asthma. Lancet 1992; 339: 569–572.

32. Khot A, Burn R. Seasonal variation and time trends of deaths from asthma in England and Wales 1960–82. BMJ 1984; 289:233–234.

33. Cadet B, Robine JM, Leibovici D. Dynamic of asthma mortality in France: Seasonal variation and peaking of mortality in 1985–87. Rev Epidemiol Sante Publ 1994; 42:103–118.

34. Weiss KB. Seasonal trends in US asthma hospitalizations and mortality. JAMA 1990; 263:2323–2328.

35. Committee on Asthma Death (Japanese Society of Pediatric Allergy and Clinical Immunology). Asthma Death Committee Report '95. Jap J Ped All Clin Immunol 1995; 9:54–66.

36. Matsui T. Asthma death and b_2-agonists. In Shinomiya K (Ed). Current Advances in Pediatric Allergy and Clinical Epidemiology. Selected proceedings from the 32nd Annual Meeting of the Japanese Society of Pediatric Allergy and Clinical Immunology. Tokyo: Churchill Livingstone, 1996, pp. 161–164.

37. Beasley R, Nishima S, Pearce N, Crane J. β-agonist therapy and asthma mortality in Japan. Lancet 1998; 351:1406–1407.

38. Toogood JH, Jennings BH, Baskerville JC, Lefcoe NM. Aerosol corticosteroids. In Weis EB, Stein M. (Eds), Bronchial asthma: Mechanisms and therapeutics (3rd ed.). Boston: Little, Brown & Co, 1993, pp. 818–841.

39. Ernst P, Spitzer WO, Suissa S, Cockroft D, Habbick B, Horwitz RI, Boivin JF, McNutt M, Buist AS. Risk of fatal and near-fatal asthma in relation to inhaled corticosteroid use. JAMA 1992; 268:3462–3464.

The Role of Air Pollution on Allergic Airway Disease

Robert J Davies*

Keywords: Air pollution, allergy, epithelial cells, cytokines, airway responsiveness

There is a wealth of epidemiological evidence indicating that air pollutants such as ozone (O_3), nitrogen dioxide (NO_2), sulphur dioxide (SO_2) and diesel exhaust particles (DEP) exacerbate rhinitis, asthma and chronic obstructive pulmonary disease. The evidence that air pollutants are a contributory cause of the increased prevalence of allergic disease is less strong and largely circumstantial. O_3 and SO_2 but not NO_2 or DEP have direct effects on lung function at concentrations encountered during episodes of pollution. O_3, NO_2, and SO_2 have been shown, either alone or in combination, to increase the airway response to inhaled allergen indicating that they can play a key role in exacerbating allergic airway disease. The fact that this effect persists for at least 48 h after exposure is highly suggestive of pollutant induced airway inflammation. The airway epithelial cell appears to be pivotal in inducing inflammation after exposure to pollutants through release of cytokines which can attract and prolong the life of eosinophils, and upregulate adhesion molecules on both the vascular endothelium and the epithelium. Therapeutic agents such as corticosteroids can abrogate this effect. DEP's not only induce airway inflammation but also have profound inhibitory effects *in vitro* on ciliary beat frequency and the permeability of the epithelium. In addition DEPs have been shown to have a specific adjuvant effect on the production of IgE against relevant bystander allergens. A clearer understanding of the signal transduction pathways by which air pollutants initiate inflammation at the level of the epithelial cell may lead to novel therapeutic interventions.

Air Pollution

Studies have demonstrated that the increase that has occurred in atmospheric concentrations of NO_2 and O_3 are associated with symptoms of rhinitis, chronic cough, phlegm, decreased morning peak flow, emergency room visits and increased hospitalization due to asthma in asthmatic adults and children, and that the effects of these pollutants may predominate after 1–2 days. Similarly, studies of respirable particulate matter have demonstrated that increased levels of PM_{10} are also associated with worsening peak flow, increased inhaler usage, respiratory symptoms and emergency room visits, and more recently cardiopulmonary and lung cancer mortality [1].

Although epidemiological studies, particularly from the developed countries, suggest that the increase in the prevalence of allergic disease such as asthma may be associated with air pollution resulting from increased use of liquid petroleum fuel, the findings from these studies have been difficult to interpret due to confounding effects of cigarette smoke, exposure to allergens, meteorological conditions and socioeconomic factors [2]. Additionally, these studies have investigated the effects of only the major pollutants individually, without taking into account the potential additive and/or synergistic effects of combinations of pollutants which are more relevant.

However, studies from Japan have demonstrated that the incidence of rhino-conjunctivitis in residents living alongside old cedar tree-lined main roads with heavy traffic all day long was much higher than that in residents living in the cedar forest but with less traffic, despite the cedar pollen counts being similar in both areas [3]. These studies suggest that the disparity in the incidence of rhino-conjunctivitis in the different areas may be a result of vehicle exhaust pollution, which was the predominating factor in areas with high incidence. Early studies from Germany, particularly by von Mutius and colleagues, demonstrated that allergic conditions such as hay fever were more common in West German cities than in East German cities, where chronic bronchitis was more prevalent, and suggested that this was likely to be a consequence

* Asthma and Allergy, London Bridge Hospital, London, UK

of the different types of air pollutants predominating in West and East Germany [4]. Recent studies from Germany have demonstrated that whilst the prevalence of atopic diseases has not altered significantly in Hamburg (West Germany), there has been a significant increase in the prevalence of these diseases in Erfurt (East Germany), suggesting that there is a converging tendency of self-reported asthma and asthma symptoms [5]. Overall, however, the differences in the respiratory conditions have largely disappeared following unification of East and West Germany and it has been suggested that this is likely to be a result of both the change in air pollution patterns and living habits in the former East Germany [6].

Luczynska and colleagues have investigated skin sensitivity to a panel of indoor and outdoor allergens in 10–11-year-old school children living in Tower Hamlets and Eltham, two areas of London segregated on the basis of their socio-economic status and traffic pollution and demonstrated that the prevalence of skin sensitivity to house dust mite, grass pollen and cockroach allergen was higher in Tower Hamlets, the more deprived and polluted of the two areas [7].

The Effects of Exposure to Air Pollutants on Lung Function

Laboratory based studies have shown inconsistent effects of NO_2 exposure on lung function and non-specific bronchial responsiveness. In one study, NO_2 at low concentration (400 ppb) did not affect lung function in normals but caused bronchoconstriction and increased bronchial responsiveness in asthmatics [8]. In contrast, numerous studies have agreed in finding significant effects of O_3, in both asthmatics and non-asthmatics, who appear to be equally sensitive to the effects of this pollutant gas. Studies of O_3 inhalation have also demonstrated that this agent produces concentration- and exposure time-related changes in symptoms and lung function, including an increase in airway resistance, a reduction in lung volumes and an increase in airway responsiveness to bronchoconstrictor agents. In a recent study, Seal and colleagues [9] investigated the lowest O_3 concentrations and the minimum exposure time required to cause significant changes in either pulmonary function or respiratory symptoms in healthy male volunteers exposed to 0–240 ppb O_3 for 0–6.8 h. Although cough

was induced at a minimum concentration of 180 ppb O_3, significant adverse changes in FEV_1 were induced at a minimum concentration of 240 ppb O_3. Furthermore, a minimum exposure time of 6.8 h to O_3 was required to see these changes. Other studies have demonstrated that there is rapid adaptation to continuing exposure to ozone.

Studies involving inhalation of sulphur dioxide (SO_2) have demonstrated that this gas also leads to bronchoconstriction in both normal healthy and asthmatic subjects and that deep breathing and intermittent exercise may potentiate this effect. Although the response to SO_2 inhalation is variable in individuals, concentrations of SO_2 that have little or no effect on normal healthy subjects can produce marked symptomatic bronchoconstriction in patients with asthma.

Some studies have demonstrated that the effects of SO_2 on lung function are potentiated by prior exposure to either NO_2 or O_3, and therefore suggest that exposure to combinations of pollutants is likely to be more harmful than exposure to individual pollutants [10].

The Enhancing Effect of Air Pollutants on Airway Responsiveness to Inhaled Allergen

Recent studies have indicated that exposure to pollutants such as O_3, NO_2 and a combination of NO_2 and SO_2 may increase the airway responsiveness of asthmatics to inhaled allergen.

Ball and colleagues [11] have exposed 15 asthmatics at rest for 1 h to either air or 0.12 pm O_3, in randomized manner, and evaluated the effect of this exposure on the airway response of these individuals to inhaled allergen. Contrary to the findings of Molfino and colleagues these authors demonstrated that pre-exposure to O_3 did not significantly decrease the concentration of allergen required to elicit a 15% decrement in FEV_1 (PC_{15}), compared with pre-exposure to air. These authors have suggested that although the difference in their findings and those of Molfino and colleagues may be as a consequence of methodological differences and differences in the subject groups used, these are more likely to be as a consequence of repeated exposure to allergen, resulting from insufficient randomization, prior to exposure to air and O_3.

Recent studies by Jörres and colleagues [12],

however, have demonstrated that prior exposure for a longer period and to a higher concentration of O_3 does indeed increase the airway responsiveness to inhaled allergen/methacholine in allergic individuals. These authors exposed groups of intermittently exercising allergic asthmatics, allergic rhinitics without asthma and healthy subjects for 3 h to 250 ppb O_3 or filtered air, in randomized manner, followed by challenge with doubling concentrations of methacholine or allergen, until the FEV_1 dropped by 20% from baseline. Exposure to O_3 itself significantly decreased the lung function in all groups of individuals, as indicated by decreased baseline FEV_1, compared with exposure to filtered air. Pre-exposure for 3 h to 250 ppb O_3 also increased the bronchial responsiveness to allergen in both the asthmatic and rhinitic subjects, as indicated by significant decreases in the amounts of allergen required to reduce the mean FEV_1 by 20% from baseline, compared with pre-exposure for 3 h to filtered air. Furthermore, pre-exposure to O_3 significantly increased the airway responsiveness to methacholine in the asthmatic patients, but not the patients with rhinitis nor the healthy subjects.

Employing a slightly different experimental format, Tunnicliffe and colleagues [13] have investigated the effect of randomized exposure at rest for 1 h to either air, 100 ppb NO_2 or 400 ppb NO_2, followed by challenge with a pre-determined dose of house dust mite (HDM) allergen required to produce a 15% fall in FEV_1, in mild asthmatics. Although exposure to 400 ppb NO_2 did not significantly alter the baseline FEV_1 in these individuals, this significantly increased the airway response to inhaled allergen during both the immediate and late phase, when compared with exposure to air.

We have investigated the effect of randomized exposure for 6 h to either air, 400 ppb NO_2, 200 ppb SO_2 or a combination of the two pollutants, followed by inhalation of increasing concentrations of *Dermatophagoides pteronyssinus* allergen, on lung function and airway responsiveness in non-exercising mild asthmatic patient volunteers to [14]. Compared with exposure to air, exposure to neither NO_2, SO_2, nor the combination of the two pollutants significantly altered FEV_1 or forced vital capacity (FVC). Although exposure to NO_2 and SO_2 decreased the mean allergen concentration required to cause a 20% fall in FEV_1 ($PD_{20}FEV_1$) by 41.2% and 32.2%, respectively, these were not significantly different compared with exposure to air. In contrast, exposure to the combination of the two pollutants significantly decreased the mean allergen

$PD_{20}FEV_1$ by 60.5%, compared with exposure to air.

In view of the epidemiological evidence that the clinical effects of air pollutants may be lagged by 1–2 days, we investigated the possibility that such a lag effect may be reproducible under strictly controlled laboratory conditions and studied the time course over which the airway response enhancing effects of pollutants may persist [15]. Non-exercising mild asthmatic patient volunteers were exposed in randomized manner for 6 h to either air or 400 ppb NO_2 + 200 ppb SO_2. Following exposure to air the individuals underwent challenge immediately with *Dermatophagoides pteronyssinus* allergen. Following exposure to 400 ppb NO_2 + 200 ppb SO_2 the individuals underwent randomized allergen challenge either immediately, 24 h or 48 h later. Exposure to the combination of NO_2 + SO_2 significantly decreased the mean allergen $PD_{20}FEV_1$ by 37.0%, 63.0% and 49.0%, immediately, 24 h and 48 h after exposure, respectively, compared with exposure to air. Additionally, the mean allergen $PD_{20}FEV_1$ at 24 h after exposure was significantly lower, when compared to that immediately after exposure to the pollutant mixture, suggesting that the enhanced airway response to inhaled allergen in asthmatic individuals, resulting from exposure to pollutants, was likely to be lagged over a period of 24–48 h and was maximal 24 h after exposure. Our recent studies with O_3 and NO_2 have shown that short exposures to high concentrations of these pollutant gases have a greater effect on the airway response to inhaled allergen than lower concentrations for a longer period of time.

Increased Airway Responsiveness to Inhaled Allergen Following Exposure to Pollutants

Although there is only circumstantial evidence to suggest a link between an increase in the prevalence of allergic airway disease and an increase in air pollution, there is little doubt that exposure to certain air pollutants enhances the airway response to inhaled allergens in susceptible individuals. However, the mechanisms underlying these effects are not fully understood.

Some studies have suggested, that air pollutants

may promote sensitization and subsequent development of allergic disease, by modulating the allergenicity of airborne allergens. Behrendt and colleagues have demonstrated that pollen collected from roadsides with heavy traffic and other areas with high levels of air pollution are covered with large numbers of airborne particulates (< 5 mm in size), and that incubation of pollen for 2–5 h in aqueous solutions prepared from these particulates led to morphological alterations in pollen and extravasation of allergens with altered antigenicity [16]. More recently, Knox and colleagues have investigated the interaction between respirable diesel exhaust particles (DEP; 30–60 nm diameter) and purified rye-grass pollen allergens Lol p 1 and Lol p 5 and demonstrated that Lol p 1 binds strongly to the DEP [17]. Collectively, these studies suggest that air pollutants may modulate allergenicity of the pollen allergens and also act as environmental triggers for exacerbation of allergic airway disease, particularly during episodes of increased air pollution in the pollen season.

Human and animal studies have suggested that pollutant exposure may increase synthesis of IgE. A study of 363 healthy non-atopic children, under the age of 12 years, demonstrated that the degree of air pollution in the areas where these children lived was significantly correlated with an increase in their mean total serum IgE levels. Diaz-Sanchez and colleagues [18] have investigated the effects of nasal challenge with 0.30 mg DEP on the local immune response of healthy volunteers and shown that this led to a four- to five-fold increase in the amounts of IgE, but not IgG, IgA, or IgM, measured in nasal lavage of these subjects, 4 days after challenge. Additionally, these authors demonstrated that the number of IgE secreting cells and the levels of ε mRNA coding for specific IgE proteins were increased approximately 20–25 fold following challenge with DEP. Recently, these authors investigated the effect of DEP on the synthesis of cytokines known to influence the production of IgE and lead to allergic reactions in the nasal mucosa of subjects allergic to ragweed allergen. These studies have demonstrated that the levels of mRNA for interleukins (IL)-2, 4, 5, 6, 10 and 13 and interferon γ (IFN-γ) were increased and readily detectable in the nasal mucosal cells of these individuals, 18 h after intranasal challenge with DEP. Interestingly, the enhancement in cytokine mRNA following challenge with DEP was considerably greater than that noted following allergen challenge alone and the levels of mRNAs for IL-4, 5, 6, 10 and 13 were

increased even further when allergen and DEP challenges were applied simultaneously. In contrast the levels of IL-2 were unchanged, whilst the levels of IFN-γ mRNA were decreased suggesting that DEP upregulated the activity of Th2-like lymphocytes. More recently, these authors have investigated the ability of DEP to act as an adjuvant to antigen in ragweed sensitive individuals undergoing nasal provocation challenges with either DEP, the ragweed allergen Amb a I or a combination of DEP and Amb a I [19]. Nasal washes were performed 18 h, as well as 4 and 8 days after challenge and analyzed for total and ragweed specific IgE. Challenge with ragweed allergen led to an increase in both total and ragweed-specific IgE in the nasal lavage fluid. Although challenge with DEP also led to an increase in total, but not ragweed specific IgE, a combined challenge with DEP and ragweed allergen increased the levels of ragweed specific IgE 16-fold, compared to levels seen after ragweed challenge alone.

In vitro studies by the same group of authors have demonstrated that the effects of DEP may at least partly be as a result of the polyaromatic hydrocarbons (PAHs) present on the DEP. Takenaka and colleagues have investigated the effect of PAHs extracted from DEP on IgE production in human peripheral blood mononuclear cells (PBMCs) or purified tonsillar B cells. These authors demonstrated that although PAH extract itself did not induce *de novo* IgE synthesis by either cell type pretreated with either anti-IL-4 or anti-CD40 monoclonal antibody (mAB), the extract enhanced the IgE production from these cells by 20–360%, when the cells were treated simultaneously with IL-4 and CD40, suggesting that PAHs were possibly acting by modifying on-going transcriptional programs related to IgE production, rather than inducing such programs *de novo*. Similarly, animal studies have demonstrated that specific IgE to ovalbumin and platinum salts is increased when the animals are exposed to O_3 or DEP compared to air [20].

Several studies have suggested that pollution-induced airway epithelial damage and impaired mucociliary clearance may allow easier penetration and access of inhaled allergens to cells of the immune system. Studies investigating the pathophysiological effects resulting from inhalation of O_3 have demonstrated that this agent leads to epithelial damage and an increased inflammatory response in the upper and lower airways, as indicated by leakage of lactate dehydrogenase, albumin and total protein, and increase in neutrophils, eosinophils, mononuclear

17

cells, fibronectin, α-1-antitrypsin, interleukins-6 and 8, granulocyte-monocyte colony stimulating factor (GM-CSF) and prostaglandin E2, in nasal lavage (NAL), proximal airway lavage (PAL) and bronchoalveolar lavage (BAL). Basha and colleagues have demonstrated that although there were no significant differences in spirometric values and symptom scores between asthmatics and healthy volunteers, after exposure for 6 h to 200 ppb O_3, there were significant increases in IL-6, IL-8 and PMN numbers in BAL fluid obtained 18 h post-exposure in asthmatics only [21]. These studies suggest that O_3 may preferentially increase the production of cytokines and inflammatory cells in asthmatics, possibly leading to an acute exacerbation at a later stage. Sandström and colleagues have investigated the effects of NO_2 inhalation in healthy non-smoking and lightly exercising individuals and demonstrated that this agent increases the numbers of lymphocytes, lysozyme-positive alveolar macrophages and mast cells in BAL. More recently, this group demonstrated that exposure for 20 minutes to 1.5–3.5 ppm NO_2 significantly reduced the mucociliary activity in healthy non-smoking volunteers [22]. Peden and colleagues have investigated the effect of prior exposure for 2 h to either air or 400 ppb O_3 on subsequent allergen-induced changes in the nasal mucosa of perennially allergic asthmatic patients and demonstrated that exposure to O_3 significantly increased the allergen-induced release of eosinophil cationic protein (ECP) in nasal lavage of these individuals, without significantly affecting the numbers of eosinophils, 4 h after allergen challenge [23]. These results suggest that exposure to O_3 may "prime" the eosinophils to subsequent activation by inhaled allergen. Similarly, we have exposed seasonal allergic rhinitics for 6 h to either 400 ppb NO_2 or air ± allergen challenge, following 30 minutes after exposure, and have evaluated the changes in nasal airway resistance (NAR) and presence of inflammatory mediators in nasal lavage [24]. Although exposure to NO_2 alone did not significantly alter the NAR or increase the concentration of ECP, tryptase or myeloperoxidase in nasal lavage, exposure to NO_2 prior to allergen challenge significantly increased the concentration of ECP, but not tryptase or myeloperoxidase, compared with exposure to air. Our findings are in accordance with those of Peden and colleagues and suggest that acute exposure to NO_2 may also "prime" the eosinophils for subsequent activation by allergen in seasonal allergic rhinitics.

In order to investigate whether treatment with steroids can alter the inflammatory response in the nasal airways under these conditions, we have investigated seasonal allergic rhinitics randomized to receive either topical fluticasone propionate aqueous nasal spray (FP) 200 mg once daily or matched placebo for 4 weeks in a double blind, crossover design. Analysis of ECP in lavage samples of these individuals, demonstrated that this was significantly increased following exposure to NO_2 + allergen, when the individuals were treated with placebo. In contrast, there was a much smaller effect of exposure to NO_2 + allergen challenge on ECP levels when these individuals were treated with FP. The difference in changes of ECP levels between placebo and FP treatments was significant suggesting that FP may down-grade NO_2 + allergen-induced eosinophil activation in allergic rhinitics.

More recently, we have investigated the effect of prior exposure to O_3 on allergen-induced inflammatory cell changes in the lower airways of mild asthmatics randomized to receive either inhaled FP 500 mg bd or matched placebo for 4 weeks. Following treatment, individuals in both groups underwent randomized exposure for 1 h to either air or 120 ppb O_3, followed by bronchoscopy and saline challenge in the right upper lobe anterior segmental orifice and allergen challenge in the right middle lobe medial segmental orifice. Bronchoscopy was repeated after 24 h and bronchial biopsies were obtained from the challenge sites. After a 4 weeks' washout period, treatment with FP or placebo was repeated and biopsy samples were obtained after prior exposure for 1 h to the alternate atmosphere of air or 120 ppb O_3. Immunohistochemical analysis of the biopsy tissue demonstrated that prior exposure for 1 h to O_3 did not significantly increase the numbers of neutrophils, EG1-, or EG2-staining cells, when compared with exposure to air. However, allergen challenge following exposure to either air or ozone significantly increased the numbers of EG2-staining cells in the placebo-treated group, an effect that was markedly reduced in patients receiving FP.

Although there are no equivalent inhalation studies investigating the effects of respirable particulates in humans, preliminary studies in rats and mice have demonstrated that exposure by inhalation for 30 minutes to concentrations of 10^5 to 5×10^5 ultrafine particles/cm^3 can lead to (1) acute pulmonary inflammation, (2) severe haemorrhagic pulmonary oedema with increased numbers of PMNs in lung lavage samples collected within 4 h of exposure, and (3) significantly increased concentrations of IL-1β, IL-6, TNF-α, inducible nitric oxide synthase and manganese superoxide dismutase, in the lung lavage samples. Additionally, these studies demonstrated that the ultrafine particles could be translocated to epithelial, interstitial and endothelial sites showing marked cell membrane injuries and cell necrosis. It has been proposed that the ultrafine particles are inhaled as singlet particles and are deposited in the alveolar region of the lung, where rather than being phagocytized by alveolar macrophages they penetrate into and interact with the alveolar epithelial, interstitial and endothelial cells. This leads to the release of pro-inflammatory mediators and subsequent infiltration by large numbers of activated PMNs which contribute further to oxidative lung injury.

Airway Epithelial Cells in the Development of Pollution-Induced Airway Disease

There is increasing evidence that airway epithelial cells may play a pivotal role in the pathogenesis of allergic airways disease, since they can express and synthesize a variety of inflammatory cytokines and adhesion molecules including IL-1β, IL-6, IL-8, IL-16, GM-CSF, tumour necrosis factor-α (TNF-α), regulated on activation, normal T cell expressed and secreted (RANTES) and intercellular adhesion molecule-1 (ICAM-1), which influence the activity of eosinophils and lymphocytes, which play important roles in the allergic reaction [25–26]. RANTES, IL-8 and GM-CSF in combination are chemoattractant for eosinophils and GM-CSF plays an important part in delaying apoptosis of eosinophils. Studies from our laboratory have recently shown that exposure of human bronchial epithelial cells to 400–800 ppb NO_2, in vitro, leads to increased epithelial permeability and damage of these cells, decreased ciliary activity, and release of pro-inflammatory mediators, including LTC_4, GM-CSF, TNF-α and IL-8 [27]. Similarly, Rusznak and colleagues have demonstrated that exposure of these cells for 6 h to ambient concentrations of 10–50 ppb O_3, well below the WHO safety guidelines, induced significant release of IL-8, GM-CSF, TNF-α and soluble (s)ICAM-1, of which release of GM-CSF, TNF-α and sICAM-1 could be blocked by treatment of the cells with 10–5M nedocromil sodium [28]. Additionally, these authors demonstrated that exposure to O_3 led to significant epithelial cell damage at concentrations above 100 ppb O_3.

However, recent studies have demonstrated that there are differences in the ability of epithelial cells of atopic and non-atopic individuals, to synthesize different amounts and and/or profiles of pro-inflammatory cytokines, and suggest that genetic pre-disposition and manifestation of the symptoms of allergic airway disease in the atopic individuals may, at least in part, be a consequence of these differences.

Studies of epithelial cells cultured from nasal tissue of non-atopic non-rhinitic subjects, patients with allergic rhinitis and patients with nasal polyps have demonstrated that the epithelial cells from rhinitics and individuals with nasal polyps synthesize significantly greater quantities of GM-CSF and IL-8, than cells of healthy non-atopic non-rhinitic individuals [29]. More recently we have demonstrated that epithelial cells cultured from nasal biopsies of atopic non-rhinitic and atopic rhinitic patients release significantly greater amounts of IL-8, GM-CSF and TNF-α than the epithelial cells from non-atopic, non-rhinitic volunteers and that this release of cytokines particularly RANTES is significantly enhanced during the pollen season [29]. Preliminary studies of epithelial cells cultured from bronchial biopsies of well characterized groups of asthmatic and non-asthmatic subjects in our laboratory have also demonstrated that bronchial epithelial cells of atopic asthmatics release significantly greater amounts of constitutive IL-8, GM-CSF, RANTES and sICAM-1, than the cells of non-atopic non-asthmatics .

Collectively, these studies suggest that genetic pre-disposition and manifestation of the symptoms of allergic airway disease in atopic individuals may, at least in part, be a consequence of increased expression, synthesis and release of specific pro-inflammatory mediators from their airway epithelial cells, both constitutively and following exposure to external factors such as allergens and pollutants.

Address for correspondence:

Prof. Robert J Davies
Asthma and Allergy
London Bridge Hospital
Emblem House
27 Tooley Street
London SE1 2PR
UK
Tel. +44 171 815-2930
Fax +44 181 355-9632

References

1. Pope CA 3rd, Thun MJ, Namboodiri MM, Dockery DW, Evans JS, Speizer FE, Heath CW, Jr. Particulate air pollution as a predictor of mortality in a prospective study of US adults. Am J Respir Crit Care Med 1995; 151:669–674.

2. Pauli G, Kopferschmitt MC, Spirlet F, Charpin D. Air pollutants and allergic sensitisation, In P Chanez, J Bousquet, FB Michel, P Godard (Eds), From genetics to quality of life. Hogrefe & Huber Publisher, Göttingen 1996, pp. 80–89.

3. Ishizaki T, Koizumi K, Ikemori R, Ishiyama Y, Kushibiki E. Studies of prevalence of Japanese cedar pollinosis among residents in a densely cultivated area. Annals of Allergy, 1987; 58:265–270.

4. von Mutius E, Fritzsch C, Weiland SK, Roll G, Magnussen H. Prevalence of asthma and allergic disorders among children in united Germany. BMJ 1992; 305: 1395–1399.

5. Heinrich J, Richter K, Magnussen H, Wichmann HE. Do asthma and asthma symptoms in adults already converge between East and West Germany. Am J Respir Crit Care Med 1996; 153(4):A856.

6. Wichmann HE. Possible explanation for the different trend of asthma and allergy in east and west Germany. Clin Exp Allergy 1996; 26:621–623.

7. Luczynska CM, Walker LA, Burney PGJ. Skin sensitivity in school children in two different areas of London. Eur Respir J 1995; 8(19):350s (abstract).

8. Bylin G, Hedenstirna G, Linduall T, Sundin B. Ambient nitrogen dioxide concentrations increase bronchial responsiveness in subjects with mild asthma. Eur Respir J 1988; 1:606–612.

9. Seal E, McDonnell WF, House DE. Pulmonary function and symptom response of resting humans exposed to low concentrations of ozone for 6.8 h. Am J Respir Crit Care Med 1996, 153(4):A303 (abstract).

10. Koenig JQ, Covert DS, Hanley QS, Belle GV, Pierson WE. Prior exposure to ozone potentiates subsequent response to sulphur dioxide in adolescent asthmatic subjects. Am Rev Respir Dis 1990; 141:377–380.

11. Ball BA, Folinsbee LJ, Peden DB and Kehrl HR. Allergen bronchoprovocation of patients with mild allergic asthma after ozone exposure. J Allergy Clin Immunol 1996; 98:563–572.

12. Jörres R, Nowak D, Magnussen H. Effect of ozone exposure on allergen responsiveness in subjects with asthma or rhinitis. Am J Respir Crit Care Med 1996; 153:56–64.

13. Tunnicliffe WS, Burge PS, Ayres JG. Effect of domestic concentrations of nitrogen dioxide on airway responses to inhaled allergen in asthmatic patients. Lancet 1994; 344:1733–1736.

14. Devalia JL, Rusznak C, Herdman MJ, Trigg CJ, Taraf H, Davies RJ. Effect of nitrogen dioxide and sulphur dioxide on the airway response of mild asthmatic patients to allergen inhalation. Lancet 1994; 344: 1668–1671.

15. Rusznak C, Devalia JL, Davies RJ. The airway response of asthmatic subjects to inhaled allergen after exposure to pollutants.Thorax 1996; 51:1105–1108.

16. Behrendt H, Becker WM, Friedrichs KH, Darsow U, Tomingas R. Interaction between aeroallergens and airborne particulate matter. Int Arch Allergy Immunol 1992; 99:425–428.

17. Knox RB, Suphioglu C, Taylor P, Peng JL, Bursill LA. Asthma and air pollution: Major grass pollen allergen binds to diesel exhaust particles (DECP). J Allergy Clin Immunol 1996; 97(1), 378 (abstract).

18. Sanchez D, Dotson AR, Takenaka H, Saxon A. Diesel exhaust particles induce local IgE production *in vivo* and alter the pattern of IgE messenger RNA isoforms. J Clin Invest 1994; 94:1417–1425.

19. Diaz-Sanchez D. The role of diesel exhaust particles and their associated hydrocarbons in the induction of allergic airway disease. Allergy 1997; 52(38):52–56.

20. Takenaka H, Zhang K, Diaz-Sanchez D, Tsien A, Saxon A. Enhanced human IgE production results from exposure to the aromatic hydrocarbons from diesel exhaust: Direct effects on B-cell IgE production. J Allergy Clin Immunol 1995; 95:103–115.

21. Basha MA, Gross KB, Gwizdala CJ, Haidar AH, Popovich J Jr. Bronchoalveolar lavage neutrophilia in asthmatic and healthy volunteers after controlled exposure to ozone and filter purified air. Chest 1994; 106:1757–1765.

22. Sandström T, Sternberg N, Eklund A, Ledin M-C, Bjemer L, Kolmodin-Hedman B, Lindström K, Rosenhall L, Ångström T. Inflammatory cell response in bronchoalveolar lavage fluid after nitrogen dioxide exposure of healthy subjects: A dose-response study. Eur Respir J 1991; 3:332–339.

23. Peden DB, Setzer RW Jr, Devlin RB. Ozone exposure has both a priming effect on allergen-induced responses and an intrinsic inflammatory action in the nasal airways of perennially allergic asthmatics. Am J Respir Crit Care Med 1995; 151:1336–1345.

24. Wang J, Devalia JL, Duddle JM, Hamilton SA, Davies RJ. The effect of exposure for 6 h to nitrogen dioxide (NO_2) on early phase nasal response to allergen challenge in patient with a history of seasonal allergic rhinitis. J Allergy Clin Immunol 1995; 96:669–676.

25. Devalia JL and Davies RJ. Airway epithelial cells and mediators of inflammation. Respir Med 1993; 87: 405–408.

26. Wang JH, Devalia JL, Xia C, Sapsford RJ, Davies RJ. Expression of RANTES by human bronchial epithelial cells *in vitro* and *in vivo* and the effect of corticosteroids. Am J Respir Cell Mol Biol 1996; 14:27–35.

27. Devalia JL, Campbell AM, Sapsford RJ, Rusznak C, Quint D, Godard PH, Bousquet J, Davies RJ. Effect of nitrogen dioxide on synthesis of inflammatory cytokines expressed by human bronchial epithelial cells *in vitro*. Am J Respir Cell Mol Biol 1993; 9:271–279.

28. Rusznak C, Devalia JL, Sapsford RJ, Davies RJ. Ozone-induced release of inflammatory mediators from human bronchial epithelial cells *in vitro* and the influence of nedocromil sodium. Eur Respir J 1996; 9:2298–2305.

29. Calderón MA, Devalia JL, Prior AJ, Sapsford RJ and Davies RJ. A comparison of cytokine release from epithelial cells cultured from nasal biopsy specimens of atopic patients with and without rhinitis and non-atopic subjects without rhinitis. J Allergy Clin Immunol 1997; 99:65–76.

The Prediction and Prevention of Childhood Asthma

John O Warner*

Keywords: Childhood asthma, BAL, airway inflammation, antenatal sensitization, allergen avoidance

Much work has still to be conducted to establish which are the key predictors of childhood asthma that might facilitate early intervention strategies to prevent the development of the disease. Hitherto, there are no reliable markers, and furthermore, there is relatively little evidence that any interventions truly prevent disease. From bronchoscopic lavage and biopsy studies in childhood asthma, there is a suggestion that the airway immunopathology is well established by the time the disease first manifests. Therefore, effective disease modifying intervention will need to be established before children show the first symptoms. The combination of allergen avoidance and the use of cetirizine have at least in certain circumstances been shown to reduce subsequent prevalence of disease.

The accepted definition of asthma in children and adults has incorporated the concept of airway inflammation as being the cardinal feature of the condition. Thus bronchial hyperresponsiveness, intermittent airflow limitation and symptoms of cough and wheeze are the consequence of the inflammation. The definition states that eosinophils and mast cells are key cellular components in the inflammatory process which distinguish it from infection induced inflammation [1]. There is now very good evidence that over 5 years of age, the immunopathology of asthma is similar if not identical [2]. However with decreasing age, it becomes progressively more difficult to apply the definition to recurrent coughing and wheezing as it manifests in the young. Indeed recurrent wheeze in infants which affects at least a third of all children very frequently does not evolve into atopic asthma, though such infants may be more prone to late onset adult chronic obstructive pulmonary disease [3].

Markers of Established Asthma

There are now many studies which have given evidence that eosinophil activation is present in childhood asthma and correlates with other markers of disease activity such as lung function and bronchial hyperresponsiveness [4]. Furthermore, bronchoalveolar lavage studies from asthmatic children have demonstrated an excess of eosinophils [5, 6, 7]. There is a correlation between eosinophil numbers and the degree of bronchial hyperresponsiveness [5]. We have also been able to show differences in levels of soluble intercellular adhesion molecule 1 (sICAM-1) and interferon-γ (IFN-γ) in lavage from asthmatic children compared to those with other airway abnormalities, including sepsis due to cystic fibrosis [2]. Furthermore, the severity of asthma is assessed by frequency of symptoms correlated with the degree of increase in sICAM. We have, in addition, shown that young children with respiratory symptoms that went on to have established asthma, had far higher numbers of activated eosinophils in the lamina propria of bronchial biopsies and increased deposition of collagen below the basement membrane than those who do not develop asthma.

There was no correlation with the severity of the above two abnormalities and the duration of symptoms before biopsy. It is perhaps, therefore, not surprising that long term follow-up studies of childhood asthmatics have shown that irrespective of treatment, those with infrequent episodic disease retain normal lung function [8] and those with severe disease tend to have abnormal lung function and increased bronchial hyperresponsiveness from the outset [9]. Thus mild remains mild and severe usually remains severe, irrespective of treatment. This almost certainly is because all of the changes that constitute the immunopathology of the disease are well established by the time of the first symptoms and subsequent intervention is unlikely to have any impact.

---

* University of Southampton/Southampton General Hospital, Southampton, Hampshire, UK. © 1999 John O Warner.

Early Markers of Asthma

At least a third of all infants have wheezing episodes associated with viral respiratory infections. The majority are totally asymptomatic between episodes and have no other trigger to symptoms. Upwards of 80% of these infants will outgrow their problem [10]. Thus respiratory syncytial virus induced bronchiolitis is commonly associated with recurrent wheeze for several years after the acute infection. However, there is little evidence that such children have a higher risk than normal of subsequently having atopic asthma [11]. Epidemiological studies have shown that low birth weight, maternal smoking during pregnancy, poor socio-economic circumstances and having older siblings are all risk factors for increased respiratory morbidity but not asthma in infancy [12]. A common feature of the effects of maternal smoking in pregnancy and low birth weight is the presence of diminished small airway calibre. This suggests that the predominant cause of wheezing in infancy is simply having smaller small airways. This has been confirmed by studies of neonatal lung function in large cohorts that have been followed through the first years of life. Those that go on to have recurrent but transient wheezing in infancy, have lower lung function prior to first symptoms [13]. Infants born to mothers who smoke during pregnancy also have decreased lung function compared with those born to non-smoking mothers [14]. As low birth weight has also been associated with a higher probability of lung disease in late adult life [3], there is therefore a link between infant wheeze and obstructive disease in later life with an asymptomatic period in mid life. However, such individuals do not have evidence of airway inflammation characteristic of asthma and, therefore, must clearly be excluded from future consideration in relation to early intervention.

No studies have yet investigated the evolution of airway inflammation in those infants who become asthmatics. We have recently found that amongst infant wheezers there is a significant increase in neutrophil numbers. It is remarkable that the neutrophil count correlated rather well with clinical severity of symptoms of disease [6]. As neutrophils are associated with more severe asthma in adults, one might ask the question whether they might not contribute significantly to the initiation of airway inflammation that leads to asthma? However, at present they provide no information that might facilitate early intervention to prevent the development of asthma. More follow-up studies are required.

Other studies have attempted to use circulating markers of airway inflammation to get some idea of evolution of disease. Thus the Oslo birth cohort study has shown that in infant wheezers compared with matched controls, there is a higher probability of salbutamol responsiveness which correlates well with the level of eosinophil cationic protein in the serum as a marker of eosinophil activation. One might predict that bronchodilator responsive individuals with eosinophil activation would be asthmatics. However, we await the follow-up studies to see whether this will show that non-invasive monitoring will provide prediction of airway disease which might facilitate the intervention strategies [15].

At present, the clinician is left with making a judgement on the basis of a presence or absence of atopy in infant wheezers. If this is associated with a family history of atopic asthma, then there is a 50–60% chance of asthma evolving. Other markers that are being investigated include circulating soluble interleukin-2 receptor levels that we have found correlate with ongoing wheezing in both atopics and non-atopics.

When Does Airway Inflammation Appear?

The above observations suggest that airway inflammation in atopic asthmatics appears before the onset of symptoms and may well probably evolve from very early infancy. This assertion is supported by observations from the Perth cohort study that identified bronchial hyperresponsiveness at 4 weeks of age in infants born to atopic parents. Given the correlation between hyperresponsiveness and eosinophilic inflammation in asthmatics, this implies that the inflammation was already present at 4 weeks of age, again sometimes years before first symptoms [16]. Thus attention is focusing on an ever earlier age and may be even on the antenatal period.

Antenatal Sensitization

We have ever increasing evidence that allergic sensitization occurs antenatally. Whether or not this has any effect on the airways before birth remains to be established.

Many studies have now identified that the neonate is not immunologically naïve but is capable of mounting significant immune responses to environmental allergens. This can only have occurred as a result of antenatal sensitization. Thus peripheral blood mononuclear cell sensitivity to allergens in neonatal bloods has predicted subsequent development of atopic disease [17, 18, 19]. Indeed, we now have evidence that the allergen specific reactivity is present in the peripheral circulation of fetuses from 22 weeks of gestation onwards [20]. The studies also suggest that there is a characteristic of the cytokine production of sensitized cells which is particularly associated with subsequent atopic disease, the hallmark being reduced IFN-γ production. However, it is clear that there is a relative inability for IFN-γ production by stimulated PBMCs from all neonates but this defect is greater in those from atopic families and who subsequently develop atopy [18, 21]. Nevertheless, there is a universal skewing of the initial T-lymphocyte response towards a Th2 cytokine profile in all newborns [22] and subsequent atopic infants appear to be defective in production of not only Th1 cytokines but also those associated with a Th2 response. This suggests that the characteristic of the immune response of the eventual atopic is that of sensitization with either an immaturity of cytokine release or alternatively some form of suppression [23].

A number of attempts have been made to introduce allergen avoidance, both ante- and post-natally. Most are focused on food allergens. The general consensus hitherto has been that antenatal avoidance achieves nothing, though most have only introduced the avoidance in the third trimester of pregnancy which is after sensitization has occurred. However postnatal avoidance, particularly focusing on breastfeeding, has been associated with a reduced prevalence of food allergy and atopic dermatitis in the first two years of life. Only one study has shown any sustained effects thereafter with an impact on asthma [24]. The others have shown no preventive effect for airway disease [25, 26].

Antenatal Allergen Exposure and Sensitivity

We have evidence that antigen exposure from 22 weeks gestation and onwards via the mother to the fetus is capable of switching on a fetal immune response that initially is characterized by a profile of Th2 cytokine activity. How this influences the subsequent development of allergic disease remains to be seen. It is likely that both dose and timing of antigen exposure will be critical to the characteristic of the response. Thus, there is some limited evidence that very high allergen exposure of the mother during pregnancy will induce an IgG antibody which may well be protective of fetal sensitization, whereas intermediate level exposure will promote sensitization and allergy, and only total exclusion from exposure will be associated with an absence of sensitization. Great caution will, therefore, be required before making any recommendations on allergen avoidance antenatally. It may be more appropriate in the long term to consider some form of immune modulation. Clearly, however, it is relevant to avoid the adjuvantising effects of such factors as environmental tobacco smoke. Such interventions may be classed as primary prophylaxis.

Secondary Prophylaxis

Secondary prophylaxis is that form of intervention that is introduced after sensitization has occurred but before there is any evidence of disease. This might reasonably be considered in individuals who have evidence of atopic sensitization but not yet asthma. One prime target is the baby with atopic dermatitis.

There are two studies that have investigated a pharmacotherapeutic intervention to prevent the development of asthma in infants with atopic dermatitis. The first employed ketotifen or placebo for 1 year in 110 infants and showed a considerably reduced prevalence of asthma over that 1-year period in those on the active treatment. Unfortunately, however, there was no follow-up and the sedative effects of the antihistamine mitigated against its uptake for secondary prophylaxis [27].

More recently, a much larger study has been conducted in similar infants comparing cetirizine with a placebo. This study also demonstrated a significant reduction in prevalence of asthma over 18 months of active treatment compared with placebo in those with evidence of sensitivity to house dust mite and/or grass pollen, which constituted 20% of the total population recruited [28]. As house dust mite and pollen sensitivity were also the strongest predictors of subsequent asthma in atopic dermatitis, this suggests that the effect may be long lasting. Uniquely this study has already shown that 6 months after the treatment had been stopped, the effect was still sustained suggesting true prevention. Longer term follow-up is required to establish the full cost benefits of this intervention. However, it provides a marker for future studies to investigate alternative pharmacotherapeutic strategies in this situation.

For secondary and tertiary prophylaxis, allergen avoidance would seem to be a reasonable strategy despite the recent rather negative meta-analysis in relation to house mite avoidance. Unfortunately this latter study failed to identify that many of the trials had not reduced levels of mites and were, therefore, unlikely to have any impact on the disease [29]. Further analysis of those studies that had achieved a reduction in mite levels showed that they were efficacious. Certainly the precedence created by studying occupational allergic asthma suggests that early removal from offending allergens can achieve total resolution, where more prolonged exposure would lead to chronic irreversible changes and ongoing disease even in the absence of continuing allergen exposure [30].

Address for correspondence:

Prof. John O Warner
Centre Block, Room CG56
Southampton General Hospital
Southampton
Hampshire SO9 4XY
UK
Tel. +44 1703 796160
Fax +44 1703 796378

References

1. Global Strategy for Asthma Management and Prevention. NHLBI/WHO workshop report. Publication No. 95–3659, 1995. National Institutes of Health, Bethesda, MD, USA.

2. Warner JO, Warner JA, Clough JB, Rao R, Marguet C, Pohunek P, Roche W. Markers of allergy and inflammation. Pediatr Allergy Immunol 1998; 9(Suppl. 11):53–57.

3. Barker DJP. Editor. Fetal and infant origins of adult disease. London, BMJ, 1992.

4. Rao KR, Frederick JM, Enander I, Gregson RK, Warner JA, Warner JO. Airway function correlates with circulating eosinophil but not mast cell markers of inflammation in childhood asthma. Clin Exp Allergy 1996; 26:789–793.

5. Ferguson AC, Whitelaw M, Brown H. Correlation of bronchial eosinophil and mast cell activation with bronchial hyperresponsiveness in children with asthma. J Allergy Clin Immunol 1992; 90:606–613.

6. Marguet C, Jouen-Boedes F, Dean TP, Warner JO. Bronchoalveolar cell profiles in children with asthma, infantile wheeze, chronic cough or cystic fibrosis. Am J Respir Crit Care Med, in press.

7. Stevenson EC, Turner G, Heaney LG, Schock BC, Taylor R, Gallagher T, Ennis M, Shields MD. Broncho-alveolar lavage findings suggest two different forms of childhood asthma. Clin Exp Allergy 1997; 27:1027–1035.

8. Oswald H, Phelan PD, Lanigan A, Hibbert M, Carlin JB, Bowes G, Olinsky A. Childhood asthma and lung function in mid adult life. Pediatr Pulmonol 1997; 23:14–20.

9. Gerritsen J, Koeter GH, Postma DS, Schouten JP, Van Aalderen WMC, Knol K. Airway responsiveness in childhood as a predictor of the outcome of asthma in adulthood. Am Rev Respir Dis 1991; 143:1468–1469.

10. Lewis S, Richards D, Bynner J, Butler N, Britton J. Prospective study of risk factors for early and persistent wheezing in childhood. Eur Respir J 1996; 8: 349–356.

11. Landau LI. Bronchiolitis and asthma: Are they related? Thorax 1994; 49:293–296.

12. Von Mutius E, Martinez FD, Fritzsch C, Nicolai T, Roell G, Thiemann HH. Prevalence of asthma and atopy in two areas of West and East Germany. Am J Respir Crit Care Med 1994; 149:358–364.

13. Martinez FD, Morgan WJ, Wright AL, Holberg C, Taussig LM. Initial airway function is a risk factor for recurrent wheezing respiratory illness during the first three years of life. New Engl J Med 1991; 143:312–316.

14. Hanrahan JP, Tager IB, Segal MR. The effect of maternal smoking during pregnancy on early infant lung function. Am Rev Respir Dis 1992; 145:1129–1135.

15. Lødrup-Carlsen KC, Ragnhild H, Ahlstedt S, Carlsen K-H. Eosinophilic cationic protein and tidal flow volume loops in children 0–2 years of age. Eur Respir J 1995; 8:1148–1154.

16. E, Stick SM, Arnott J, Turner DJ, Young S, Landau LI, Le Soeuf PN. Bronchial responsiveness and lung function in recurrently wheezy infants. Am Rev Respir Dis 1991; 144:1012–1015.

17. Kondo N, Kobayashi Y, Shinoda S et al. Cord blood lymphocyte responses to food antigens for the prediction of allergic disorders. Arch Dis Child 1992; 67:1003–1007.

18. Warner JA, Miles EA, Jones AC et al. Is deficiency of IFN-γ production by allergen triggered cord blood

cells a predictor of atopic eczema? Clin Exp Allergy 1994; 24:423–430.

19. Kondo N, Kobayashi Y, Shimoda S et al. Reduced IFN-γ production by antigen stimulated cord blood mononuclear cells is a risk factor for allergic disorders – 6-year follow-up study. Clin Exp Allergy 1998; 28:1340–1344.

20. Jones AC, Miles EA, Warner JO et al. Fetal peripheral blood mononuclear cell proliferative responses to mitogenic and allergenic stimulae during gestation. Pediatr Allergy Immunol 1996; 7:109–116.

21. Tang MLK, Kemp AS, Thorburn J, Hill DJ. Reduced IFN-γ secretion in neonates and subsequent atopy. Lancet 1994; 344:983–985.

22. Prescott SL, Macaubas C, Holt BJ. Transplacental priming of the human immune system to environmental allergens: Universal skewing of initial T-cell responses towards the Th2 cytokine profile. J Immunol 1998; 160:4730–4737.

23. Williams TJ, Jones CA, Miles EA et al. Fetal and neonatal IL-13 production during pregnancy and at birth, and subsequent development of atopic symptoms. J Clin Invest (submitted).

24. Saarinen UM, Kajosaari M. Breastfeeding as prophylaxis against atopic disease: Prospective follow-up study until 17 years. Lancet 1995; 346:1065–25.

25. Zeiger RS. Secondary prevention of allergic disease: an adjunct to primary prevention. Pediatr Allergy Immunol 1995; 6:127–138.

26. Hide DW, Matthews S, Tariq S, Arshad SH. Allergen avoidance in infancy and allergy at 4 years of age. Allergy 1996; 51:89–93.

27. Iikura Y, Naspitz CK, Mikawa H, Talaricoficho S, Baba M, Sole D, Nishima S. Prevention of asthma by ketotifen in infants with atopic dermatitis. Ann Allergy 1992; 68:233–236.

28. ETAC Study Group. Allergic factors associated with the development of asthma and the influence of cetirizine in a double blind, randomised, placebo-controlled trial. First results of ETAC. Pediatr Allergy Immunol 1998; 9:116–124.

29. Gotzsche P-C, Hammarquist C, Burr M. House dust mite control measures in the management of asthma: Meta-analysis. Br Med J 1998; 317:1105–1110.

30. Paggiaro PL, Vagaggini B, Bacci E et al. Prognosis of occupational asthma. Eur Respir J 1994; 7:761–767.

Asthma Epidemiology: Old and New Issues

Jonathan M Samet*

Keywords: Asthma, atopy, epidemiology, exposure, prevalence

Epidemiology, the scientific method used to investigate health and disease in populations, has long held a central role in research on asthma. Epidemiologic evidence has described the natural history of asthma, characterized by environmental determinants of disease development and exacerbation, and provided an indication of the genetic basis of the disease through demonstration of familial aggregation. Key questions for asthma researchers include:
– Why does prevalence of asthma vary markedly throughout the world?
– Why does the occurrence of asthma vary over time and what is driving the current increase?
– Will risk factor reduction affect the occurrence of asthma?
– What are the genes that determine risk for asthma?
– Why does the asthma mortality rate vary over time and across countries? What is the role of therapeutic agents in risk for asthma mortality?
– Can the natural history of asthma be modified by environmental modifications or therapeutic interventions?

Introduction

Epidemiology, the scientific method used to investigate health and disease in populations, has long held a central role in research on asthma. Epidemiologic evidence has described the natural history of asthma, characterized environmental determinants of disease development and exacerbation, and provided an indication of the genetic basis of the disease through the demonstration of familial aggregation. At the century's end, the scientific literature includes thousands of reports on the findings of epidemiologic studies. In 1999, a literature search using Medline and the key words of "asthma" and "epidemiology" identified 1,089 citations in English. Studies based in epidemiologic approaches are in progress throughout the world addressing hypotheses related to natural history, risk factors, and genetics. The identification of risk factors for childhood asthma, such as early life exposures to allergens, has prompted the initiation of intervention trials to test if the development of asthma can be slowed.

The evidence on asthma from epidemiologic studies has been summarized in numerous reviews and monographs (see [1–3] for summaries of this literature). In brief, the incidence of the disease has been described in several, population-based studies [2]. Peak incidence occurs before age 10 years and then falls before rising again across the middle-aged years of life. Fortunately, death from asthma is relatively uncommon, but deaths do occur and routine vital statistics have shown substantial fluctuations that have not been readily explained [4]. Asthma prevalence has been described in many countries and also documented over time in a number of countries. The prevalence data convincingly show marked geographic variation and, in some populations, remarkably high prevalence estimates, ranging up to 20% [2]. Asthma risk has been associated with a number of factors, including allergen exposure, maternal smoking during pregnancy and childhood exposure to tobacco smoke, respiratory infections, occupational agents, and air pollution. Its genetic basis is indicated by the demonstration of familial aggregation and its association with atopy, also a genetically determined condition.

In spite of the voluminous epidemiologic evidence on asthma, key questions remain unanswered and calls for further research are persistent and increasingly urgent as the prevalence of the disease rises without seeming explanation. These questions are summarized below:
– Why does the prevalence of asthma vary markedly throughout the world?
– Why does the occurrence of asthma vary over time and what is driving the current increase?

* Johns Hopkins University, Baltimore, MD, USA

- Will risk factor reduction affect the occurrence of asthma?
- What are the genes that determine risk for asthma?
- Why does the asthma mortality rate vary over time and across countries? What is the role of therapeutic agents in risk for asthma mortality?
- Can the natural history of asthma be modified by environmental modifications or therapeutic interventions?

Answering these questions will require a substantial commitment to research on asthma and a decades-long research program. This review will address each of these questions in turn, commenting briefly on the current epidemiologic evidence and then turning to potential research approaches. First, I review the methods used by epidemiologists in investigating asthma.

Epidemiologic Approach to Asthma

The tools of the epidemiologist for investigating asthma include a set of general study designs and the more specific respiratory questionnaires and lung function tests that are used to determine if asthma is present and to characterize the asthma phenotype. The study designs used by epidemiologists are both observational and experimental, depending on whether the exposure status of study participants is that occurring naturally or is determined by the investigator. The key observational designs include the cross-sectional study or survey, the cohort study, and the case-control study [5]; all have been applied to the study of asthma. The cross-sectional design involves the collection of data on the presence of disease and on risk factors at one point in time. This design has been widely applied to determine the frequency of asthma, as in the International Study of Asthma and Allergies in Childhood (ISAAC) [6]. Associations with risk factors can also be investigated using the cross-sectional design, but the associations are subject to potentially complicated biases [3]. The persons with asthma at any particular time are those "survivors" with the diagnosis who have neither died nor lost the asthma phenotype; furthermore, there may also be temporal ambiguity between environmental exposures and asthma risk because the presence of

asthma may have prompted environmental changes.

For this reason, the cohort and case-control designs are more appropriate for investigating risk factors for asthma. The cohort study involves the follow-up of persons over time with the ascertainment of new cases of disease; risk can then be estimated in relation to relevant exposures, whether characterized at the start of follow-up or over time as the exposures vary. Well-known cohort studies include, for example, the birth cohort study initiated in Tucson, Arizona [7], and the study conducted in the United Kingdom on early-life exposure to house dust mite and asthma and wheezing onset [8]. The case-control study involves the comparison of exposures of asthma cases with those of appropriately selected, comparable controls. This design has been infrequently applied to the study of asthma, although it represents a statistically efficient and feasible approach. Infante-Rivard [9] applied this design in an investigation of risk factors for incident childhood asthma in Montreal, Canada. Incident cases were identified at the time of urgent care visits and appropriate controls were selected from the same venue. Exposures were assessed by questionnaire and environmental measurements.

The key experimental design is the randomized clinical trial, widely applied for assessing therapeutic agents, but also appropriate for evaluating preventive interventions, such as allergen avoidance. In fact, randomized controlled trials of allergen avoidance and risk for allergic diseases have already been conducted [10]. Additional, more specialized designs based around families are used by genetic epidemiologists to explore the genetic basis of asthma [11].

In research on asthma, epidemiologists use a variety of standardized data collection tools: Respiratory symptom and disease questionnaires, exposure questionnaires, spirometry, measures of airways responsiveness, and indexes of atopy–skin testing, and levels of specific and total IgE. These tools have evolved over decades of use and recommendations for standardized application have been made by a number of groups [3].

One persistent obstacle in epidemiologic research on asthma has been the seeming impossibility of defining the disease in an operationally useful manner. Numerous definitions have been offered and criteria applied by researchers have been variable [2, 12]. This problem has been the topic of several symposia and numerous commentaries. The 1971 Ciba symposium [13] ended with the conclusion that asthma could not be defined; little progress towards a useful definition had been made by the 1996 Ciba symposium on the rising trends in asthma [1]. Newer definitions have incorporated the latest concepts of pathogenesis, but there are no counterpart criteria for application by epidemiologists. Burney's proposal [14] to study the elements of the asthma phenotype, without necessarily applying a unifying disease definition, seems appropriate for facilitating research and comparability across investigations. I now turn to the key questions to be addressed in epidemiologic research.

Why Does the Prevalence of Asthma Vary Markedly Throughout the World?

A remarkably high degree of variation in asthma prevalence around the world has been documented [2]. In the ISAAC study, for example, there was an approximately 20-fold range in prevalence rates of self-reported asthma [6]. Within countries, variation in prevalence has also been shown. In the United States, prevalence tends to be higher in inner-city children, compared with children in the suburbs [15]. Potential explanations for the variation include (1) methodologic issues such as differential responses to survey instruments and varying rates of asthma diagnosis by health care providers; (2) differing rates of exposure to causal factors; and (3) differences in the genetic liability to asthma. The use of standardized methodology, as in the ISAAC study, suggests that the variation cannot be attributed to methodologic factors alone.

The more interesting hypotheses needing follow-up relate to the potential contributions of environmental and genetic factors to these differences. Large databases, like the ISAAC study, can be analyzed in a second-stage to assess determinants of variation. Follow-up surveys of environmental exposures directed at populations with the highest and lowest rates should also offer insights into the role of environmental factors in determining asthma occurrence. Undoubtedly, gene–environment interactions are critical in determining the development of asthma. While we presently lack understanding of the genetic basis of asthma, DNA could reasonably be collected from populations at vary-

ing risk with recognition that genetic probes for asthma will become available.

Why Does the Occurrence of Asthma Vary Over Time and What Is Driving the Current Increase?

The trend of rising asthma over the last decade, particularly in children, is of grave public health concern. With prevalence rates reaching 20% among children in some countries, there is a well-recognized urgency in identifying the responsible factors. Thoughtful analyses indicate that the rise cannot be attributed solely to diagnostic trends and emphasis has been placed on the role of the environment, construed in its broadest sense [16, 17].

The rapidity of the rise in asthma can only be explained by changing environmental exposures. Numerous speculations have been offered to explain the increase: (1) changes in housing that have increased exposures to indoor air pollutants and allergens; (2) changes in early life respiratory illness experience leading to a change in immunophenotype; (3) inactivity with less exercise; and (4) dietary changes [16, 18, 19]. These hypotheses are based in the descriptive and somewhat anecdotal and patchy information on changes in these factors over recent decades. As outdoor air quality has generally improved over recent decades, outdoor air pollution has generally been considered as unlikely to play a role in the recent rise.

These speculative hypotheses remain untested. Having observed the rise in asthma over the last several decades, we now lack prospectively collected data to test reasonable hypotheses. The requisite information would include the frequency of exposure to various risk factors over time and estimates of the effects of these risk factors acting alone or in concert on risk for asthma. The lack of this information is a strong rationale for implementing a properly designed surveillance system. In some countries, data systems provide tracking of asthma prevalence and of morbidity through medical care surveys and hospitalization data. In the United States, for example, the Centers for Disease Control and Prevention and the Council of State and Territorial Epidemiologists have reviewed surveillance data and offered a proposal for strengthening the surveillance now in place [20]. Any surveillance program, however, needs to go beyond simply counting events and add information on established and putative risk factors. Nested case-control studies, conducted periodically over time, offer an efficient strategy for tracking the effects of risk factors. The Surveillance, Epidemiology, and End Results (SEER) Program of the US National Cancer Institute, started over 25 years ago, represents a useful model. The population-based cancer registries that comprise the Program have proved invaluable for monitoring the occurrence of cancer in the United States and following up leads for risk factors.

Will Risk Factor Reduction Affect the Occurrence of Asthma?

Epidemiologic studies have identified a number of risk factors for asthma, although some ambiguity remains concerning whether some of these factors increase incidence or severity (or both). Exposures to tobacco smoke and to indoor allergens can be modified and trials of exposure reduction in at-risk children could prove informative, both as to the potential benefits of environmental modification and as further evidence of the causal role of these or other factors. The planning and implementation of intervention studies seems timely. Indoor allergens [18] and tobacco smoke [21] have been repeatedly associated with asthma and further observational studies seem unlikely to be informative with regard to the potential for prevention.

What Are the Genes that Determine Risk for Asthma?

The last decade has seen an unanticipated leap in our capability of exploring the genetic basis of disease. With sound evidence that asthma is familial, the genes that determine risk for asthma are being aggressively investigated [22]. Bleecker et al. [22] describe the general approach of first defining the phenotype(s) of interest, identifying families or populations for study, investigating the mode of inheritance with segregation analysis, performing linkage analysis to identify chromosomal regions

of interest, characterizing and mapping the regions of interest to localize genes, and then assessing gene function. A number of groups are investigating the genetic basis of asthma and the results of several genome-wide searches have been reported [23, 24]. Surprisingly, however, in spite of the clear evidence for familial aggregation, a consistent set of linkages has not yet been achieved.

This line of investigation may be bedeviled by the unsolved challenge of defining asthma and characterizing the asthma phenotype. Definitions and study criteria for asthma have varied widely across studies [12]. Additionally, gene–environment interactions are almost certainly of importance and the genetic studies have only limited data on environmental exposures, particularly at the time of asthma onset. The first wave of studies of asthma genetics needs to be brought to completion before further research directions can be established. To the extent possible, epidemiologic studies of asthma should include the collection of genetic material for future analysis.

Why Does the Asthma Mortality Rate Vary Over Time and Across Countries?

While deaths from asthma occur, these deaths are generally considered to be preventable and their occurrence is viewed as a sentinel event for follow-up and identification of the responsible factors. Since the rise in asthma mortality in a number of countries during the 1960s, asthma mortality has been closely tracked in many countries. A further increase in asthma mortality began in some countries in the 1970s; the increase was particularly dramatic in New Zealand [4]. The 1960s epidemic of asthma deaths and the subsequent rise and fall of asthma mortality in some countries during the 1970s and 1980s have been well documented and the causes investigated using descriptive approaches and more formal methods for the later epidemic. The descriptive analyses have also shown substantial variation across countries in rates of asthma mortality [3, 4].

Many hypotheses have been offered concerning the two epidemics of asthma deaths; a leading and partially proven hypothesis indicts therapeutic agents (see below) [4]. However, research is still needed on the determinants of asthma mortality within particular countries and on the substantial variation across countries. Studies are needed that explore the comparative accuracy of the death certificate diagnosis of asthma across countries and also over time. Standardized case-control studies, assessing risk factors for asthma death in various countries, should also be designed. As for the occurrence of asthma, comprehensive surveillance is needed for risk factors for asthma deaths.

What Is the Role of Therapeutic Agents in Risk for Asthma Mortality?

Based on the descriptive, clinical characterization of the asthma deaths in the United Kingdom during the 1960s, the hypothesis was advanced that inhaled β-agonists may have been responsible [25]. While this hypothesis was not formally tested using the appropriate design, a case-control study of asthma deaths, the epidemic waned after the withdrawal from the market of a particularly potent isoproterenol inhaler [4]. An ecological analysis further supported this hypothesis [26]. Questions concerning the safety of β-agonists were again raised when asthma mortality rose dramatically in New Zealand in the 1970s [4, 27]. A series of case-control studies in New Zealand showed increased risk for death associated with use of fenoterol, which had been introduced into New Zealand in the 1970s. A case-control study of fatal and near-fatal asthma in the province of Saskatchewan, Canada, showed increased risk for fenoterol and for other β-agonists [28].

There has been substantial debate concerning the interpretation of these studies. Do the associations represent a specific effect of fenoterol or a class effect of β-agonists generally? A further methodologic complexity is the bias referred to as confounding by indication; that is, persons with more severe asthma are more likely to receive the more potent medication and at greater doses, in comparison with persons having less severe asthma. Controlling for this type of bias is difficult and full control may not be possible, leaving open the possibility that residual bias may partially explain the association between fenoterol or other drugs and risk for asthma death.

Without pronouncing on the still-heated debate over the risks of fenoterol, the occurrence of two epidemics of mortality among persons having a common disease reinforces the need for surveillance for the causes of asthma deaths and for the adverse consequences of therapeutic agents for asthma. Case-control studies offer one approach. The Sasketchewan study provides a useful model for another: Using large, administrative databases to synthetically carry out cohort studies with linkage methods. Asthma therapy is evolving with the introduction of new therapeutic agents and more powerful formulations of long-used medications. Care is increasingly guideline driven. Comprehensive and sustained monitoring is needed to track the consequences, both beneficial and adverse, of asthma therapy.

Conclusions

Epidemiologic research has provided invaluable insights into the etiology of asthma and its natural history. Risk factors have been identified and prevention trials have been implemented. Lacking adequate epidemiologic surveillance, however, we are ill-equipped to explain the changing picture of incidence and mortality or to track the effects of therapy on outcome of asthma. Comprehensive surveillance is an urgent priority.

The pathogenesis of asthma has been intensely investigated for several decades. Contemporary investigative methods continue to elucidate the complex interplay of cells and cytokines that produce inflammation in asthma. We are also explaining the genetic basis of this response. Ultimately, this work will need to be placed within a population context, using epidemiologic approaches.

Address for correspondence:

Jonathan M Samet, MD, MS
School of Hygiene and Public Health
Johns Hopkins University
615 North Wolfe Street, Suite W6041
Baltimore, MD 21205-2179
USA
Tel. +1 410 955-3286
Fax +1 410 955-0863
E-mail jsamet@jhsph.edu

References

1. Ciba Foundation Symposium. The rising trends in asthma. Chadwick DJ, Cardew G (Eds). Chichester: John Wiley & Sons, 1997.

2. Wiesch D, Samet JM. Epidemiology and natural history of asthma. In Middleton E, Reed CE, Ellis EF, Adkinson NF, Yunginger JW, Busse WW (Eds), Allergy: Principles and practice (5th ed.), Chapter 2. St. Louis: Mosby-Year Book, Inc., 1998, pp. 799–815.

3. Pearce N, Beasley R, Burgess C, Crane J. Asthma epidemiology. Principles and methods. New York/Oxford: Oxford University Press, 1998.

4. Beasley R, Pearce N, Crane J. International trends in asthma mortality. In Chadwick DJ, Cardew G (Eds), The rising trends in asthma. Chichester: John Wiley & Sons, 1997, pp. 140–150.

5. Gordis L. Epidemiology. Philadelphia: W.B. Saunders, 1996.

6. Beasley R, Keil U, Von Mutius E, Pearce N, ISAAC Steering Committee. Worldwide variation in prevalence of symptoms of asthma, allergic rhinoconjunctivitis, and atopic eczema: ISAAC. Lancet 1998; 351:1225–1232.

7. Martinez FD, Wright AL, Taussig LM, Holberg CJ, Halonen M, Morgan WJ. Asthma and wheezing in the first six years of life. The Group Health Medical Associates. N Engl J Med 1995; 332(3):133–138.

8. Sporik R, Holgate ST, Platts-Mills TA, Cogswell JJ. Exposure to house-dust mite allergen (Der p I) and the development of asthma in childhood. A prospective study. N Engl J Med 1990; 323(8):502–507.

9. Infante-Rivard C. Childhood asthma and indoor environmental risk factors. Am J Epidemiol 1993; 137(8): 834–844.

10. Arshad SH, Matthews S, Gant C, Hide DW. Effect of allergen avoidance on development of allergic disorders in infancy. Lancet 1992; 339(8808):1493–1497.

11. Khoury MJ, Beaty TH, Cohen BH. Fundamentals of genetic epidemiology. New York: Oxford University Press, 1993.

12. Wiesch D, Samet JM, Meyers DA, Bleecker ER. Classification of the asthma phenotype in genetic studies. In Liggett SB, Meyers DA (Eds), The genetics of asthma. New York: Marcel Dekker, Inc., 1996, pp. 421–438.

13. Ciba Foundation Study Group. Identification of asthma. Edinburgh: Churchill Livingstone, 1971.

14. Burney P. Interpretation of epidemiological surveys of asthma. In Chadwick DJ, Cardew E (Eds), The rising trends in asthma. Chichester: John Wiley & Sons, 1997, pp. 111–121.

15. Crain EF, Weiss KB, Bijur PE, Hersh M, Westbrook L, Stein RE. An estimate of the prevalence of asthma and wheezing among inner-city children. Pediatrics 1994; 94(3):356–362.

16. Woolcock AJ, Peat JK. Evidence for the increase in asthma worldwide. In Chadwick DJ, Cardew G (Eds), The rising trends in asthma. Chichester: John Wiley & Sons, 1997, pp. 122–134.

17. Weiss KB, Gergen PJ, Wagener DK. Breathing better or wheezing worse? The changing epidemiology of asthma morbidity and mortality. In Omenn GS, Lave LB (Eds), Annual review of public health, Chapter 14. Palo Alto: Annual Reviews Inc., 1993, pp. 491–513.

18. Platts-Mills TAE, Sporik RB, Chapman MD, Heymann PW. The role of domestic allergens. In Chadwick DJ, Cardew G (Eds), The rising trends in asthma. Chichester: John Wiley & Sons, 1997, pp. 173–185.

19. Weiss ST. Diet as a risk factor for asthma. In Chadwick DJ, Cardew G (Eds), The rising trends in asthma. Chichester: John Wiley & Sons, 1997, pp. 244–253.

20. Mannino DM, Homa DM, Pertowski CA, Ashizawa A, Nixon LL, Johnson CA, Ball LB, Jack E, Kang DS. Surveillance for asthma – United States, 1960–1995. MMWR 1998; 47(2):1–30.

21. Schwartz J, Slater D, Larson TV, Pierson WE, Koenig JQ. Particulate air pollution and hospital emergency room visits for asthma in Seattle. Am Rev Respir Dis 1993; 147:826–831.

22. Bleecker ER, Postma DS, Meyers DA. Genetic susceptibility to asthma in a changing environment. In Chadwick DJ, Cardew G (Eds), The rising trends in asthma. Chichester: John Wiley & Sons, 1997, pp. 90–99.

23. Daniels SE, Bhattacharrya S, James A, Leaves NI, Young A, Hills MR, Faux JA, Ryan GF, Lathrop GM, Musk AW, Cookson WOCM. A genome-wide search for quantitative trait loci underlying asthma. Nature 1996; 383(19):247–250.

24. The Collaborative Study on the Genetics of Asthma. A genome-wide search for asthma susceptibility loci in ethnically diverse populations. Nature Genetics 1997; 15(4):389–392.

25. Speizer FE, Doll R, Heaf P. Observations on recent increase in mortality from asthma. Br Med J 1968; 1(5588):335–339.

26. Stolley PD, Schinnar R. Association between asthma mortality and isoproterenol aerosols: A review. Prev Med 1978; 7(4):519–538.

27. Pearce N, Hensley MJ. Epidemiologic studies of β agonists and asthma deaths. Epi Rev 1998; 20(2):173–186.

28. Spitzer WO, Suissa S, Ernst P, Horwitz RI, Habbick B, Cockcroft D, Boivin JF, McNutt M, Buist AS, Rebuck AS. The use of β-agonists and the risk of death and near death from asthma. New Engl J Med 1992; 326(8):501–506.

The Pros and Cons of Evidence-Based Guidelines for Asthma Management

John O Warner*

Keywords: Childhood asthma, evidence-based medicine, management guidelines

It is entirely appropriate to promote quality guidelines for the management of childhood asthma. However, these should be developed using a combination of evidence-based systematic reviews of the literature, with the judicious use of other non-randomized or controlled published evidence and the opinions and clinical experience of respected experts. The involvement of patients and their representatives as well as other professional bodies is clearly important as well as representation from all levels of medical care. Guidelines can only be practical and applicable if they not only present the evidence base but also are sufficiently flexible, clearly expressed and applicable in all target populations. Thus, evidence-based medicine contributes significantly to guidelines but is not the 'be all and end all', and should not be allowed to dictate the final management profile, unless the very broad definition of EBM suggested by Sackett [1] is employed.

The pros and cons of evidence-based medicine have been well rehearsed in the medical literature. However, it is important to have a grasp of the concepts involved in this relatively new approach to the evaluation of management of disease.

The general concept of evidence-based medicine is that it involves a combination of systematic reviews of medical literature, mega randomized trials and meta-analysis. However, it is worthwhile examining the definition of evidence-based medicine given by the great doyen of this discipline, D.L. Sackett [1]: "The conscientious, explicit and judicious use of current best evidence in making decisions about the care of individual patients. It requires the integration of clinical expertise, external evidence, and patients' values and expectations." This is a far broader idea which tends to encompass the best intentions implicit in the publication of many guidelines for the management of asthma. Clearly, however, there should be a league table of grades of evidence to be employed in any guide-lines. A grading of evidence has been suggested by the USA Agency for Health Care Policy & Research [2]. Thus the types of evidence may be classified in the following order:

1. Evidence obtained from meta-analysis of randomized controlled trials.
2. Evidence obtained from at least one large randomized controlled trial.
3. Evidence obtained from at least one large well designed controlled study without randomization.
4. Evidence obtained from at least one other type of well designed quasi-experimental study.
5. Evidence obtained from well designed non-experimental descriptive studies such as comparative studies, correlation studies and case control studies.
6. Evidence obtained from expert committee reports or opinions and/or clinical experience of respected authorities.

Most would only accept (1) and (2) in making any emphatic recommendation on management, while the other levels of evidence would indicate the need for randomized controlled studies but may, in the short term before completion and publication of trials, be used to guide management though not to be taken as an absolute given.

Clearly these criteria for an evidence base do not take into account clinical judgement and experience; qualitative factors; attitudes of patients and their carers; and demands related to individual clinical consultations. Furthermore, they are encumbered by inevitable publication bias which sometimes excludes the negative controlled randomized study. It bypasses at least to a certain extent clinical advice, unless category (6) in the listing is accepted and it facilitates a take-over of the clinical consultation by technocrats and managers.

Thus in designing clinical guidelines, clearly the priority should be to access the evidence base that is available and to ensure that this has been correctly interpreted so that when followed, can lead to improvements in health. It is also important to establish whether the outcomes would be the same when employed in different clinical circumstances. It is, therefore, quite inappropriate to make recommendations on gold standard management guidelines for asthma in a developing country that has no access to what are often more expensive medications. Furthermore there are some situations in which, for instance, inhaled therapy is not an acceptable option to patients, either because of age or attitudes.

Ideally in drawing up guidelines, a multi-professional group should be involved. These should represent primary, secondary and tertiary medical care as well as other professional bodies, patients and their advocates. Guideline development, therefore, requires an intensive input from trained and experienced reviewers and the process is labour-intensive and inevitably expensive. Sadly, such resource is usually not available and, therefore, most published guidelines on the management of asthma have been based on the judgement of a select group of self-avowed experts. Most attempt to access an evidence base but in the end rely predominantly on best established practice and expert opinion. To what extent the outcome would differ if a more thorough and comprehensive review of the knowledge base had been conducted, is a moot point. One suspects that there would not be a great deal of difference. However, future publication of guidelines will need to indicate where recommendations are based on good published evidence and where it is based on conventional wisdom.

backed up by recently published data from randomized controlled trials wherever possible. However, concern was expressed about inappropriate extrapolation of such studies from adults with asthma to wheezing in young children and also from older asthmatic children to wheezing infants. It is in making these distinctions that fundamental problems arise in interpreting the evidence base.

Previous publications of paediatric asthma guidelines had been criticized on the basis that they might be employed by technocrats and managers to dictate to the clinician how individual asthmatics should be managed. Furthermore, concern was expressed that they would be used in a court of law as a means to condemn doctors who, for reasons which may have been perfectly appropriate in individual cases, had not followed the guidelines[4]. It was never the intention of the individuals involved with the publication of guidelines that they should be written in tablets of stone, demanding adherence from all clinicians. The use of the word "guidelines" clearly indicates that they are to be viewed as an aid to clinical practice but to be interpreted only in the light of individual clinical situations and the individual clinician's judgement.

Clearly not all clinicians managing childhood asthmatics will have the luxury of being able to devote vast amounts of time to evaluation of the evidence base and, therefore, the production of guidelines will have considerable value in improving standards of care. Furthermore, they will hopefully also produce some degree of consistency of approach to management between the various levels of care. Many of the problems that arose in the past in the inconsistent management of childhood asthmatics were because there was no consistency of approach by nurse specialists, pediatricians and chest physicians [5].

Pediatric Asthma Guidelines

The most recent Pediatric Asthma Consensus guidelines were evolved by 42 participants, representing 23 countries from around the world [3]. The primary aim set by the participants was to develop clinically sound and practical guidelines for the management of childhood asthma that could be implemented in different health care systems and with a reasonable chance of achieving compliance. It was agreed that the guidelines should be based on best established practise and expert opinion,

Definition of Asthma

The ideal definition of a disease will be based on a clear understanding of the underlying aetio-pathology. Despite improved understanding of the pathology, physiology, immunology and even the genetic basis for asthma in childhood, we still do not know the basic mechanisms underlying the development of the disease. Furthermore, we have little information on the immunopathology in the airways of infant wheezers, many of whom do not subsequently develop asthma. Thus, the definition has varied depending on the purposes for which it was being sought.

Epidemiologists have tended to use the symptom of wheeze as being the cardinal feature, while the clinician will tend to include persistent cough, particularly at night and precipitated by a range of standard triggers; the immunologists will use an objective evaluation of allergic status; the physiologists, evidence of variable airflow limitation; and the pathologists, the presence of "eosinophilic bronchitis."

Defining asthma is clearly an interesting intellectual exercise but can only be of value to the practising clinician if it gives some idea of prognosis and can help identify which is the most appropriate therapeutic approach, having the maximum chance of being efficacious and the minimum of producing side-effects. Indeed, on this basis it would seem far more appropriate to consider the sensitivity and specificity of measurements which predict outcome and therapeutic response, rather than to review very large controlled clinical trials. The latter tend to lump heterogeneous groups of patients, some of whom clearly are responders and others are not. Furthermore, some have a higher propensity for side-effects. Thus the true evidence base for management of any disease and certainly asthma, will only be available when the science of prediction has improved appreciably. One suspects that the new discipline of pharmacogenetics will have a great deal to contribute to this area.

Natural History of Childhood Asthma

There is a commonly held misconception that early intervention in the management of asthma will in some way alter the natural history of the condition. There is no evidence base for this idea. Indeed, the 28-year follow-up of children with infrequent episodic asthma demonstrated that they had normal lung function as adults, irrespective of any therapeutic intervention, with the majority not receiving inhaled steroids [6]. Conversely, the follow-up into adulthood of childhood asthmatics in Holland demonstrated that the predictors of abnormal lung function and bronchial hyperresponsiveness as an adult were abnormal lung function and bronchial hyperresponsiveness as a child irrespective of treatment

[7]. Thus one might conclude that mild is always mild and severe may well remain severe, again irrespective of therapy. Under such circumstances, current therapeutic recommendations must be based on short-term efficacy and benefits to quality of life rather than on any misguided view about potential for cure.

Previous published guidelines have tended to set unrealistic aims in relation to supposed cure of asthma or prevention of so-called irreversible airway obstruction. There has been inappropriate extrapolation of therapeutic practice and evidence, from older children with established asthma to children with infrequent episodic disease or to infant wheezers [8]. It is perhaps more important at this stage in the science and art to emphasise that there is no cure for asthma and the goals of the treatment should be to achieve maximum improvement in lifestyle and lung function with minimal side-effects of treatment. For the overwhelming majority of patients, this still achieves a normalization of lifestyle, and optimal growth and development. However, for some this is not possible.

Monitoring

Thoracic physicians have emphasized the importance of the use of peak flow meters to give accurate information on this very variable disease. Less attention has been paid to interval lung function which is deemed to be unhelpful because of the variability of the disease. However interval spirometry, particularly using flow volume loops, can give very important information on the severity of disease. Thus, children with infrequent episodic asthma would be expected to have normal spirometry during healthy periods, whereas the persistent asthmatic will always have some abnormalities on spirometry. This, in turn, will help guide management decisions, the former not requiring inhaled steroids, whilst in the latter, inhaled steroids should be considered mandatory.

Furthermore, it is important to emphasise that peak flow meters can give very spurious information and may also interfere with therapeutic compliance. It is difficult enough to train children to use an inhaler effectively without confusing them with the addition of a peak flow meter. Far more value might be achieved by accurate and continuous monitoring of compliance with inhaler usage rather than peak flow. Unfortunately studies published on the value of peak flow monitoring have tended to recruit patients with good compliance and are not based on an intention to "monitor and treat" analysis. Without this, it is impossible to generalise on the importance of such monitoring and, indeed, significant doubts have been expressed about its value in recent publications [9].

The most important monitoring remains key clinical questions related to sleep disturbance, β-agonist requirement, morning cough and wheeze, breakthrough symptoms with viral infections, and the degree of exercise induced problems. For the overwhelming majority of children, answers to these questions will accurately identify the status of the asthma. Other investigations, such as measurement of bronchial hyperresponsiveness or seeking markers of allergic inflammation, such as eosinophil cationic protein or exhaled nitric oxide, have yet to be shown to have any significant clinical value [10]. There is currently a considerable interest in monitoring other modalities, such as quality of life which certainly instinctively seems appropriate and important, but has yet to establish its place as a clinical tool [11].

Therapeutic Interventions

Allergen Avoidance

There is overwhelming evidence that allergy is an important prerequisite for the development and persistence of asthma. Thus allergen avoidance seems to be a worthy strategy to pursue. However, the only meta-analysis published on house mite avoidance measures suggests that this is ineffective [12]. Scrutiny of the analysis indicates that a number of different mite avoidance strategies were lumped together in order to achieve sufficient power for the analysis. It is clear that some modalities are relatively ineffective, such as the use of acaracides and allergen denaturants, whereas others such as using bed covers clearly have efficacy [13]. Thus conclusions drawn from the meta-analysis are very likely to be false and indicate the shortcomings of one component of evidence-based medicine.

Education

It is self-evident that good patient and family education is an important component of management of any chronic condition. Inadequate knowledge is certainly associated with increased morbidity. However, there are precious few studies which have indicated that morbidity can be improved by any educational strategy. It is easy to improve knowledge but less effects can be achieved in terms of modifying behaviour. Nevertheless, most would consider guidelines to be incomplete without making some recommendations on educational strategies [14].

Pharmacotherapy

Most guidelines present the pharmacotherapeutic recommendations in the form of an algorithm or step-up schedule starting with inhaled β_2-agonists for infrequent episodic asthma and progressing to inhaled corticosteroids for persistent disease. This presupposes that asthma is a progressive problem, requiring a progression of treatment. However clinical experience and, indeed, long term follow-up studies suggest that most asthmatics remain true to character. In other words, those with severe disease present with severe problems and those with infrequent episodic disease remain with mild problems throughout life. Thus, treatment may be better defined in terms of "horses for courses," namely ring-fenced specific therapeutic approaches for each severity category. The key is to identify the patients in the correct category which, again, focuses on accurate initial assessment rather than on "trial and error" therapeutic approaches. The danger with the latter is that the patient ends up receiving an excess of treatment inappropriately. The only reason this does not happen more frequently is that the patients are often wiser than their physicians and will step down and even withdraw treatment when they believe they have improved. Additional protection from side-effects is probably achieved by the gross inefficiency of most inhalation delivery systems and the poor inhalation technique employed by many patients. These issues tend not to be adequately addressed in the big randomized controlled clinical trials but must have a profound influence on outcome.

New Treatments

At present, the range of drugs available to treat asthma in childhood which have established efficacy are relatively limited. They include long and short acting β_2-specific agonists, oral theophyllines, sodium cromoglycate, nedocromil sodium and inhaled steroids. Indeed, many restrict their treatment to β_2-agonists, inhaled and oral steroids. The leukotriene receptor antagonists are beginning to find a place and, of course, oral corticosteroids are reserved for acute exacerbation. There are, however, a wide array of other drugs that have potential value. These include antihistamines for infant wheezers, immunotherapy in some special circumstances, while a host of new potential approaches are beginning trials, including the use of anti-IgE antibodies, and finally for very severe disease, the use of cyclosporin and other forms of immune suppression. In patients with severe brittle asthma; poor compliance with inhaled therapy; or atypical disease, there must be no bar to the use of speculative approaches to therapy, even in the absence of an evidence base.

Address for correspondence:

Prof. John O Warner
Centre Block, Room CG56
Southampton General Hospital
Southampton
Hampshire SO9 4XY
UK
Tel. +44 1703 796160
Fax +44 1703 796378

References

1. Sackett DL. Apply overviews and meta-analyses at the bedside. J Clin Epidemiol 1995; 48:61–66.

2. Scottish Intercollegiate Guideline Network. Clinical guidelines, criteria for appraisal for national use, 1995.

3. Warner JO, Naspitz CK, Cropp GJA. Third International Pediatric Consensus statement on the management of childhood asthma. Pediatr Pulmonol 1998; 25:1–17.

4. Godfrey S. Management of asthma: A consensus statement. Arch Dis Child 1990; 64:1760 (Letter).

5. Henry RL, Milner AD. Specialist approach to childhood asthma: Does it exist? Br Med J 1983; 287:260–261.

6. Oswald H, Phelan PD, Lanigan A, Hibbert M, Conlin JB, Bowes G, Olinsky A. Childhood asthma and lung function in mid adult life. Pediatr Pulmonol 1997; 23:14–20.

7. Gerritsen J, Koeter GH, Postma DS, Schouten JP, Van Aalderen WMC, Knol K. Airway responsiveness in childhood as a predictor of the outcome of asthma in adulthood. Am Rev Respir Dis 1991; 143:1468–1469.

8. Pedersen S, Warner JO, Price JF. Early use of inhaled steroids in children with asthma. Clin Exp Allergy (Debate) 1997; 27:995–1006.

9. Brand PLP, Duiverman JW, Van Essen-Zandvliet EEM, Kerrebijn KF and the Dutch CVSLD Study Group. Peak flow variation in childhood asthma: Correlation with symptoms, airways obstruction, hyperresponsiveness during long term treatment with inhaled corticosteroids. Thorax 1999; 54:103–107.

10. Van Rensen ELJ, Straathof KCM, Veselie-Charvat MA, Zwinderman AH, Bel EH, Sterk PJ. Effect of inhaled steroids on airway hyperresponsiveness, sputum eosinophils and exhaled nitric oxide levels in patients with asthma. Thorax 1999; 54:403–408.

11. Juniper EF, Guyatt GH, Feeny DH. Measuring quality of life in the parents of children with asthma. Quality Life Res 1996; 5:27–34.

12. Gotzsche PC, Hammarquist C, Burr M. House dust mite control measures in the management of asthma: Meta-analysis. Br Med J 1998; 317:1105–1110.

13. Ehnert B, Lau-Schadendorf S, Weber A, Buettrer P, Schou C, Wahn U. Reducing domestic exposure to dust mite allergen reduces bronchial hyper-reactivity in sensitive children with asthma. J Allergy Clin Immunol 1992; 90:135–138.

14. Global strategy for asthma management and prevention. NHLBI/WHO Workshop Report. Publ. No. 95–3659. Nat. Inst. Health, Bethesda, MD, USA, 1995.

Asthma Education – What Does This Mean and Does it Work?

Martyn R Partridge*

Keywords: Asthma, patient education, compliance, self management

Recent systematic reviews of patient education and self management advice in adults have suggested that such interventions have beneficial effects on a variety of outcomes. The most efficacious interventions are those which include the issuing of a detailed written self-treatment (action) plan. In adults there is no evidence to suggest that such plans are better if based on peak flow monitoring, as opposed to symptoms alone, but because some patients are unable to subjectively perceive worsening of airway calibre, plans based on both objective and subjective monitoring are usually offered.

There is less information available about the efficacy of patient education regarding self management in children but some good studies have suggested that a nurse interventim (which includes issuing of self management advice) to those admitted to hospital with asthma, can reduce the rate of subsequent readmissions.

A recent systematic review of the literature on patient education and self management concluded that self management education about asthma which involved self monitoring by either peak flow or symptoms, regular medical review and a written action plan, improves health outcomes for adults with asthma. Asthma education which allowed patient adjustment of medications based on a written action plan was shown to be more efficacious than asthma self management which did not [1]. Armed with this information we need to tease out more about what asthma education should involve in day to day clinical care and whether the same applies to children as to adults and how we deliver such care.

Table 1 summarises the important components of a successful approach to patient education and self management and we need to continually remind ourselves of the importance of good communication within consultations. International guidelines on the management of asthma stress the importance of the development of meaningful part-

Table 1.

The important components of a successful patient education and self management programme are:
– Good communication between patient and health professional
– Addressing fears and concerns as they arise
– Acknowledging attitudes to medication
– Negotiating goals
– Offering (tailored) reinforcing education materials
– Assessing the patients or parents desire to take control
– Access to group support where appropriate
– Appropriate skills in monitoring their condition

nerships between health professionals and those with asthma (or the parents of those with asthma).

Communication: Every one of the world's 300 million asthmatics brings to this common condition a different personality, different past life's experiences, different fears and concerns and different goals and expectations. We need to recall this before "sending" messages and the most important opening question we can ask of our patients is "What is it you want of me" or "What is it I can do for you." Taking this approach is less likely to lead to a situation where there are barriers to our subsequent educational efforts – barriers such as those listed in Table 2. Understanding how prevalent are feelings of denial of the diagnosis is important. In one qualitative study patients invited for interview because they had a diagnosis of asthma and had been on preventative asthma therapies for over a year frequently expressed comments about having been called in error [2]. "She said it's bronchial asthma I have so I'm bronchial not asthmatic," or "I've been chesty for years but now they have stuck the label 'asthma' on me but I don't feel any different." Even those with asthma who accept the

* Chest Clinic, Whipps Cross Hospital, London, UK, and Chief Medical Adviser, UK National Asthma Campaign

Table 2. Potential barriers to education.

Denial of diagnosis
Denial of severity of condition
Misconceptions about nature of the disease
Belief that relieving medicines are best
Feeling of stigma
"Drugs cause side effects"
Steroid phobia
Anxiety re lack of control
Depression
Cultural preconceptions

Table 3. Summary of what patients "need" to know about their asthma.

The diagnosis and how it was made
How to use an inhaler
The difference between relievers and preventers
How to use a peak flow meter
Signs and symptoms that suggest worsening asthma
and what to do if present
When and where they will be followed up

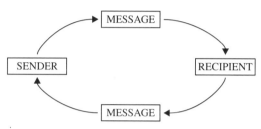

Figure 1. Fundamental to each consultation is the realisation that communication involves a sender, a message and a recipient. Too often the doctor sends and doesn't listen, and too often the message is inadequately tailored to the needs of the individual recipient.

diagnosis may nevertheless not accept its implications. Many express a dislike of the need for regular therapy and not specifically a dislike of steroids [3]. Others have goals which differ from those of the health professional. Guidelines may tell us that the aim of treatment is the abolition of symptoms but a patient who is fearful of steroids may "trade" some symptoms for the possibility of reduced therapy. In these circumstances it is for us to elicit these goals and when one individual's goal veers too far from a safe approach, we need to negotiate a new goal. Figure 1 reminds us clearly that within good communication there is a sender, a message and a recipient and as health professionals we need to remember that understanding the recipient is a priority and this should come before sending any messages or offering information.

What Information Do Those With Asthma Need to Know?

Information clearly needs to be tailored to the recipient and should reflect their "wants" rather than our perception of what they "need" to know. Use of open ended questions can help the tailoring of proffered information but guidelines suggest to us certain information which all those with asthma should probably know (Table 3). How we reinforce these messages is similarly important for we know that much that we offer a patient is forgotten shortly after the consultation ends. In one study of doctor/patient consultations on approximately half the occasions the doctor did not tell the patient how to take the medication, or how long to take the medication for and on no occasions did the doctor check the patient's understanding of what had gone before [4]. Simply writing down for patients the details of their medication has been shown to improve recall [5], and in a paediatric situation to increase adherence to a correct sequence of treatment changes [6]. In another study of patients being discharged from hospital, giving patients written information about their discharge medication similarly improved their ability to recall information about medication regimens and purpose some months later [7].

These studies illustrate how tailoring information to individual patients may increase knowledge – in this case about their medication, but the giving of information about the disease, whilst possibly increasing knowledge, will not necessarily influence subsequent behaviour or outcomes [8]. However it is important to realise that "no proven benefit" does not necessarily imply that an intervention is of no value for it may serve as an essential substrate for other activities. For example, the giving of a booklet may not by itself alter behaviour but it may enhance a patient's satisfaction with their health professional such that the patient is subsequently more receptive to advice. We also need to recognise that how we give such core printed information may be important. For example, it may be preferable for the patient to receive written information from the doctor with the advice "You may wish to read this and write down any resulting questions so that we may discuss them next time" rather than the patient just helping themselves to the leaflet from a rack in the waiting room.

It is also important to recognise that nowadays health professionals represent just one source of information amongst many, and in addition to conflicting or supporting information received from family, friends or role models, the patient or parent may have downloaded information of variable quality from the web. It may therefore be helpful to ask "Have you received information from any source which has left you with questions you wish to ask me." Sometimes eliciting patients' fears, concerns and "questions for the doctor" in written format prior to the consultation [9] is also helpful (Figure 2).

Personalizing Information and Self Treatment Action Plans

The Global Strategy for the Management and Prevention of Asthma [10] recommends a six-part approach to asthma management with Part 1 being Patient Education, about which they say: "The aim of patient education, which is a continual process, is to provide the patient with asthma, and the patient's family with suitable information and training so that the patient can keep well and adjust treatment according to a medication plan developed with the health professional. The emphasis must be on the development of an ongoing partnership amongst health care professionals, the patient and the patient's family."

Self-management is a term that does not always mean the same to every person and does not always mean the same when applied to different diseases.

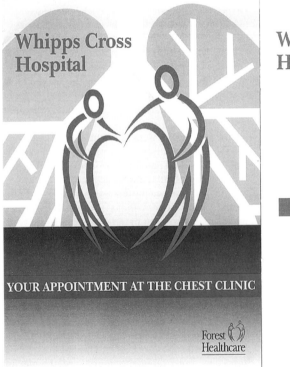

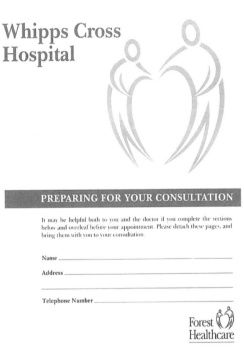

Figure 2. An example of a booklet which is sent to the patient before a clinic appointment and which contains information of value to the patient regarding whereabouts of the clinic, what to bring with them and advice as to what may happen during their attendance at the clinic. The middle four pages contain space for the patient to fill in their past medical history and includes a section entitled "Questions for the doctor."

ZONE 1

Your asthma is under control if

it does not disturb your sleep

it does not restrict your usual activities

and

your peak flow readings are above _____

ACTION

Your preventer is

You should normally take

_____ puffs/doses

_____ times every day (using a spacer),

even when you are feeling well

Your reliever is

You should normally only take it when yor are

short of breath, coughing or wheezing, or before exercise

Your other medicines are

_____

ZONE 2

Your doctor or nurse may decide not to use this zone

Your asthma is getting worse if

you are needing to use you

_____

(reliever inhaler) more than usual

you are waking at night with asthma symptoms

and

your peak flow readings have fallen to between

_____ and _____

ACTION

increase your usual medicines

increase your

_____

(preventer inhaler) to

_____

Continue to take your

_____

(reliever inhaler) to relieve your asthma symptoms

Figure 3. An example of the content of a self-management plan used for adults and produced by the UK National Asthma Campaign.

For some diseases self-management involves predominant changes in lifestyle (e. g., arthritis, obesity and hypertension), and here generic advice regarding the value of weight reduction and regular instruction may be offered by lay people (or those with the condition) and could even be generic and offered to those with several different conditions at the same time. For other conditions, for example, diabetes and asthma, lifestyle change such as diet, exercise and allergen avoidance are equally important but the main self motivated intervention is altering prescribed medication to maintain control of the condition and prevent deterioration to a crisis level. Under these circumstances it seems best that

ZONE 3

Your asthma is severe if

you are getting increasingly breathless

you are needing to use your

_____

(reliever inhaler) every

_____ hours or more often

and

your peak flow readings have fallen to

between _____ and _____

ACTION

Take

____ prednisolone (steroid) tablets

(strength _____ mg each) and then

_____

_____

Discuss with your doctor how and when to stop taking the tablets

Continue to take your

_____

(reliever and preventer inhales) as prescribed

ZONE 4

It is a medical alert/emergency if

your symptoms cotinue to get worse

and

your peak flow readings have fallen to below

_____

Do not be afraid of causing a fuss.

Your doctor will want to see you urgently.

ACTION

get help immediately

Telephone your doctor straightaway on

_____

or call ambulance

Take

____ prednisolone (steroid) tablets

(strength _____ mg each) immediately

Continue to take your

_____

(reliever/inhaler) as needed, or every

five to ten minutes until the ambulance arrives

Figure 3 (continued).

self-management (in this case predominantly self treatment) is best supervised or given in a co-management manner with the health professional.

Most self treatment plans involve a mixture of advice based upon symptoms and (for adults and older children) advice based upon the individuals personal best known peak flow. Plans such as those shown in Figures 3 and 4 have threshold levels for action when peak flow is 80%, 70% and 50% of the patient's best known peak flow. Some studies have varied these action levels to 85%, 70% and 50% [11], whilst others have used 70%, 50% and 30% which clearly permits much greater deterioration before the patient adjusts their treatment.

Table 4. A possible symptom-based self-management plan (from [14]).

1. When you feel normal continue maintenance treatment with:
    a) bronchodilators as needed
    b) inhaled steroids twice daily
2. If you catch a cold or start to feel tight or awake at night with wheezing or have a persistent cough:
    a) double the dose of inhaled steroid until you return to normal, then reduce to your usual maintenance dose of inhaled steroids
    b) Use bronchodilators two puffs every 4 hours as needs
3. If the effect of your bronchodilators lasts only 2 hours and you find doing your normal activities make you short of breath:
    a) Start Prednisolone tablets, 40mg daily
    b) Continue this dose for at least one week until symptoms have normalised, then reduce Prednisolone by 5mg daily until stopped
4. If the effect of your bronchodilators lasts only 30 minutes or you have difficulty talking:
    a) Consult family physician immediately
    b) If unavailable call Ambulance (999 / 911), or
    c) Go directly to hospital emergency department

In the adult out patient studies of Ignacio-Garia and Gonzalez-Santos [12] and Lahdensuo et al. [11] self treatment plans similar to that shown in the figure were given within the context of a randomized controlled clinical trial, and in both significant improvement in asthma control and use of health service resources were seen at 6 months and 12 months respectively, following the patients being given self treatment advice. In the second of these studies [11] this improved control was achieved despite the self-management group using less steroid tablets than the control group and this implies either that the lesser step of doubling inhaled steroids at the first sign of deterioration prevents decline to the point where steroid tablets are needed, or that giving control to the patient enhances compliance with routine treatment. In this study patients were shown to have complied with advice to start steroid tablets on over three-quarters of the occasions that their clinical condition or peak flow suggested that they should do so. Such high rates of compliance with self treatment plans were not shown by Klein and van der Palen [13], but 65% of patients using a peak flow based plan complied with self treatment in the study by Turner and colleagues [14].

How long does the effect of self treatment advice last after it is given? Clearly most such advice is reinforced and the advice continually adjusted according to the clinical situation during follow up of patients, but within the published trials we can see retention of benefit at 12 months in the Finnish study [11]. More recently the New Zealand group have published further long term results [15]. Patients were enrolled in a 6 month asthma education-al programme which involved the issuing of self treatment advice written for them on a credit card sized plan, and asthma outcomes and use of health service resources were evaluated in the 12 months before they were recruited to the programme and for 2 years afterwards. Significant improvements were seen in symptoms suffered, in emergency visits to general practitioners and in visits to emergency departments and hospital admissions, and this benefit was maintained up to 2 years after the end of the 6 month programme. They showed that compliance with the use of peak flow monitoring (as opposed to monitoring of symptoms and bronchodilator usage) was very variable with less than a quarter of patients reporting daily monitoring of peak flow although this increased to 73% reporting daily recordings of peak flow when unwell. In other studies peak flow monitoring has not been thought to contribute to management [16, 17] but these studies included a number of children and young asthmatics and for some time it has been recognised that symptoms or even spirometry may be better at detecting imminent decline in asthma control in children. [18].

Turner and colleagues performed a randomized controlled clinical trial comparing peak flow based and symptoms based plans for adult patients with asthma attending a primary care clinic [14]. If using a symptom based plan it is important that we have an understanding of the sort of specific advice that should be given and the advice given in this study is reproduced in the Table 4. These results showed that both symptom based, and peak flow based self-management plans were associated with significant

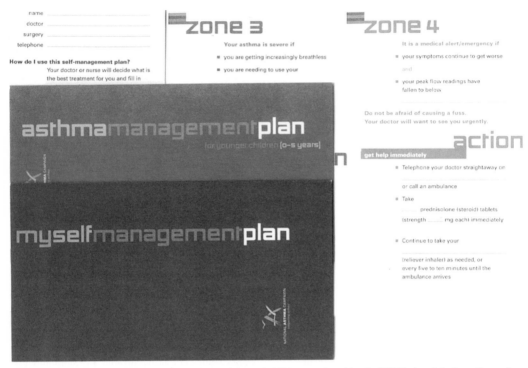

name
doctor
surgery
telephone

How do I use this self-management plan?
Your doctor or nurse will decide what is
the best treatment for you and fill in

zone 3

Your asthma is severe if

• you are getting increasingly breathless

• you are needing to use your

asthmamanagement**plan**
for younger children [0–5 years]

myselfmanagement**plan**

zone 4

It is a medical alert/emergency if

• your symptoms continue to get worse

and

• your peak flow readings have
fallen to below

Do not be afraid of causing a fuss.
Your doctor will want to see you urgently.

action

get help immediately

• Telephone your doctor straightaway on

or call an ambulance

• Take

prednisolone (steroid) tablets
(strength .... mg each) immediately

• Continue to take your

(reliever inhaler) as needed, or
every five to ten minutes until the
ambulance arrives

Figure 4. Example of simple "Action Plans" for adults and children produced by the UK National Asthma Campaign.

improvement in spirometry, bronchial hyperre-sponsiveness and quality of life and that there was no detectable advantage in the use of peak flow monitoring.

Unfortunately, this study did not ascertain patient preference and in two other studies adult patients and parents of children have reported satisfaction with objective monitoring [19]. This study also used low peak flow thresholds for action (decline to 70% before increasing inhaled steroids and to 50% before starting steroid tablets], and it is just possible that days lost from work or unscheduled doctor visits might have been reduced more with higher thresholds.

On the available evidence therefore there is a real question mark over whether self-treatment plans should be based on peak flow recordings. There is no evidence of an improved outcome associated with their use and a lot of evidence that the patients only monitor their peak flow when their symptoms suggest the need. Many doctors intrinsically hold on to the desire for patients to monitor themselves objectively because of the knowledge that failure to measure peak flow by doctors has clearly been shown to be associated with under-estimation of se-verity, and because numerous studies have now shown that some adults and child patients with asthma have a limited ability to perceive when their airway calibre is severely compromised [20, 21, 22]. However detection of this group is difficult. Resistive loading, and hypoxic and bronchial challenge studies to detect poor perception are not commonly used in clinical practice and we have limited understanding as to whether perception of asthma is a stable state.

The remaining questions relate to whether the same conclusions regarding self treatment plans apply to children as to adults, who should administer such plans and who represents the subgroups most in need of such plans. In one study in an inner city children's hospital, children admitted to hospital with acute severe asthma were allocated to either traditional care or to a visit by a specialist asthma nurse [23]. During a single educational intervention lasting up to 40 minutes, the nurse went over the circumstances that had led to the child's admission, and used that scenario as an opportunity to explain how in future different interventions designed to reduce the risk of deteriorating asthma could be employed. This spoken advice was backed up by written advice, a self-treatment plan and where appropriate, peak flow monitoring. During a follow up period of 2–14 months there was a significant reduction in the readmission rate in the intervention group compared to the conventionally managed patients.

In conclusion, it therefore appears that offering both adults and children self treatment plans within the context of a wider patient education programme and within the context of a partnership between health professional and patient where good communication is practised, is associated with reduced suffering from asthma.

Address for correspondence:

Martyn R Partridge, MD, FR-CP
Consultant Physician
Chest Clinic, Whipps Cross Hospital
London, E11 1NR
UK
Tel. +44 181 535-6675
Fax +44 181 535-6709
E-mail mrp@wxhchest.demon.co.uk

References

1. Gibson PG, Coughlan J, Wilson AJ, Abramson M, Bauman A, Hensley MJ, Walters EH. Self management education and regular practitioner review for adults with asthma (Cochrane Review). In the Cochrane Library, Issue 1 1999. Oxford Update software.

2. Adams S, Pill R, Jones A. Medication, chronic illness and identity- the perspective of people with asthma. Soc Sci Med 1997; 45:189–201.

3. Osman LM. Predicting patient attitudes to asthma medication. Thorax 1993; 48:827–830.

4. Falvo D, Tippy P. Communicating information to patients – patient satisfaction and adherence as associated with residents skills. J Fam Prac 1988; 26:643–647.

5. Raynor DK, Booth TG, Blenkinsopp, A. Effect of computer generated reminder charts on patients compliance with drug regimens. Br Med J 1998; 306: 1158–1161.

6. Pedersen S. Ensuring compliance in children. Eur Respir J 1992; 5:143–145.

7. Sandler DA, Heaton C, Gainer ST, Mitchell JR. Patients and general practitioners satisfaction with information given on discharge from hospital, audit of new information card. Br Med J 1989; 299:151–1513.

8. Gibson PG, Coughlan J, Wilson AJ, Abramson M, Bauman A, Hensley M, Walters EH. The role of limited information in asthma patient education (Cochrane Review). In the Cochrane Library 1998. Oxford update software.

9. Partridge MR, Roberts CM. Eliciting fears and concerns and maximising consultation time: The use of a posted pre clinic questionnaire. Patient Educ Counselling 1994; 23:589.

10. Global Initiative for asthma. Global strategy for asthma management and prevention (NHLBI/WHO Workshop report). National Institutes of Health, National Heart Lung & Blood Institute, Publication Number 95-3659, Bethesda, Maryland 1995.

11. Lahdensuo A, Haahtela T, Herrala J, Kava T, Kiviranta K, Kunsisto P, Permaki E, Boussa J, Saarelainen S, Svahn T. Randomised comparison of guided self-management and traditional treatments of asthma over one year. Br Med J 1996; 312:748–752.

12. Ignacio-Garcia J, Gonzalez-Santos P. Asthma self-management education programme by home monitoring of peak expiratory flow. Am J Respir Care Med 1995; 151:353–359.

13. Van der Palen J, Klein JJ, Rovers MN. Compliance with inhaled medication and self treatment guidelines following a self-management programme in adult asthmatics. Eur Respir J 1997; 10:652–657.

14. Turner MO, Taylor D, Bennett R, Fitzgerald JM. A randomised trial comparing peak expiratory flow and symptom self-management plans for patients with asthma attending a primary care clinic. Am J Respir Crit Care Med 1998; 157:540–546.

15. D'Souza WJ, Tekaur H, Fox C, Harper M, Gennell T, Ngatvere M, Wickens K, Crane J, Pearce N, Beasley R. Long term reduction in asthma morbidity following an asthma self-management programme. Eur Respir J 1998; 11:611–616.

16. Chang Yeung M, Chang JH, Mantreda J, Ferguson A, Becker A. Changes in peak flow, symptoms score, and the use of medication during acute exacerbations of asthma. Am J Respir Crit Care Med 1996; 154:889–893.

17. Uwyyed K, Springer C, Avital A, Bar-Yishay E, Godfrey S. Home recording of PEF in young asthmatics: Does it contribute to management? Eur Respir J 1996; 9:872–879.

18. Sly PD, Cahill P, Willet K, Burton P. Accuracy of mini peak flow meters in indicating changes in lung function in children with asthma. Br Med J 1994; 308:572–574.

19. Lloyd BW, Ali MH. How useful do parents find home peak flow monitoring for children with asthma. Br Med J 1992; 305:1128–1129.

20. Kikuchi Y, Okabe S, Tamura G, Hi-da W, Homma M, Shirad K, Takishima T. Chemosensivity and percep-

tion of dyspnoea in patients with a history of near fatal asthma. N Engl J Med 1994; 330:1329–1334.

21. Kendrick AH, Higgs CMB, Whitfield MJ, Laslo G. Accuracy of perception of severity of asthma: Patients treated in general practices. Br Med J 1993; 307:422–424.

22. Kifle Y, Seng V, Davenport PW. Magnitude estimation of inspiratory resistive loads in children with life threatening asthma. Am J Respir Crit Care Med 1997; 156:1530–1535.

23. Madge P, McColl J, Paton J. Impact of a nurse led home management training programme in children admitted to hospital with acute asthma. A randomised controlled clinical trial. Thorax 1997; 52:223–238.

Natural History of Asthma

Malcolm R Sears*

Keywords: Asthma, natural history, epidemiology, atopy, persistence, remission

Early childhood wheezing is common, and may persist, particularly if there is a family history of asthma and atopy, and personal development of atopy. Remission of early childhood wheezing is common among those whose symptoms relate to small airways and exposure to maternal cigarette smoke. Of all children with recurrent wheezing, about two-thirds remit in adolescence or as adults. Factors predicting persistence include a family history of asthma and atopy, severity of early childhood asthma, frequency of attacks, atopy especially to indoor allergens, persistent airway hyperresponsiveness, female gender, and personal smoking. Remission of adult asthma is uncommon, occurring primarily in younger subjects with milder disease treated early in its course. Many adults develop largely irreversible airflow limitation. Mortality, while uncommon, has gradually increased in many countries until recently. Excessive use of potent short-acting β-agonists may increase the degree of airway responsiveness and the severity of disease, a likely explanation for two epidemics of asthma mortality in young people. Other risk factors for mortality include poverty, race, poorly controlled asthma, and inadequate access to good health care.

Until recently, there was a relative dearth of information about the natural history of asthma or wheezing in very early life as most studies had examined the progression or remission of asthma from mid childhood to adult life. However, a longitudinal study in Tucson, Arizona, has provided considerable insight into the likelihood of development and persistence of asthma in the first six years of life [1]. In this study, 1,246 children born to parents enrolled in a health maintenance organization were studied through questionnaires completed by the parents. Subgroups of children within this birth cohort had measurements of serum IgE both at birth and at age 9 months, and pulmonary function testing in infancy and at age 6 years. The children were followed up at age 3 and 6 years, with respect to symptomatic status and pulmonary function. Follow-up data were available on 826 children at age 6 years. During the first six years of life, only 51% remained free of wheezing symptoms, while 20% developed wheezing before the age of 3 years but remitted by age 6 years, 15% had not had wheezing before age 3 but developed wheezing by age 6, while 14% developed wheezing before age 3 with persisting symptoms to age 6. Hence, although 49% of children had reported wheezing in the first 6 years of life, only 29% were still wheezing at age 6 years, indicating that close to half of early childhood wheezing remitted. Those with remission by age 6 years were found to have lower lung function both at age one year and at 6 years, and to be more frequently exposed to maternal cigarette smoke, but were not more likely to have features of atopy including high IgE levels, positive skin tests, or a family history of asthma. In contrast, those whose wheezing persisted through early childhood to age 6 were more likely to have a family history of maternal asthma, elevated serum IgE at one year and 6 years of age, and abnormal lung function at age 6 years although not at age one year. Hence, factors indicating likelihood of persistence were both genetic and environmental, linked with atopy, whereas early wheezing followed by remission was more closely associated with small airways and cigarette smoke exposure rather than family allergy.

Natural History of Childhood Asthma

The natural history of childhood asthma, including the pattern of remission and persistence through to adulthood, has been examined in a number of studies. These include follow-up from office or university clinic practices, and a small number of longitudinal population studies. The most reliable studies of the natural history of asthma are those which use an unselected cohort of subjects among

* Asthma Research Group, McMaster University, Hamilton, Ontario, Canada

whom the incidence and prevalence of asthma is determined, and the features of asthma re-examined periodically over time. Less than ten longitudinal studies have been conducted in this manner. Those children seen in office or specialty clinic practice are more likely to have severe asthma than children identified with asthma in a population-based study. This selective recruitment of a less well population in clinics and hospitals leads to higher rates for persistence on follow-up, and risks for persistence which differ in some respects from those found in follow-up of population-based cohorts.

Follow-Up from Office and Specialist Practices

An early study of outcome of childhood asthma was conducted in Boston, Massachusetts, comprising a 20 year follow-up of subjects diagnosed as having asthma in childhood [2]. At review, 11 of 449 children had died, 4 of asthma, giving a mortality rate of 0.5 per 1,000 asthmatics per annum. Of 114 children whose asthma seemed related to animal exposure, only 17% were symptom free or "cured" as adults, whereas among 36 individuals with food related asthma, 44% were cured, as were 57% of 21 subjects whose asthma was related to pollen allergy. Of 199 children with mixed atopic or unidentified etiology of asthma, 25% were well as adults, 11% were well provided they avoided known trigger factors, 30% had mild asthma but suffered from hay fever as adults, and 30% had persistent asthma, which in 17% of the whole sample was severe. Overall, about half of the group with atopic asthma in childhood had persistent symptoms as adults.

Blair reviewed 267 children initially diagnosed and treated for asthma in London, UK, when less than 12 years of age [3]. At 20-year follow-up, of 244 children were available for review, 28% were fully asymptomatic, 24% had minimal symptoms, 27% had experienced remission for 3 years or more but had relapsed as adults, while 21% had had persistent asthma since childhood. Risk factors for persistence included the presence of other atopic disease, the family history of asthma, and the severity of asthma in childhood [4].

Several follow-up studies from specialist clinics have been conducted in Denmark and the Netherlands, where characteristics of children with asthma assessed in a university clinic setting were carefully documented. Of 119 children aged 6 to 14 years seen at a university clinic in The Netherlands between 1966 and 1969, 101 were available for review after 16 years [5]. At both surveys, investigations included symptom questionnaires, skin allergy testing, spirometry and methacholine challenge testing. Only 43% of this cohort of children had persisting symptoms as adults, and only 29% showed histamine responsiveness as compared with 82% in childhood. The severity of symptoms, and the degree of airway responsiveness if present, was less in adults than it had been in childhood. Low lung function in childhood and increased airway responsiveness were predictive of persistence of asthma into adulthood, although surprisingly atopy was not. However, 95% of the cohort were atopic as children, and this likely obscured any ability to define a differential risk between atopic and nonatopic children.

In a separate study of another cohort of 406 children aged 8 to 12 years seen at the same outpatient clinic between 1972 and 1976, who were followed up at age 25 years, 259 were available for full assessment [6]. Of these, 76% had persistent symptoms as adults, more in women than men (85% versus 72%). Over half of the childhood asthmatics took asthma medication regularly or intermittently as adults. Persistence to adulthood was predicted in part by the severity of symptoms in childhood, lung function as measured by FEV_1 in childhood, and childhood airway responsiveness.

In a Copenhagen study 70 of 85 children who had been seen at a hospital clinic when aged 5 to 15 years were assessed 10 to 12 years later [7]. Overall there was improvement in both atopic and nonatopic asthmatics, with decreased severity of symptoms and improved lung function. However, 86% had had symptoms within the previous 12 months as adults, and most required treatment. The severity of lung function abnormality in childhood was a predictive factor for the outcome in both the atopic and nonatopic subjects.

Natural History of Asthma in Longitudinal Population Studies

Several longitudinal studies of populations selected randomly from a local community have reported follow-up assessments of asthma on one or more occasions over time periods varying from 6 to 28 years. The sample sizes, the means of obtaining the cohort, the frequency of review and the methods of investigations have varied considerably. However, several findings are common to these studies.

In Scotland, 2,511 children were selected in 1962 as a 1 in 5 sample of primary school children in Aberdeen. Parental interview together with spirometry identified 121 with confirmed asthma, and a further 167 who had wheezing with infections. Twenty-five years later, 65% of those diagnosed as asthmatic in childhood, together with 67% of those wheezing with infections, and 59% of 167 control children without wheezing or asthma were reviewed using questionnaire, lung function assessment and airway responsiveness measurements [8]. A history of childhood asthma was associated with adult wheezing with an odds ratio of 14.4, and with sputum production with an odds ratio of 3.3, as well as with a lower FEV_1 and greater airway responsiveness compared with normals. Those with childhood wheezing not diagnosed as asthma at that time had an odds ratio for wheezing as adults of 3.8, and had less severe symptoms, with essentially normal lung function and airway responsiveness as adults. Predictors for adult wheezing included the original symptom group, atopy, and smoking as adults.

One of the longest studies of the natural history of childhood asthma commenced in 1969 in Australia, when a random sample of Grade 2 children in Melbourne schools was assembled [9]. This cohort included every 7 year old child with diagnosed asthma or with "wheezy bronchitis" (more than 5 episodes per year of wheezing associated with infection), every second child with "mild wheezy bronchitis" (less than 5 episodes per year associated with infection), and every twentieth normal child. This cohort was followed up at ages 10, 14, 21, 28, and 35 years, with 86% cohort retention at age 35.

The study sample was "enriched" at age 10 with the addition of 67 children with more severe asthma to provide data for outcome of severe asthma. This complicates assessment of the reported data, but it is possible to extract sufficient data to look at trends in the original randomly selected population sample. Among these, at age 35, 20% had persistent symptoms of wheezing while a further 15% had symptoms occurring less than one per week in the previous three months, so that in total 35% had wheezing symptoms [10]. Among those who were initially classified as having "asthma" at age 7, 50%

had frequent or persistent symptoms and only 30% were entirely asymptomatic. Among those with "wheezy bronchitis" whether having more or less than 5 episodes per year, two thirds were asymptomatic as adults. Hence, the likelihood of persistence of childhood wheezing symptoms was strongest in those already given the diagnosis of asthma at age 7. Risk factors for persistence of childhood symptoms to age 35 included multiple episodes occurring before the age of two years, the presence of eczema and of atopy, and low lung function in childhood.

In a separate Australian study, 8,600 children age 7 years living in Tasmania in 1968 were assessed by questionnaire and spirometry [11]. Of this population, 16.2% reported asthma. The cohort was followed up some 20 years later with a 74% response rate among 1000 asthmatics and 1000 normals selected from the initial cohort. Among those who had asthma reported at age 7, 25.6% had asthma as young adults. Of those who were asymptomatic at age 7, 10.0% now had asthma. Current frequent asthma as adults was reported by 5.4% and 2.1% respectively of those symptomatic or asymptomatic in childhood. Current adult asthma was more likely to associate with a later age of onset, a greater total number of attacks and more frequent attacks. Risk factors for persistence of childhood asthma into adulthood included not only their own personal history of childhood asthma, but being female, having eczema, low lung function as children, and a family history of asthma.

A longitudinal study was commenced in the UK in 1958 with a birth cohort of 18,559 children born in one week in March [12]. These children have been reviewed at age 7, 11, 16, 23, and 33 years with respect to respiratory illness. At age 7, 18.2% reported asthma or wheeze ever, but by age 11 the prevalence of reported symptoms ever had decreased to 12.0% and by age 16 to 11.5%. The prevalence of current asthma or wheezing (in the last 12 months) at ages 7, 11, 16, and 23 was respectively 8.1%, 4.6%, 3.3% and 4.0%. There was substantial attrition in this study, and only 31% of the initial birth cohort contributed information at all surveys from age 7 to 33 years. The incidence of asthma between age 17 and age 33 was associated with cigarette smoking and a history of hayfever, with weaker independent associations with female sex and histories of eczema and migraine [13]. Relapse of asthma at age 33 after earlier remission of childhood wheezing was more likely among atopic subjects and current smokers. Among the 1,880 subjects who reported asthma or wheezing between birth and age 7, the prevalence of wheezing attacks in the previous year was 50% at age 7 (i. e., half had already gone into remission), 18% at age 11, 10% at age 16, 10% at age 23, followed by significant relapse with 27% reporting symptoms at age 33.

In Dunedin, New Zealand, a longitudinal study of 1037 children was commenced involving a cohort of children born between April 1972 and March 1973 and still residing in the province of Otago at age 3 years [14]. Respiratory assessments have been performed at age 9, 11, 13, 15, 18, and 21 years, together with measurements of spirometry, airway responsiveness to methacholine, and allergy including skin testing and IgE measurements. At each age the prevalence of diagnosed asthma was substantially less than the prevalence of recurrent wheezing. Atopy (defined as one or more positive skin test weals ≥ 2 mm diameter) was found in 44% of the population at age 13, and 60% at age 21. The prevalence of airway responsiveness (methacholine $PC_{20} \leq 8$ mg/ml or > 10% response to salbutamol in obstructed children) decreased with age from 18% at age 9 to become stable at 8–10% of the population between age 13 and 21. In this cohort, factors associated with persistence of asthma or recurrent wheezing symptoms from the time of onset to age 21 include sensitization to house dust mite and cat, airway responsiveness, and to a small extent, current cigarette smoking at age 18 and 21 years [15].

Factors Predisposing to Persistence of Childhood Asthma

Family History

In most studies, a family history of asthma (particularly if accompanied by a strong family history of atopy) is the dominant risk factor for development of childhood asthma and personal atopy and for persistence of asthmatic symptoms [16, 17]. Those studies not finding strong associations with family history of allergic disease are those in which virtually all subjects were atopic on entry to the study making it difficult to show a difference in persistence between atopic and nonatopic children [5].

Atopy

The great majority of studies, especially those based on a population sample, have shown that personal atopy is a risk factor for persistence of asthma. Remission occurs less frequently in those with more marked degrees of atopy [11, 13, 15].

Environmental Exposures

It seems highly likely that persistent allergen exposure is a risk factor for persistent symptoms, but epidemiologically based data supporting this hypothesis, with documentation of levels of exposure correlated with the risk of persistence, are meager. Among clinical studies of children and young adults attending emergency rooms for management of troublesome asthma, atopy to indoor allergens including house dust mite and cockroach is very common, and high exposure levels have been found in their homes [18].

Personal smoking has been shown to be a risk factor for persistence of childhood respiratory symptoms to adulthood in a number of studies. Among Aberdeen children, those who took up smoking in adolescence and adulthood had more symptoms and lower lung function, but did not have more airway hyperresponsiveness, than nonsmokers [8]. Personal smoking as an adult was a significant risk factor for adult wheezing but not for airway responsiveness. In the UK national cohort, relapse of asthma at age 33 after prolonged remission of childhood wheezing more commonly occurred among current smokers [13]. Persistence of symptoms to age 21 in the New Zealand cohort was also associated with smoking [15].

Severity of Childhood Asthma

Virtually all studies, whether from population-based cohorts studied longitudinally or from office or specialist clinic follow-up studies, have indicated that the greater the severity of childhood asthma, the more likely it is to persist [2, 4–8, 10, 11, 13, 15]. This is true whether severity is measured by their frequency of episodes in childhood, lung function abnormality, or the severity of airway responsiveness.

Gender

Childhood asthma is more common among boys than girls, probably because the prevalence of atopy is higher among boys than girls, but persistence of childhood asthma into adulthood is more common in females in virtually all longitudinal series [10, 11, 13, 15]. The prevalence of current asthma changes from male dominance to female dominance at about the age of puberty. This phenomenon is less evident among studies following clinic populations, again because the cohort that is being followed is selected by the entry of more males with troublesome asthma in childhood, but even then there is a greater likelihood of persistence among females [5–7].

Does Treatment Affect the Natural History of Childhood Asthma?

This cannot be answered with certainty. Among the Melbourne cohort, Martin et al. considered that the prognosis of childhood asthma to adulthood was not influenced by management of childhood asthma [19]. This may reflect the noninterventional nature of that epidemiological study, and almost certainly reflects the enrichment of the population cohort by subjects with more severe asthma, together with high levels of smoking found in that cohort. One would expect that adequate treatment of childhood asthma would attenuate the prevalence and severity of adult disease. Studies such as those of Agertoft and Pedersen examining the influence of inhaled corticosteroid therapy in children with substantial improvement noted in those children who received early rather than later corticosteroid therapy suggests that early intervention could reduce the likelihood of persistence to chronic adult asthma [20].

Natural History of Adult Onset Asthma

There are remarkably few data examining the course and prognosis of adult asthma, and the effects of treatment. In Scandinavia, there was a very low incidence of remission of adult asthma, in that only 3% of those reporting current asthma in 1986 were asymptomatic on review 10 years later [21]. Studies of occupational asthma as a prototype of

adult asthma show frequent persistence of both symptoms and abnormal pulmonary function and airway hyperresponsiveness, even when the subjects are removed from exposure, although the outcome does depend on the duration of exposure and the sensitizing agent [22].

Among a cohort of younger adults in The Netherlands, retested 25 years after their initial investigations for asthma, 40% had no symptoms in later adult life, but the majority still showed airway hyperresponsiveness with only 21% not being hyperresponsive [23]. Remission of asthma was more likely to occur in younger subjects, in those with less severe disease at initial study, and in those in whom treatment was initiated relatively early after the onset of asthma. In contrast, among older subjects residing in Tucson, Arizona, who were aged over 65 years at enrolment, the remission rate for asthma over a 7-year follow-up period was less than 7% [24].

Reed has recently reviewed aspects of the natural history of asthma in adults [25]. Collectively, studies of adult asthma generally show a quite rapid decline in lung function shortly after the diagnosis is made, with a slowing of rate of decline in subsequent years. The rate of decline is greater in older subjects, and is related to IgE levels and blood eosinophils, although paradoxically, nonatopic patients have faster overall decline in FEV_1 than atopic patients. The rate of decline is faster in smokers. In his own series of Mayo Clinic patients over age 65, the best post-bronchodilator FEV_1 was < 60% predicted in 28%, and < 70% predicted in 57%, indicating substantial loss of reversibility despite treatment in older asthmatics [25]. Interestingly, the maximum post-bronchodilator FEV_1 did not correlate with the duration of the disease.

Mortality from Asthma

The risk to an individual asthmatic of dying from asthma is very small. However, over the last three decades, there has been increasing concern about asthma mortality, particularly focused on two epidemics which increased mortality rates particularly among young people to levels 3 to 5 times those seen in the pre-epidemic years. The causes of these epidemics has been much debated but there is now general consensus that the 1960s epidemic which occurred in England and Wales, Australia and New

Zealand was linked with use of high dose isoprenalin as an adrenergic agonist used in the management of asthma [26]. The second epidemic, which was confined to New Zealand, was linked with the excessive use of a high dose β adrenergic agent, fenoterol [27]. Initially these agents were thought to increase the risk of mortality because of cardiac arrhythmias, but recent clinical trials have demonstrated that frequent use of an inhaled short-acting β-agonist may increase airway responsiveness to allergen and decrease control of asthma leading to greater severity of disease and therefore greater risk of mortality [28–31]. The abrupt decline in both mortality and morbidity as measured in hospital admissions in New Zealand adults after withdrawal of fenoterol from the therapeutic armamentarium is strong evidence that this agent was associated with an increased severity of disease which reversed quite rapidly after the drug was withdrawn [32].

In many countries there was a gradual upward trend in mortality through the 1960s to mid 1980s, which in most countries has now plateaued and begun to decline. Use of inhaled corticosteroid is thought to be a significant factor protecting against mortality, although this is only shown objectively in one case control study to date [33]. Nevertheless, the recognition that asthma can be fatal, that overreliance on β-agonists may be a direct or indirect risk factor for mortality and certainly is a marker of uncontrolled asthma which requires urgent attention, have all contributed to reducing the mortality rate from asthma. Other risk factors for mortality, especially in inner-city areas of the United States, include poverty, race, allergen exposure, discontinuity of care and lack of inhaled corticosteroid therapy [34]. Many individuals with these risk factors are in a constant state of poorly controlled asthma, and are at risk of death if they experience worsening of asthma in a situation where help is not readily accessible.

Address for correspondence:

Dr. M R Sears
Firestone Regional Chest & Allergy Unit
St. Joseph's Hospital
50 Charlton Avenue East
Hamilton, Ontario L8N 4A6
Canada
Tel. +1 905 521-6000
Fax +1 905 521-6132
E-mail searsm@fhs.csu.McMaster.ca

References

1. Martinez FD, Wright AL, Taussig LM, Holberg CJ, Halonen M, Morgan WJ. Asthma and wheezing in the first six years of life. N Engl J Med 1995; 332:133–138.

2. Rackemann FM, Edwards MC. Asthma in children: A follow-up study of 688 patients after an interval of twenty years. N Engl J Med 1952; 246:815–823.

3. Blair H. Natural history of childhood asthma. Arch Dis Child 1977; 52:613–619.

4. Blair H. Symposium: The wheezy child. Natural history of wheezing in childhood. J Royal Soc Med 1979; 72: 42–48.

5. Gerritsen J, Koeter GH, Postma DS, Schouten JP, Van Aalderen WMC, Knol K. Airway responsiveness in childhood as a predictor of the outcome of asthma in adulthood. Am Rev Respir Dis 1991; 143:1468–1469.

6. Roorda RJ, Gerritsen J, Van Aalderen WMC, Schouten JP, Veltman JC, Weiss ST, Knol K. Risk factors for the persistence of respiratory symptoms in childhood asthma. Am Rev Respir Dis 1993; 148:1490–1495.

7. Ulrik CS, Backer V, Dirksen A, Pedersen M, Koch C. Extrinsic and intrinsic asthma from childhood to adult age: A 10-year follow-up. Respir Med 1995; 89:547–554.

8. Godden DJ, Ross S, Abdalla M, et al. Outcome of wheeze in childhood. Symptoms and pulmonary function 25 years later. Am J Respir Crit Care Med 1994; 149:106–112.

9. Williams H, McNicol KN. Prevalence, natural history and relationship of wheezy bronchitis and asthma in children. An epidemiological study. Br Med J 1969; 4:321–325.

10. Oswald H, Phelan PD, Lanigan A, Hibbert M, Bowes G, Olinsky A. Outcome of childhood asthma in mid-adult life. Br Med J 1994; 309:95–96.

11. Jenkins MA, Hopper JL, Bowes G, Carlin JB, Flander LB, Giles GG. Factors in childhood as predictors of asthma in adult life. Br Med J 1994; 309:90–93.

12. Anderson HR, Pottier AC, Strachan DP. Asthma from birth to age 23: Incidence and relation to prior and concurrent atopic disease. Thorax 1992; 47:537–542.

13. Strachan DP, Butland BK, Anderson HR. Incidence and prognosis of asthma and wheezing illness from early childhood to age 33 in a national British cohort. Br Med J 1996; 312:1195–1199.

14. Silva PA. The Dunedin Multidisciplinary Health and Development Study: A 15-year longitudinal study. Pediatric Perinatal Epidemiol 1990; 4:96–127.

15. Sears MR, Wiecek E, Willan A, Flannery EM, Taylor DR, Herbison GP, Holdaway MD. Persistence, remission, and relapse of childhood asthma: A longitudinal

study from age 9 to age 21. Eur Respir J 1998; 12 (Suppl 28):401s.

16. Sears MR, Holdaway MD, Flannery EM, Herbison GP, Silva PA. Parental and neonatal risk factors for atopy, airway hyper-responsiveness, and asthma. Arch Dis Childhood 1996; 75:392–398.

17. Roorda RJ, Gerritsen J, Van Aalderen VMC, Knol K. Influence of a positive family history and associated allergic diseases on the natural course of asthma. Clin Exp Allergy 1992; 22:627–634.

18. Platts-Mills TAE, Vervloet D, Thomas WR, Aalberse RC, Chapman MD. Indoor allergens and asthma: Report of the Third International Workshop. J Allergy Clin Immunol 1997; 100:S1–S24.

19. Martin AJ, Landau LI, Phelan PD. Asthma from childhood at age 21: The patient and his disease. Br Med J 1982; 284:380–382.

20. Agertoft L, Pedersen S. Effects of long-term treatment with an inhaled corticosteroid on growth and pulmonary function in asthmatic children. Respir Med 1994; 88:373–381

21. Ronmark E, Jonsson E, Lundback B. Remission of asthma 1986–1996 – Report from the Obstructive Lung Disease in Northern Sweden study. Eur Respir J 1997; 10(Suppl 25):164s.

22. Venables KM, Chan-Yeung M. Occupational asthma. Lancet 1997; 349:1465–1469.

23. Panhuysen CIM, Vonk JM, Koeter GH, Schouten JP, van Altena R, Bleecker ER, Postma DS. Adult patients may outgrow their asthma. A 25-year follow-up study. Am J Respir Crit Care Med 1997; 155:1267–1272.

24. Burrows B, Barbee RA, Cline MG, Knudson RJ, Lebowitz MD. Characteristics of asthma among elderly adults in a sample of the general population. Chest 1991; 100:935–942.

25. Reed CE. The natural history of asthma in adults: The problem of irreversibility. J Allergy Clin Immunol 1999; 103:539–547

26. Stolley PD. Asthma mortality. Why the United States was spared an epidemic of deaths due to asthma. Am Rev Respir Dis 1972; 105:883–890.

27. Sears MR, Taylor DR. The β_2-agonist controversy. Observations, explanations and relationship to asthma epidemiology. Drug Safety 1994; 11:259–283.

28. Sears MR, Taylor DR, Print CG, Lake DC, Li Q, Flannery EM, Yates DM, Lucas MK, Herbison GP. Regular inhaled β-agonist treatment in bronchial asthma. Lancet 1990; 336:1391–1396.

29. Taylor DR, Sears MR, Herbison GP, Flannery EM, Print CG, Lake DC, Yates DM, Lucas MK, Li Q. Regular inhaled β-agonist in asthma: effect on exacerbations and lung function. Thorax 1993; 48:134–138.

30. Cockcroft DW, McPaarland CP, Britto SA, Swystun VA, Rutherford BC. Regular inhaled salbutamol and airway responsiveness to allergen. Lancet 1993; 342: 833–837.

31. Gauvreau GM, Jordana M, Watson RM, Cockcroft DW, O'Byrne PM. Effect of regular inhaled albuterol on allergen-induced late responses and sputum eosinophils in asthmatic subjects. Am J Respir Crit Care Med 1997; 156:1738–1745

32. Sears MR. Epidemiological trends in asthma. Can Respir J 1996; 3:261–268.

33. Ernst P, Spitzer W, Suissa S, Cockcroft D, Habbick B, Horwitz R, Boivin J-F, McNutt M, Buist AS. Risk of fatal and near fatal asthma in relation to inhaled corticosteroid use. JAMA 1992; 268:3462–3464.

34. McFadden ER, Warren EL. Observations on asthma mortality. Ann Intern Med 1997; 127:142–147.

Leukotriene Modifying Agents in the Treatment of Asthma

Joseph D Spahn*/**, David Fost***, Stanley J Szefler*/**/****

Keywords: Leukotriene antagonists, leukotriene synthesis inhibitors, leukotriene modifiers, montelukast, pranlukast, zafirlukast, zileuton

Leukotrienes are a class of lipid derived inflammatory mediators which appear to be involved in the pathogenesis of airway inflammation associated with asthma. Leukotriene modifying agents have been developed to either inhibit leukotriene synthesis or to antagonize the action of selective leukotrienes. Their specific role in asthma management is the subject of ongoing clinical research. Although they are slightly less effective than inhaled corticosteroids as long term controllers, they offer certain advantages such as ease of administration and a good safety profile.

Introduction

Asthma, even in its mildest form, is characterized as an inflammatory disease of the airways. Over the past 20 years, we have learned a great deal regarding the complexities of airway inflammation. Many cellular elements such as mast cells, eosinophils, Th2 lymphocytes, neutrophils, macrophages, and epithelial cells are involved as well as intercellular chemical mediators including eosinophil basic proteins, cytokines, and leukotrienes. Inflammation is thought to be directly and/or indirectly associated with the variable airflow obstruction characteristic of asthma and is manifest as recurrent wheezing, episodic chest tightness and cough. Inflammation is also linked with airway hyperresponsiveness. The leukotrienes are a specific class of lipid derived inflammatory mediators which appear to be involved in the pathogenesis of asthma. With the development of potent drugs that interfere with leukotriene production or function, there has been an increasing amount of interest in this component of the inflammatory process. This review will focus on the role leukotrienes play in the pathogenesis of asthma and the development of leukotriene modifying agents for application to asthma management.

Leukotriene Biochemistry

The leukotrienes are a group of lipid-derived mediators with a broad range of biological effects on both cells and tissues. They are members of the eicosanoid family of physiologically active substances that also include prostaglandins and thromboxanes. They are synthesized through the arachidonic acid cascade that occurs in a variety of inflammatory cells including eosinophils, mast cells, basophils, and macrophages. As depicted in Figure 1, the first step involves enzymatic cleavage of arachidonic acid from membrane phospholipids by phospholipase A_2. Arachidonic acid can then be converted to prostaglandins and thromboxanes through the action of cyclooxygenase, or to the leukotrienes through the action of 5-lipoxygenase. Of note, 5-lipoxygenase must first be activated by binding to a membrane bound protein called 5-lipoxygenase activating protein or FLAP. 5-lipoxygenase can then catalyze the conversion of arachidonic acid to the unstable intermediate 5-hydroperoxy-eicosatetraenoic acid (5-HPETE) which is subsequently converted to LTA_4. LTA_4 may be either hydrolyzed via LTA_4 hydrolase to LTB_4 or converted to LTC_4 through the action of LTC_4 synthase. LTC_4 is then transported out of the cell where it can be converted to LTD_4 or LTE_4 in the peripheral

* National Jewish Medical and Research Center, Denver, CO, USA
** University of Colorado Health Sciences Center, Denver, CO, USA
*** Dr. Fost is now at the Asthma & Sinus Center of New Jersey, USA
**** Helen Wohlberg & Herman Lambert Chair in Pharmacokinetics

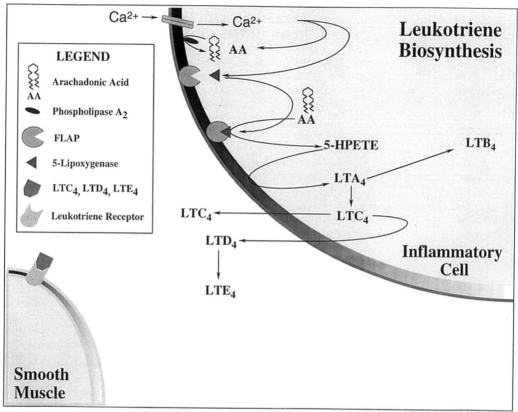

Figure 1. Diagram depicting leukotriene biosynthesis. See text for details.

circulation or tissues. The cysteinyl leukotrienes appear to bind to a single LTD_4 receptor known as $CysLT_1$. LTE_4 is a partial agonist for this receptor and it is speculated that LTC_4 must be converted to LTD_4 before binding to this receptor in humans. A separate LTC_4 receptor has been identified in animal models and it is possible that additional cysteinyl leukotriene receptors exist in humans as well. LTB_4 interacts with its own distinct receptor.

The Role of Leukotrienes in Asthma

Bronchial smooth muscle contraction and inflammation of the airways are hallmarks of asthma. Edema of the airway wall and excessive mucus production also contribute to the airflow obstruction seen in asthma. *In vitro* and *in vivo* studies have demonstrated that the leukotrienes may elicit or participate in many of these processes. *In vitro* studies with human airway tissue have shown LTC_4 and LTD_4 to be potent mucus secretagogues at concentrations as low as 1 pg/ml [1]. Intradermal injection results in an increased vascular permeability and localized tissue edema as depicted by a sustained wheal and erythema response [2].

Clinical studies of leukotrienes in asthma have revealed the following. First, leukotrienes have been measured in various body fluids including urine, nasal secretions, and bronchoalveolar lavage fluid with leukotriene concentrations consistently higher in asthmatic compared to nonasthmatic subjects [3–5]. Moreover, concentrations of the leukotrienes have been found to increase following allergen, exercise, or aspirin challenges in susceptible patients [6, 7]. Second, inhalation of leukotrienes can evoke asthmatic symptoms. For example, the inhalation of LTD_4 or LTE_4 at concentrations several log-fold less than that of histamine results in bronchospasm [8].

Inhalation of these compounds also results in increased airway hyperresponsiveness to histamine or methacholine [9, 10]. Bronchoscopy with biopsy performed before and after challenging asthmatic patients with inhaled LTE_4 has also shown a several-fold increase in eosinophils and neutrophils within the lamina propria [11].

Third, and perhaps the most clinically relevant, is the ability to block or attenuate specific asthmatic responses with anti-leukotriene drugs. The pharmacologic modulation of leukotriene synthesis or function has been shown to inhibit bronchospasm following allergen exposure [12], aspirin exposure [13], and exercise [14] in susceptible asthmatic patients. Clinical trials with anti-leukotriene drugs in asthmatic subjects have shown improvement in baseline pulmonary function as well as an acute bronchodilatory effect [15]. The clinical effects of these drugs further supports the hypothesis that the leukotrienes contribute to the pathogenesis of asthma and may help to elucidate the precise role that these mediators play in the development of this disease.

Anti-Leukotriene Medications

There are two major ways to effectively eliminate or modulate leukotriene activity. First, one can inhibit leukotriene production by developing inhibitors of either 5-lipoxygenase (e. g., zileuton) or FLAP (FLAP inhibiting drugs are still under investigation). Alternatively, one can inhibit function by developing compounds that prevent leukotrienes from binding to their receptors (i. e., receptor antagonists). There are 2 classes of leukotriene receptor antagonists. The cysteinyl leukotriene receptor antagonists (e. g., zafirlukast, montelukast) competitively block leukotriene binding to $CysLT_1$, while LTB_4 receptor antagonists block LTB_4 binding (LTB_4 antagonists are still in development). There are three leukotriene modifying agents available for use in the United States. Clinical data on the efficacy of these agents is rapidly accumulating and should help determine where these medications should be placed in the treatment regimens of asthmatic patients.

Zileuton

Zileuton (Zyflo®, Abbott) was the first leukotriene modifying agent approved for use in the United States. Approved in 1996, it remains the only 5-lipoxygenase inhibitor available for clinical use. Zileuton therapy results in improved lung function both acutely and after chronic use. The acute bronchodilatory effect appears to be significant between 1 and 2 hours post dose [16]. Zileuton would therefore not be appropriate for use as a "rescue" medication but may have an adjunctive role in the acute management of asthma exacerbations. Longer clinical trials in adults with mild to moderate asthma have shown improvements in FEV_1 and asthma symptoms, as well as decreased β-agonist use and reductions in urinary LTE_4 levels [15, 17].

Zileuton has the potential advantage of blocking LTB_4 in addition to cysteinyl leukotriene production. While the role of LTB_4 in the pathogenesis of asthma remains unclear, 5-lipoxygenase inhibitors such as zileuton may be more efficacious in certain subsets of asthmatic patients. LTB_4 is a chemoattractant for neutrophils *in vitro* [18] and LTB_4 levels in bronchoalveolar lavage fluid have been shown to correlate with the percentage of neutrophils [5]. Nocturnal asthma and sudden-onset asthma are two conditions associated with increased neutrophils in the airways [19, 20]. Recent bronchoscopic studies in patients with severe steroid dependent asthma have noted a neutrophil predominance in bronchoalveolar lavage fluid [21]. Thus, zileuton may be uniquely suited for these types of asthma. In addition, zileuton therapy has been shown to decrease LTB_4 levels in bronchoalveolar lavage fluid while improving nocturnal lung function [22].

The side effect profile for zileuton is comparable to placebo with the exception of elevation in serum ALT levels in approximately 2% of patients. As a result, monitoring of liver function is recommended at baseline, monthly intervals for the first 3 months, every 2 to 3 months for the remainder of the first year of therapy, and then periodically for patients maintained on long-term treatment. Zileuton is metabolized by the cytochrome P450 isoenzyme system and is therefore subject to interactions with other drugs metabolized by this enzyme system. Co-administration with theophylline results in an approximate doubling of serum theophylline levels necessitating a reduction in theophylline dosing and close monitoring of serum levels. Increased serum levels of warfarin, propranolol, and terfenadine have also been demonstrated when co-administered with zileuton. Drug interaction studies have shown no interaction between zileuton and prednisone or ethinyl estradiol. No formal drug interaction studies have been conducted between zileuton and cisapride, cyclosporine, calcium channel blockers, or astemizole. Clinical and drug monitoring would be reasonable with the co-administration of zileuton and cisapride, cyclosporine, calcium channel blockers, or any other medication metabolized by the cytochrome P450 enzyme system.

Because zileuton has a short serum half-life, it requires frequent dosing intervals. The recommended four times daily dosing schedule renders this medication less convenient than the leukotriene receptor antagonists that can be taken once or twice daily. Lastly, zileuton is not approved for use in children less than 12 years old.

Zafirlukast

In September 1997, zafirlukast (Accolate®, Zeneca) became the first leukotriene receptor antagonist approved for use in the United States for patients 12 years of age and older. Clinical studies performed with asthmatic subjects have demonstrated attenuation of the bronchospastic response to inhaled methacholine and aeroallergens [23, 24] following zafirlukast administration. A multicenter placebo controlled study in which adults with moderate asthma received zafirlukast for 6 weeks demonstrated improvements in asthma symptoms, nocturnal awakening, and "as needed" β-agonist use [25]. Accompanying the improvement in symptoms was a significant improvement in lung function with an 11% improvement in the mean FEV_1 compared with baseline values. Adverse effects in this study included headache, gastritis, pharyngitis, and rhinitis but were not significantly different from placebo.

Zafirlukast also influences the cytochrome P450 isoenzyme system and therefore has the potential to interact with other drugs metabolized by this isoenzyme system. Co-administration with warfarin results in an increased prothrombin time and therefore necessitates close monitoring of patients receiving both medications. Phenytoin and carbamazapine should similarly be closely monitored when used concomitantly with zafirlukast. Of note, erythromycin and theophylline appear to decrease plasma levels of zafirlukast without appreciable alterations in their own serum levels. Formal studies have not been published regarding concomitant use of zafirlukast and other drugs which interact with the cytochrome P450 system such as cisapride, cyclosporin, calcium-channel blockers, and astemizole. Nonetheless, close monitoring is reasonable

when these medications are co-administered with zafirlukast.

Zafirlukast is thought to be a safe medication with few serious adverse effects noted. Of note, a recent JAMA publication described eight cases of Churg-Strauss vasculitis, a syndrome involving severe asthma, eosinophilia, pulmonary infiltrates, sinus abnormalities, and neuropathy in asthmatic patients treated with zafirlukast [26]. All of the patients were adults with steroid dependent asthma. The onset of the vasculitis in each case occurred after the patients were placed on zafirlukast and were then successfully tapered off of oral steroids. Their symptoms improved following cessation of the zafirlukast and re-instituting oral steroids. Although controversial, it is conceivable that these patients had an underlying eosinophilic vasculitis disorder that was masked by the steroid treatment. In any case, it would be prudent either to avoid using this medication or monitor it carefully in patients with steroid dependent asthma until more information is developed on this rare medical disorder.

Montelukast

A second leukotriene receptor antagonist, montelukast (Singulair®, Merck), became available for use in February 1998. Montelukast is the only anti-leukotriene medication approved for use in children (6 years of age and older). Clinical efficacy has been demonstrated with montelukast in the treatment of mild to moderate asthma, and the side effect profile is comparable to placebo. In one of the only published studies evaluating an anti-leukotriene medication in children with asthma, Knorr et al. [27] found 8 weeks of daily montelukast administered to patients between the ages of 6 and 14 years resulted in an 8.23% increase in mean morning FEV_1 [27]. It should be noted, however, that the placebo arm of this study showed a 3.58% increase in their mean morning FEV_1. Additional outcomes reaching statistical significance included a decrease in total daily as-needed β-agonist use, asthma exacerbations and peripheral blood eosinophil counts with an improvement in AM peak expiratory flow rates and quality of life questionnaires. Daytime asthma symptoms, nocturnal awakenings, rescue corticosteroid use, and school loss were among the outcome parameters that did not reach statistical significance. Montelukast has also demonstrated effectiveness in attenuating exercise-induced asthma [28]. While the results of these trials lend further support for a role of the leukotrienes in pediatric asthma, this leukotriene antagonist appears to be slightly less efficacious than inhaled glucocorticoids, which remain the gold standard for the long-term treatment of airway inflammation in moderate to severe asthma [29].

Who Should Be Using Leukotriene Modifiers

The newly revised National Asthma Education and Prevention Program Expert Panel Report 2: Guidelines for the Diagnosis and Management of Asthma [30] categorizes asthma medications into two major classes, long-term control medications and quick-relief medications. The former class generally includes medications with anti-inflammatory properties while the quick relief medications are generally rapid onset bronchodilators. A daily long-term control medication should be added to the regimen of any patient with persistent asthma. A diagnosis of mild persistent asthma should be given when asthma symptoms occur more than twice a week (but less than once a day), nocturnal symptoms more than twice a month, and 20% to 30% diurnal variability in peak expiratory flow rates. Appropriate medications at this level of severity would include low dose inhaled corticosteroid, cromolyn or nedocromil, or sustained release theophylline. The Expert Panel Report 2 states that the position of the leukotriene modifiers in asthma therapy is not fully established but they may be considered for use as daily long-term control medication in patients with mild persistent asthma.

Potential Advantages of the Leukotriene Modifiers

The leukotriene modifiers have several potential advantages over the other long-term control medications. First, leukotriene modifiers are administered orally and therefore do not require patients to master techniques of more complicated delivery systems such as metered dose inhalers. Oral medications also require much less time to administer inhaled to metered dose inhalers and nebulized delivery systems. These advantages would be expected to increase patient adherence to the medication regimen, particularly with chronic treatment. Second, the leukotriene modifiers (especially the receptor antagonists) have an excellent safety profile. They lack the systemic adverse effects associated with inhaled corticosteroids such as potential effects on growth velocity, osteoporosis or ocular disorders as well as the more serious gastrointestinal, cardiovascular, and central nervous system toxicities of theophylline. In addition, the leukotriene modifiers do not require serum level monitoring which further simplifies their clinical use. Given that these compounds are nonsteroidal, yet display some anti-inflammatory effects, they can be used in patients unwilling to take inhaled steroids due to "steroid phobia." The leukotriene modifiers may be beneficial in the long-term treatment of mild persistent asthma in patients who might otherwise remain under-treated due to any of these issues. Other potential applications of these medications include the following:

1. An alternative to inhaled glucocorticoid therapy in patients who are unable to take inhaled medications.
2. A supplement to inhaled controller medications to reduce need for high dose inhaled glucocorticoid therapy.
3. A medication with a different mechanism of action could have an additive effect with other medications in improving the overall response to treatment.
4. They may offer the opportunity to individualize the approach to therapy as we begin to understand the differences in asthma pathophysiology among patients. Perhaps some patients have a primary leukotriene mediated disease process.

Of note, the Expert Panel Report 2 does not define a role for the leukotriene modifiers in the treatment of moderate or severe asthma. Pranlukast, a leukotriene receptor antagonist which is not yet available in the United States, has been shown to be beneficial in reducing asthma exacerbations in moderate to severe asthmatics following reduction of high dose inhaled glucocorticoid therapy [31]. Compared to placebo, patients on pranlukast were able to tolerate a 50% reduction in inhaled glucocorticoid dose while maintaining FEV_1, morning and evening peak expiratory flow rates, and daily asthma symptom scores at or above baseline values. Two markers of inflammation, serum eosinophil cationic protein and exhaled nitric oxide, rose in the placebo group while remaining stable in the group receiving the leukotriene antagonist. Leukotriene modifiers may therefore have a role as steroid sparing agents in moderate to severe asthma patients. It is not clear whether leukotriene modifying agents could prevent potential irreversible changes due to inflammation associated with asthma, and it is not clear whether any medication, other than possibly inhaled glucocorticoids [32–37] could be helpful in alleviating this component of asthma pathogenesis.

Aspirin Sensitivity. Aspirin (ASA) idiosyncrasy, or the tendency to develop bronchospasm and/or rhinitis following the ingestion of ASA, can be a major problem in some adults with asthma. The pathogenesis of aspirin sensitive asthma appears to involve the overproduction of leukotrienes secondary to shunting of arachidonic acid to the 5-lipoxygenase pathway due to blockage of the cyclooxygenase pathway, or by reduction of the inhibition of leukotriene production caused by the prostaglandins. Other nonsteroidal anti-inflammatory drugs which block the cyclooxygenase pathway have also been shown to elicit similar responses in select patients. Leukotriene modifiers have been shown to attenuate the fall in FEV_1 and the rise in urinary LTE_4 which occur following ASA challenges [13]. Leukotriene modifiers may therefore have a role in the treatment of patients with a history of ASA sensitivity.

Exercise-Induced Asthma. Exercise induced asthma is a common trigger in both adult and pediatric asthmatics. Bronchospasm following exercise has been shown to occur in the majority of asthmatic children, and in a sizable minority of nonasthmatic allergic children [38]. As previously discussed, leukotrienes are potent bronchoconstrictors with elevated urinary LTE_4 levels noted following exercise challenges in some asthmatic children [39]. Consequently, these medications can play a role in the prevention of exercise-induced bronchospasm [14, 28]. Leukotriene receptor antagonists and 5-lipoxygenase inhibitors have been shown to attenuate exercise-induced bronchospasm in asthmatic subjects when given orally on a daily basis. Further, inhalation of a leukotriene receptor antagonist has been shown to be comparable to inhaled cromolyn in attenuating exercise induced bronchospasm [40]. Further studies will need to be done to determine the role of the leukotriene modifiers in the treatment of these important subsets of asthma.

Future Directions

The advent of pharmacologic agents that specifically target leukotriene formation and function may help to define the roles of these agents in other inflammatory conditions. Leukotrienes are thought to play a role in the pathogenesis of rhinitis and chronic sinusitis as well as chronic urticaria. Case reports of patients with such conditions responding to leukotriene modifiers are accumulating and clinical studies will inevitably follow [41, 42]. Although the leukotriene modifying agents may possess some anti-inflammatory effects, studies are needed to show reductions in airway inflammation and resolution of airway changes secondary to inflammation. Lastly, head-to-head studies comparing the efficacy and safety of the leukotriene modifiers and inhaled glucocorticoids have yet to be published. Studies such as these are greatly needed as we attempt to position this new class of asthma medications.

Conclusions

We now know that chronic mucosal inflammation of the airways plays a prominent role in the immunopathogenesis of asthma. Appreciation of this inflammatory process in the pathogenesis of asthma has led to an increased emphasis on the use of long term anti-inflammatory medications for the treatment of persistent asthma. Leukotriene modifiers are a new class of targeted therapy for use in patients with asthma. These medications may modify both airway inflammation and airway tone. They are safe and easy to administer. The currently available leukotriene modifiers have limited efficacy and would therefore not be expected to replace inhaled corticosteroids as monotherapy for moderate to severe asthma but may be useful as a supplement to more potent anti-inflammatory medications. Patients with mild persistent asthma may be successfully controlled with a leukotriene modifier combined with an as needed β_2-agonist. Inhaled glucocorticoids have the potential advantage of altering the progression of disease associated with chronic inflammation, but this remains to be verified in long-term clinical studies. The leukotriene modifiers may also be particularly useful in patients with aspirin idiosyncrasy and exercise induced bronchospasm. Ongoing studies should help define the precise role of the current and future leukotriene modifiers in the treatment of asthma and other inflammatory disorders.

Acknowledgments

The authors wish to thank Maureen Plourd-Sandoval for assistance in preparing this manuscript. This study was supported in part by Public Health Services Research Grants HL36577 and General Clinical Research Center Grant 5 MO1 RR00051 from the Division of Research Resources, and an American Lung Association Asthma Research Center Grant.

Address correspondence to:

Stanley J Szefler, MD
National Jewish Medical and Research Center
1400 Jackson St., Rm. J209
Denver, CO 80206
USA
Tel. +1 303 398-1193
Fax +1 303 270-2189
E-mail szeflers@njc.org

References

1. Marom Z, Shelhamer JH, Bach MK, Morton DR, Kaliner M. Slow-reacting substances, leukotrienes C4 and D4, increase the release of mucus from human airways *in vitro*. Am Rev Respir Dis 1982; 126:449.

2. Soter NA, Lewis RA, Corey EJ, Austen KF. Local effects of synthetic leukotrienes (LTC4, LTD4, LTE4, and LTB4) in human skin. J Invest Dermatol 1983; 80:115.

3. Drazen JM, O'Brien J, Sparrow D, Weiss ST, Martins MA, Israel E, Fanta CH. Recovery of leukotriene E4 from the urine of patients with airway obstruction. Am Rev Respir Dis 1992; 146:104.

4. Lam S, Chan H, LeRiche JC, Chan-Yeung M, Salari H. Release of leukotrienes in patients with bronchial asthma. J Allergy Clin Immunol 1988; 81:711.

5. Wardlaw AJ, Hay H, Cromwell O, Collins JV, Kay AB. Leukotrienes, LTC4 and LTB4, in bronchoalveolar lavage in bronchial asthma and other respiratory diseases. J Allergy Clin Immunol 1989; 84:19.

6. Wang D, Clement P, Smitz J, Derde MP. Concentrations of chemical mediators in nasal secretions of patients with hay fever during natural allergen exposure. Acta Otolaryngol (Stockh) 1994; 114:552.

7. Kumlin M, Dahlen B, Bjorck T, Zetterstrom O, Granstrom E, Dahlen SE. Urinary excretion of leukotriene E4 and 11-dehydro-thromboxane B2 in response to bronchial provocations with allergen, aspirin, leukotriene D4, and histamine in asthmatics. Am Rev Respir Dis 1992; 146:96.

8. Smith LJ, Geller S, Ebright L, Glass M, Thyrum PT. Inhibition of leukotriene D4-induced bronchoconstriction in normal subjects by the oral LTD4 receptor antagonist ICI 204,219. Am Rev Respir Dis 1990; 141:988.

9. Kaye MG, Smith LJ. Effects of inhaled leukotriene D4 and platelet-activating factor on airway reactivity in normal subjects. Am Rev Respir Dis 1990; 141:993.

10. Arm JP, Spur BW, Lee TH. The effects of inhaled leukotriene E4 on the airway responsiveness to histamine in subjects with asthma and normal subjects. J Allergy Clin Immunol 1988; 82:654.

11. Laitinen LA, Laitinen A, Haahtela T, Vilkka V, Spur BW, Lee TH. Leukotriene E4 and granulocytic infiltration into asthmatic airways. Lancet 1993; 341:989.

12. Taylor IK, O'Shaughnessy KM, Fuller RW, Dollery CT. Effect of cysteinyl-leukotriene receptor antagonist ICI 204.219 on allergen-induced bronchoconstriction and airway hyperreactivity in atopic subjects. Lancet 1991; 337:690.

13. Israel E, Fischer AR, Rosenberg MA, Lilly CM, Callery JC, Shapiro J, Cohn J, Rubin P, Drazen JM. The pivotal role of 5-lipoxygenase products in the reaction of aspirin-sensitive asthmatics to aspirin. Am Rev Respir Dis 1993; 148:1447.

14. Reiss TF, Hill JB, Harman E, Zhang J, Tanaka WK, Bronsky E, Guerreiro D, Hendeles L. Increased urinary excretion of LTE4 after exercise and attenuation of exercise-induced bronchospasm by montelukast, a cysteinyl leukotriene receptor antagonist. Thorax 1997; 52:1030.

15. Israel E, Rubin P, Kemp JP, Grossman J, Pierson W, Siegel SC, Tinkelman D, Murray JJ, Busse W, Segal AT, et al. The effect of inhibition of 5-lipoxygenase by zileuton in mild-to-moderate asthma. Ann Intern Med 1993; 119:1059.

16. Israel E, Rubin P, Pearlman H, Cohn J, Drazen JM. 5-lipoxygenase inhibition by zileuton causes acute bronchodilation in asthma. Ann Intern Med 1992; 145:A16.

17. Israel E, Cohn J, Dube L, Drazen JM. Effect of treatment with zileuton, a 5-lipoxygenase inhibitor, in patients with asthma. A randomized controlled trial. Zileuton Clinical Trial Group. JAMA 1996; 275:931.

18. Palmblad J, Malmsten CL, Uden AM, Radmark O, Engstedt L, Samuelsson B. Leukotriene B4 is a potent and stereospecific stimulator of neutrophil chemotaxis and adherence. Blood 1981; 58:658.

19. Sur S, Crotty TB, Kephart GM, Hyma BA, Colby TV,

Reed CE, Hunt LW, Gleich GJ. Sudden-onset fatal asthma. A distinct entity with few eosinophils and relatively more neutrophils in the airway submucosa? Am Rev Respir Dis 1993; 148:713.

20. Martin RJ, Cicutto LC, Smith HR, Ballard RD, Szefler SJ. Airways inflammation in nocturnal asthma. Am Rev Respir Dis 1991; 143:351.

21. Wenzel SE, Szefler SJ, Leung DY, Sloan SI, Rex MD, Martin RJ. Bronchoscopic evaluation of severe asthma. Persistent inflammation associated with high dose glucocorticoids. Am J Respir Crit Care Med 1997; 156:737.

22. Wenzel SE, Trudeau JB, Kaminsky DA, Cohn J, Martin RJ, Westcott JY. Effect of 5-lipoxygenase inhibition on bronchoconstriction and airway inflammation in nocturnal asthma. Am J Respir Crit Care Med 1995; 152:897.

23. Rosenthal R, Lavins BJ, Hanby LA. Effect of treatment with safirlukast (Accolate®) on bronchial hyper-responsiveness in patients with mild-to-moderate asthma. J Allergy Clin Immunol 1996; 97:250A.

24. Findlay SR, Barden JM, Easley CB, Glass M. Effect of the oral leukotriene antagonist, ICI 204,219, on antigen-induced bronchoconstriction in subjects with asthma. J Allergy Clin Immunol 1992; 89:1040.

25. Spector SL, Smith LJ, Glass M. Effects of 6 weeks of therapy with oral doses of ICI 204,219, a leukotriene D4 receptor antagonist, in subjects with bronchial asthma. ACCOLATE Asthma Trialists Group. Am J Respir Crit Care Med 1994; 150:618.

26. Wechsler ME, Garpestad E, Flier SR, Kocher O, Weiland DA, Polito AJ, Klinek MM, Bigby TD, Wong GA, Helmers RA, Drazen JM. Pulmonary infiltrates, eosinophilia, and cardiomyopathy following corticosteroid withdrawal in patients with asthma receiving zafirlukast. JAMA 1998; 279:455.

27. Knorr B, Matz J, Bernstein JA, Nguyen H, Seidenberg BC, Reiss TF, Becker A. Montelukast for chronic asthma in 6- to 14-year-old children: A randomized, double-blind trial. Pediatric Montelukast Study Group. JAMA 1998; 279:1181.

28. Bronsky EA, Kemp JP, Zhang J, Guerreiro D, Reiss TF. Dose-related protection of exercise bronchoconstriction by montelukast, a cysteinyl leukotriene-receptor antagonist, at the end of a once-daily dosing interval. Clin Pharmacol Ther 1997; 62:556.

29. van Essen-Zandvliet EE, Hughes MD, Waalkens HJ, Duiverman EJ, Pocock SJ, Kerrebijn KF. Effects of 22 months of treatment with inhaled corticosteroids and/or β2-agonists on lung function, airway responsiveness, and symptoms in children with asthma. The Dutch Chronic Non-Specific Lung Disease Study Group. Am Rev Respir Dis 1992; 146:547.

30. National Asthma Education and Prevention Program Expert Panel. Report 2: Guidelines for the diagnosis and management of asthma. In National Institutes of Health, National Heart, Lung and Blood Institute, 1997, Pub. No. 97.

31. Tamaoki J, Kondo M, Sakai N, Nakata J, Takemura H, Nagai A, Takizawa T, Konno K. Leukotriene antagonist prevents exacerbation of asthma during reduction of high-dose inhaled corticosteroid. The Tokyo Joshi-Idai Asthma Research Group. Am J Respir Crit Care Med 1997; 155:1235.

32. Haahtela T, Jarvinen M, Kava T, Kiviranta K, Koskinen S, Lehtonen K, Nikander K, Persson T, Selroos O, Sovijarvi A, et al. Effects of reducing or discontinuing inhaled budesonide in patients with mild asthma. N Engl J Med 1994; 331:700.

33. Agertoft L, Pedersen S. Effects of long-term treatment with an inhaled corticosteroid on growth and pulmonary function in asthmatic children. Respir Med 1994; 88:373.

34. Selroos O, Pietinalho A, Lofroos AB, Riska H. Effect of early vs. late intervention with inhaled corticosteroids in asthma. Chest 1995; 108:1228.

35. Overbeek SE, Kerstjens HA, Bogaard JM, Mulder PG, Postma DS. Is delayed introduction of inhaled corticosteroids harmful in patients with obstructive airways disease (asthma and COPD)? The Dutch CNSLD Study Group. Chest 1996; 110:35.

36. Olivieri D, Chetta A, Del Donno M, Bertorelli G, Casalini A, Pesci A, Testi R, Foresi A. Effect of short-term treatment with low-dose inhaled fluticasone propionate on airway inflammation and remodeling in mild asthma: A placebo-controlled study. Am J Respir Crit Care Med 1997; 155:1864.

37. Laitinen A, Altraja A, Kampe M, Linden M, Virtanen I, Laitinen LA. Tenascin is increased in airway basement membrane of asthmatics and decreased by an inhaled steroid. Am J Respir Crit Care Med 1997; 156:951.

38. Kawabori I, Pierson WE, Conquest LL, Bierman CW. Incidence of exercise-induced asthma in children. J Allergy Clin Immunol 1976; 58:447.

39. Kikawa Y, Miyanomae T, Inoue Y, Saito M, Nakai A, Shigematsu Y, Hosoi S, Sudo M. Urinary leukotriene E4 after exercise challenge in children with asthma. J Allergy Clin Immunol 1992; 89:1111.

40. Robuschi M, Riva E, Fuccella LM, Vida E, Barnabe R, Rossi M, Gambaro G, Spagnotto S, Bianco S. Prevention of exercise-induced bronchoconstriction by a new leukotriene antagonist (SK&F 104353). A double-blind study versus disodium cromoglycate and placebo. Am Rev Respir Dis 1992; 145:1285.

41. Kukhta AL, Bratton DL, Chan KH, Wood RP, Langmack EL, Westcott JW, Wenzel SE, Liu AH. Leukotriene pathway modifiers: Are they the newest line of therapy for chronic sinusitis?: Case reports. J Allergy Clin Immunol 1998; 101:S252A.

42. Spector S, Tan RA. Antileukotrienes in chronic urticaria [letter]. J Allergy Clin Immunol 1998; 101:572.

ECP and Other Markers of Inflammation

Kai-Håkon Carlsen*

Keywords: Asthma, inflammation markers, children, ECP, EPX, NO in exhaled air, ICAM-1

Inflammation can be characterized by measuring inflammatory products in serum, urine, and in secretions from different locations of the respiratory tract. These products of the inflammatory processes may indicate different cells participating in the process and different stages of the inflammatory process. Some of these products are common to several types of inflammation, others may be specific to the cell type that is the source of the product; and some may characterize the inflammatory phase in which the inflammatory products are produced or released. The inflammatory processes occur locally in the respiratory tract, and the availability of the different factors in blood may differ.

Inflammation markers may indicate early unspecific stages of airway inflammation, such as the soluble adhesion molecule s-ICAM-1. Increased levels of such inflammatory products are not specific to asthma, but also occur in other inflammatory processes such as chronic lung disease of newborns.

Eosinophil inflammation products such as eosinophil cationic protein (ECP) and eosinophil protein-X (EPX) are among the markers most thoroughly studied. It has been found that increased serum resp. urinary levels of these proteins are present in active asthma, and that they are reduced by antiinflammatory treatment such as inhaled steroids. They may also be increased in other atopic conditions such as atopic dermatitis. As a diagnostic tool, inflammation markers have thus far not been optimal, with estimated positive likelihood ratios values of 2–4.

Measurement of nitric oxide (NO) in exhaled air as a marker of airway inflammation specific to asthma has created much interest. Further clarification is needed.

Airway inflammation is presently considered to be the most important characteristic of bronchial asthma, with several different cells being involved, among which the eosinophil is the most important. As wheezing may have several different causes (and the prognosis of early wheezers probably differs according to cause(s) [1]), it is conceivable that airway inflammatory processes may differ according to cause. Thus, the inflammatory processes in early childhood wheezing may differ from those of bronchial asthma in later childhood, which have been much better studied.

A richer understanding of airway inflammatory processes, especially in asthma, has been obtained recently, and this process continues through ongoing intensive research. Inflammation can be characterized by measuring inflammatory products in serum, urine, and secretions from different locations of the respiratory tract. These products of the inflammatory processes may indicate the different cells participating in the process and different stages of the inflammatory process. Some of these products are common to several types of inflammation, whereas others may be specific to the cell type that is the source of the product. Some may characterize the inflammatory phase in which the inflammatory products are produced or released. The inflammatory processes occur locally in the respiratory tract, and the availability of the different factors in the blood may differ. Under some circumstances, living cells must be obtained for stimulation in cell cultures to obtain measurable levels.

Different cells release different mediator substances upon stimulation. Some of the mediator substances are virtually specific to cells of origin, others may be released from several different cells. Examples are histamine and tryptase from the mast cell and the basophil granulocyte, eosinophil cationic protein (ECP), eosinophil protein X (EPX) (also called eosinophil-derived neurotoxin [EDN]) and major basic protein (MBP) from eosinophil cells, myeloperoxidase (MPO), and human neutrophil lipokalin (HNL) from neutrophil granulocytes, and leukotrienes, especially leukotriene C$_4$ (LTC$_4$) from several different cell types. Ideally, it should be possible to characterize the inflammatory processes with regard to the activity of the participating cells.

It is also possible to analyze other inflammatory

*   Voksentoppen Children's Center and Research Institute of Asthma and Allergy, Oslo, Norway

products, being active during early phases of inflammation. This accounts for interleukins, IL-4 representing mainly the Th2 cell line, INF-γ (mainly from Th1 cells), and IL-6 and IL-8 representing general inflammatory activity. It has been difficult, though not impossible, to measure the interleukins in serum [2]; but these cytokines have mostly been measured after stimulation of cell cultures. Furthermore, it has become possible to measure other soluble inflammatory products including soluble adhesion molecules, s-ICAM-1 (soluble intercellular adhesion molecule 1 in serum). ICAM-1 is of particular interest because of its activity in the early stages of inflammation, but it has also been shown to be a major receptor of human rhino-virus [3], which has a special importance for virus-induced asthma and wheeze [4, 5].

ICAM-1

ICAM-1 is an adhesion molecule involved in the early stages of inflammation in the contact between antigen-presenting cells and T cells. Soluble ICAM-1 in serum has been measured in different respiratory disorders and may be looked upon as an unspecific marker of inflammatory activity. This adhesion molecule is of special interest to early childhood asthma, as ICAM-1 has been identified as the major human receptor for rhinoviruses [3]. Under experimental conditions, transformed bronchial epithelial cells did not increase the expression of ICAM-1 during infection with rhinovirus 14, but the production of the cytokines IL-6, IL-8 and GM-CSF did increase. By adding ICAM-1 antibodies to the cell cultures, one could prevent the increase in cytokines [6]. Furthermore, increased expression of ICAM-1 was demonstrated both on circulating T-cell subsets in asthmatics with dual response to allergen [7] and on respiratory epithelial cells in asthmatics [8]. Serum ICAM-1 was reported to be increased in atopic asthma patients [9] compared to nonatopic. Ceyhan and coworkers, on the other hand, found neither increased levels of serum ICAM-1 in asthma patients nor correlations to symptom severity, lung function, and bronchial responsiveness [10].

In premature infants with respiratory distress syndrome, elevated plasma levels of soluble ICAM-1 was found at 14 days of age in those infants developing chronic lung disease and correlated to duration of intermittent positive pressure ventilation [11]. Thus, s-ICAM-1 may be an unspecific inflammatory marker. However, it may be useful as a marker of early inflammation in different inflammatory conditions in the respiratory tract.

Interleukin-4 and Interferon-γ

IL-4 stimulates B-cell differentiation into IgE producing cells. IL-4 and interferon-γ (IFN-γ) have opposite roles in this aspect. Phytohaemagglutinin-stimulated cell cultures of mononuclear cells from peripheral blood produced significantly more IL-4 and less IFN-γ when taken from atopic asthmatic children compared to nonatopic asthmatic children and nonatopic control children [12]. IL-4 and IFN-γ are difficult to detect in sera, but they have been studied in relation to possible predictive value. Borres and coworkers followed 64 infants from birth to 18 months of age. Children who had developed atopic disease (asthma, atopic dermatitis, urticaria, allergic rhinoconjunctivitis) at 18 months of age had increased IL-4 at 3, 6, 9, and 18 months of age compared to nonatopic children, whereas IFN-γ did not differ. IFN-γ was detected in only 49 of 196 serum samples in these children [2].

Daher and coworkers reported IL-4 to be significantly higher both in wheezy babies and in atopic asthmatic children between 7 and 14 years of age compared to controls [13].

Leukotrienes (LT)

Cysteinyl leukotrienes (C_4, D_4, and E_4) are generated from arachidonic acid, a constituent of cell membrane phospholipids. Leukotrienes are powerful mediators released from a number of cells including eosinophils, neutrophils and mast cells [14]. Cysteinyl leukotrienes have been found to be low or undetectable in plasma [15], whereas LTB_4 may be analyzed in plasma. In children 5–10 years old, Sampson et al. [15] reported that LTE_4 urinary levels and plasma levels of LTB_4 were higher during acute exacerbation of asthma and one month later compared to levels in healthy children. Balfour-Lynn and coworkers [16] did not find increased levels of urinary LTE_4 during acute wheezing or after a symptom-free period of at least one week. The LTE_4 levels did not differ between RS-virus-positive and RS-virus-negative infants. The same group also reported increased levels of tumor necrosis factor-α (TNF-α) in nasal washings during acute episodes of wheeze compared to the recovery period, and in higher concentrations during RS virus infections [16]. TNF-α was not detected in serum from infants with TNF-α in their nasal secretions [16]. Previously, Volovitz and coworkers [17, 18] reported increased levels of LTC$_4$ as well as of the other leukotrienes in nasal fluid during respiratory syncytial virus infections. The cytokine TNF-α may thus stimulate cells to release leukotrienes locally in the respiratory tract during respiratory syncytial virus infections. The possible long-term implications of these findings are not known.

Tryptase

Tryptase was found in mucosal bronchial biopsies in subjects with mild to moderate asthma, and was proposed to be important for the remodelling of the airways due to the inflammatory processes [19]. Tryptase was recovered from serum during acute anaphylaxis and acute bronchial allergen provocation. However, it failed to be detected using inhaled steroids in any atopic children with moderate to severe asthma who were symptom-free for the last 3 weeks, in children with mild asthma with sporadic symptoms using only inhaled β_2-agonists, in children with acute asthma attacks being admitted to the hospital, in children with mild to moderate atopic dermatitis, and in healthy control children [20]. Hedlin and co-workers [21] could not detect tryptase in sera from cat allergic children before or during bronchial challenge. Even with the development of more sensitive methods for tryptase measurements, serum tryptase levels were not increased above reference levels in symptomatic asthmatic children between 5 and 10 years of age [22]. This suggests that serum levels of tryptase will not be useful in monitoring the chronic inflammatory processes involving mast cells and basophil cells.

Myeloperoxidase

Myelioperoxidase (MPO) is a granule protein from neutrophil leukocytes which is also found to a lesser extent in monocytes. It has been found to be a good marker of neutrophil activity in blood and other tissue fluid [23]. Kristjánsson et al. [20] found increased levels of s-MPO in symptom-free asthmatic children without antiinflammatory therapy during acute asthma. Pedersen and coworkers [24] found that s-MPO decreased during treatment with inhaled steroids in adult asthmatics. Elevated levels of s-MPO are not specific to airway inflammation from asthma, but are also found in other chronic lung disorders [25]; thus it represents an unspecific marker of airway inflammation.

In infants with acute bronchiolitis from respiratory syncytial virus, Sigurs et al. [26] found significantly higher levels of s-MPO during the acute infection than one month later, but s-MPO levels could not predict later development of asthma.

In young children less than 2 years of age with early recurrent wheezing, in contrast to s-ECP, s-MPO did not differ between wheezy subjects and control subjects [27]. No correlation was found between s-MPO and lung function or between s-MPO and the change in lung function after salbutamol inhalation [27].

No reference values of s-MPO have been published in young children. In a recent study in Oslo, s-MPO correlated to s-ECP in young healthy children without respiratory disease [24]. Significantly higher levels of s-MPO were found in healthy infants below 12 months of age than in children 12–23 months of age and children 24–41 months old. When employing inflammation markers in children of different ages, it is important to have access to age-specific reference values.

Neutrophils also release other granule proteins. Among these human neutrophil lipokalin (HNL) seems to be a specific marker of the neutrophil cell which is able to discriminate between acute viral and bacterial infections [23]. Little is known about this protein with respect to asthma in children.

Eosinophil Markers

The eosinophil cell is a key cell in the inflammatory orchestra of asthma [28]. Several markers of eosinophil inflammation have been studied with respect to bronchial asthma, but there are few studies on infants and young children. Several eosinophil mediators have been assessed regarding their possible relationship to asthma symptoms, lung function, and bronchial responsiveness. Eosinophil cationic protein (ECP), eosinophil protein X (EPX) (also called eosinophil-derived neurotoxin [EDN]), eosinophil peroxidase (EPO), and major basic protein (MBP) have been studied. ECP and EPO are considered to be unique eosinophil proteins, whereas small amounts of EPX are found in neutrophils and MBP in basophils [23].

ECP in particular has been studied extensively in children with asthma [20, 22, 29–31]. The results are somewhat conflicting, but these discrepancies may be explained by the different designs used in the studies reported and different patient characteristics. Inhaled steroids in particular influence s-ECP levels. Zimmerman and co-workers [29] reported that s-ECP varied with asthma symptoms. Ferguson et al. [32] could not support this, but in their study 14 out of 24 children with active asthma symptoms received inhaled steroids, whereas none of the nonsymptomatic children received inhaled steroids. On the other hand, Koller and coworkers [30] found that s-ECP levels varied with symptom activity, regardless of the use of inhaled steroids. Kristjánsson and coworkers found significantly increased s-ECP levels in children with acute asthma. They also found increased s-ECP levels in asymptomatic asthmatic children without inhaled steroid treatment compared to the asymptomatic children with inhaled steroids [20]. We recently reported [33] that s-ECP had a moderate effect in discriminating between active asthma and nonsymptomatic asthma by calculating positive and negative likelihood ratios for s-ECP at levels above and below 20 µg/l. These observations suggest that s-ECP may contribute to the assessment of disease control obtained by implemented therapeutic measures, also as regards antiinflammatory treatment. This is supported by the findings in a study from Oslo [33] in which s-ECP levels were higher in asthmatic children with chronic persistent asthma symptoms compared to occasional symptoms and to asymptomatic children – regardless of therapy. Thus, even if significant differences were found between the different asthma groups, the calculation of positive and negative likelihood ratios demonstrated a certain informative value by s-ECP, even though s-ECP could not discriminate between single patients in the different symptom groups. In this study, also the activity of atopic eczema was found to influence the s-ECP level.

Nasal ECP levels have been studied in infants during acute bronchiolitis. In two studies Garofolo et al. [34, 35] reported that nasal ECP albumin ratios were significantly higher during acute RS virus bronchiolitis than during pneumonia or upper respiratory tract infections or in healthy infants. On the other hand, Sigurs and coworkers [26] found nasal ECP albumen ratios to be lower during acute RS virus bronchiolitis compared to one month later. Furthermore, nasal ECP albumin ratio or s-ECP during the acute infection did not predict which children would later develop asthma.

The findings by Garofolo et al. [31] are supported by Ingram and coworkers [31], who found marked elevated ECP levels in nasal washes in 9 of 22 wheezing children below 2 years of age and in only 1 of 17 control subjects; s-ECP levels did not differ, however. Thus, in the majority of studies, wheezing illness during infancy and the first 2 years of life is characterized by raised ECP levels in the respiratory tract. In early recurrent wheezing in children below 2 years of age, Lødrup Carlsen et al. [27] reported higher s-ECP levels in patients compared to healthy control subjects. Also a close correlation was found between s-ECP and the reversibility of lung function (tidal breathing) in response to salbutamol inhalation, thus suggesting a possible predictive value of s-ECP in these young children. It is also of interest that a dose relationship was found between maternal smoking and s-ECP levels in healthy infants and children below 2 years of age [24]. Zimmerman et al. [36] reported higher s-ECP levels in atopic than in nonatopic children below the age of 5 years (mean age 1.8 years) with asthma and without previous treatment with inhaled steroids. Furthermore, they found that s-ECP decreased after starting treatment with inhaled steroids.

Eosinophil protein X (EPX) has been evaluated both in the serum and urine of asthmatic children. Rao and coworkers [22] recently reported a close correlation to s-ECP in symptomatic asthmatic children 5 to 10 years old, and a low but significant correlation between s-EPX and lung function, and between s-EPX and bronchial responsiveness [22].

Zimmerman et al. [36], from their study in preschool children with asthma, reported that s-EPX levels were higher in symptomatic than asymptomatic asthmatic atopic children, and higher in atopic children than in nonatopic.

Clough [37] reported a study of children below 3 years of age, who had been recruited within 12 weeks of their first episode of wheeze and who were followed up for 12 months. Children above 1 year of age who continued to wheeze had significantly higher s-EPX levels than those who became asymptomatic. s-EPX levels of the asymptomatic children and those less than 1 year of age at recruitment did not differ from that of control subjects [37].

Few studies have so far been published on urinary EPX (u-EPX) levels in asthmatic children. Kristjánsson and coworkers [38] reported higher u-EPX levels, higher s-EPX levels, and higher s-ECP levels in children 8 to 16 years old with atopic asthma who had not treated with inhaled steroids compared to control children. After 3 months' treatment with inhaled budesonide, u-EPX and s-ECP – but not s-EPX – decreased significantly. This corresponded to a significant increase in PEF over the 3 months. This study suggests that s-ECP and u-EPX may be used in the assessment of airway inflammation in atopic asthma in children, and for monitoring inflammatory activity. The benefit of u-EPX over the other inflammatory markers is the lack of need for blood sampling. This is particularly useful in infants and young children. However, little is known regarding the usefulness of u-EPX in infants and young children.

Nitric Oxide in Exhaled Air

Nitric oxide (NO) is produced by a number of cells in the respiratory tract, and increased concentrations of NO have been reported in exhaled air from asthmatic patients compared to healthy individuals [39]. Furthermore, a decrease in the concentration of exhaled NO was observed in asthmatic patients after starting treatment with inhaled steroids [40]. It was demonstrated by sampling through a fiberoptic bronchoscope that exhaled NO is mainly derived from the lower respiratory tract [41]. Data from infants and young children are thus far lacking, because of sampling difficulties. However, weight is put upon the need to standardize the sampling of NO also in young children. With the development of suitable sampling techniques, the measurement of exhaled NO may possibly give important information regarding early stages of airway inflammation in young children. Some data may indicate that the diagnostic value of exhaled NO in the absence of inhaled steroids is greater that the usefulness in monitoring treatment effect.

Address for correspondence:

Prof. Kai-Håkon Carlsen
Voksentoppen Children's Center and
Research Institute of Asthma and Allergy
Ullveien 14
N-0791 Oslo
Norway
Tel. +47 22 136500
Fax +47 22 136505
E-mail kaic@usit-div.uio.no

References

1. Martinez FD, Wright AL, Taussig LM, Holberg CJ, Halonen M, Morgan WJ. The Group of Health Medical Associates. Asthma and wheezing in the first six years of life. N Engl J Med 1995; 332(3):133–138.

2. Borres MP, Einarsson R, Björkstén B. Serum levels of interleukin-4, soluble CD23 and INF-γ in relation to the development of allergic disease during the first 18 months of life. Clin Exp Allergy 1995; 25:543–548.

3. Greve JM, Davis G, Meyer AM, Forte CP, Yost SC, Marlor CW, Kamarck ME, McClelland A. The major human rhinovirus receptor is ICAM-1. Cell 1989; 56:839–847.

4. Carlsen KH, Ørstavik I, Leegaard J, Høeg H. Respiratory virus infections and aeroallergens in acute bronchial asthma. Arch Dis Child 1984; 59:310–315.

5. Johnston SL, Pattemore PK, Sanderson G, Smith S, Lampe F, Josephs L, Symington P, O'Toole S, Myint SH, Tyrrell DAJ, et al. Community study of viral infections in exacerbations of asthma in 9–11 year old children. BMJ 1995; 310(6989):1225–1229.

6. Subauste MC, Jacoby DB, Richards SM, Proud D. Infection of a human respiratory epithelial cell line with rhinovirus. Induction of cytokine release and modulation of susceptibility to infection by cytokine exposure. J Clin Invest 1995; 96(1):549–557.

7. De Rose V, Rolla G, Bucca C, Ghio P, Bertoletti M, Baderna P, Pozzi E. Intercellular adhesion molecule-1 is upregulated on peripheral blood T lymphocyte subsets in dual asthmatic responders. J Clin Invest 1994; 94(5):1840–1845.

8. Manolitsas ND, Trigg CJ, McAulay AE, Wang JH, Jordan SE, D'Ardenne AJ, Davies RJ. The expression of intercellular adhesion molecule-1 and the beta 1-integrins in asthma. Eur Respir J 1994; 7(8):1439–1444.

9. Shiota Y, Wilson JG, Marukawa M, Ono T, Kaji M. Soluble intercellular adhesion molecule 1 (ICAM-1)

antigen in sera of bronchial asthmatics. Chest 1996; 109(1):94–99.

10. Ceyhan BB, Sungur M, Celikel T, Ozgun SS. Role of the adhesion molecule ICAM-1 in asthma. J Asthma 1995; 32(6):419–427.

11. Little S, Dean T, Bevin S, Hall M, Ashton M, Church M, Warner JO, Shute J. Role of elevated plasma soluble ICAM-1 and bronchial lavage fluid IL-8 levels as markers of chronic disease in premature infants. Thorax 1995; 50:1073–1079.

12. Tang ML, Coleman J, Kemp AS. Interleukin-4 and interferon-gamma production in atopic and non-atopic children with asthma. Clin Exp Allergy 1995; 25(6):515–521.

13. Daher S, Santos LM, Sole D, De Lima MG, Naspitz CK, Musatti CC. Interleukin-4 and soluble CD23 serum levels in asthmatic atopic children. J Invest Allergol Clin Immunol 1995; 5(5):251–254.

14. Chung KF. Leukotriene receptor antagonists and biosynthesis inhibitors: Potential breakthrough in asthma therapy. Eur Respir J 1995; 8(7):1203–1213.

15. Sampson AP, Castling DP, Green CP, Price JF. Persistent increase in plasma and urinary leukotrienes after acute asthma. Arch Dis Child 1995; 73(3):221–225.

16. Balfour-Lynn I, Valman HB, Wellings R, Webster ADB, Taylor GW, Silverman M. Tumour necrosis factor-α and leukotriene E4 production in wheezy infants. Clin Exp Allergy 1994; 24:121–126.

17. Volovitz B, Welliver RC, De Castro G, Krystofik DA, Ogra PL. The release of leukotrienes in the respiratory tract during infection with respiratory syncytial virus: Role in obstructive airways disease. Pediatr Res 1988; 24:504–507.

18. Volovitz B, Faden H, Ogra PL. Release of leukotriene C4 in respiratory tract during acute viral infection. J Pediatr 1988; 112:218–222.

19. Djukanovic R, Roche WR, Eilson JW, Beasly CRW, Twentyman OP, Howard PH, Holgate ST. Mucosal inflammation in asthma. State of the art. Am Rev Respir Dis 1990; 142:434–457.

20. Kristjánsson S, Shimizu T, Strannegård IL, Wennergren G. Eosinophil cationic protein, myeloperoxidase and tryptase in children with asthma and atopic dermatitis. Pediatr Allergy Immunol 1994; 5(4):223–229.

21. Hedlin G, Ahlstedt S, Enander I, Håkansson L, Venge P. Eosinophil cationic protein (ECP), eosinophil chemotactic activity (ECA), neutrophil chemotactic activity (NCA) and tryptase in serum before and during bronchial challenge in cat-allergic children with asthma. Pediatr Allergy Immunol 1992; 3:144–149.

22. Rao R, Frederick JM, Enander I, Gregson RK, Warner JA, Warner JO. Airway function correlates with circulating eosinophil, but not mast cell, markers of inflammation in childhood asthma. Clin Exp Allergy 1996; 26:789–793.

23. Venge P. The monitoring of inflammation by specific cellular markers. Scand J Clin Lab Invest Suppl 1994; 219:47–54.

24. Lødrup Carlsen KC, Halvorsen R, Carlsen KH. Serum inflammatory markers and effects of age and tobacco smoke exposure in young non-asthmatic children. Acta Paediatr 1998; 87:559–564.

25. Pettersen M, Norseth J, Carlsen KH. Eosinophil cationic protein (ECP) in allergic asthma, non-allergic asthma and other chronic lung diseases (CLD). Allergy 1993; 48:90S

26. Sigurs N, Bjarnason R, Sigurbergsson F. Eosinophil cationic protein in nasal secretion and in serum and myeloperoxidase in serum in respiratory syncytial virus bronchiolitis: Relation to asthma and atopy. Acta Paediatr 1994; 83(11):1151–1155.

27. Lødrup Carlsen KC, Halvorsen R, Ahlstedt S, Carlsen KH. Eosinophil cationic protein and tidal volume loops in children 0–2 years of age. Eur Respir J 1995; 8(7):1148–1154.

28. Bousquet J, Chanez P, Lacoste JY, Barnéon G, Ghavanian N, Enander I, Venge P, Ahlstedt S, Simony-Lafontaine J, Godard P, et al. Eosinophilic inflammation in asthma. N Engl J Med 1990; 323:1033–1039.

29. Zimmerman B, Lanner A, Enander I, Zimmerman RS, Peterson CGB, Ahlstedt S. Total blood eosinophils, serum eosinophil cationic protein and eosinophil protein X in childhood asthma: Relation to disease status and therapy. Clin Exp Allergy 1993; 23:564–570.

30. Koller DY, Herouy Y, Götz M, Hagel E, Urbanek R, Eichler I. Clinical value of monitoring eosinophil activity in asthma. Arch Dis Child 1995; 73(5):413–417.

31. Ingram JM, Rakes GP, Hoover GE, Platts-Mills TA, Heymann PW. Eosinophil cationic protein in serum and nasal washes from wheezing infants and children. J Pediatr 1995; 127(4):558–564.

32. Ferguson AC, Vaughan R, Brown H, Curtis C. Evaluation of serum eosinophilic cationic protein as a marker of disease activity in chronic asthma. J Allergy Clin Immunol 1995; 95(1 Pt 1):23–28.

33. Carlsen KH, Halvorsen R, Pettersen M, Carlsen KC. Inflammation markers and symptom activity in children with bronchial asthma. Influence of atopy and eczema. Pediatr Allergy Immunol 1997; 8(3):112–120.

34. Garofalo R, Kimpen JL, Welliver RC, Ogra PL. Eosinophil degranulation in the respiratory tract during naturally acquired respiratory syncytial virus infection. J Pediatr 1992; 120(1):28–32.

35. Garofalo R, Dorris A, Ahlstedt S, Welliver RC. Peripheral blood eosinophil counts and eosinophil cationic protein content of respiratory secretions in bronchiolitis: Relationship to severity of disease. Pediatr Allergy Immunol 1994; 5(2):111–117.

36. Zimmerman B, Enander I, Zimmerman R, Ahlstedt S. Asthma in children less than 5 years of age: eosinophils and serum levels of the eosinophil proteins ECP and EPX in relation to atopy and symptoms. Clin Exp Allergy 1994; 24(2):149–155.

37. Clough JB, Basomba A, Sastre J (Eds). Proceedings I. XVI European Congress of allergology and clinical immunology (ECACI '95). Bologna: Monduzzi Editore, 1995. Markers of atopy and asthma in infancy and early childhood, pp. 491–494.

38. Kristjánsson S, Strannegård IL, Strannegård Ö, Peterson C, Enander I, Wennergren G. Urinary eosinophil protein X in children with atopic asthma: A useful marker of antiinflammatory treatment. J Allergy Clin Immunol 1996; 97:1179–1187.

39. Alving K, Weitzberg E, Lundberg JM. Increased amounts of nitric oxide in exhaled air of asthmatics. Eur Respir J 1993; 6:1268–1270.

40. Kharitonov SA, Yates DH, Barnes PJ. Inhaled glucocorticoids decrease nitric oxide in exhaled air of asthmatic patients. Am J Respir Crit Care Med 1996; 153(1):454–457.

41. Kharitonov SA, Chung KF, Evans D, O'Connor BJ, Barnes PJ. Increased exhaled nitric oxide in asthma is mainly derived from the lower respiratory tract. Am J Respir Crit Care Med 1996; 153(6 Pt 1):1773–1780.

Orally Exhaled Nitric Oxide Levels as a Marker of Airway Inflammation in Childhood Asthma

Daniela Spallarossa*, Michela Silvestri*, Elena Battistini*, Ida L Macciò*, Bruno Fregonese*, Maurizio Biraghi**, Giovanni A Rossi*

Keywords: Nitric oxide, childhood, allergic asthma

Because nitric oxide (NO) release may be induced in bronchial epithelium by proinflammatory cytokines, it has been hypothesized that it may reflect the intensity of the inflammatory component of airway diseases. Indeed, increased NO levels in the expired air (e-NO) are present in asthma, and preliminary results suggest that this non-invasive test may be clinically useful in the management of patients with this disorder. Yet, questions have been raised concerning the technical aspects of e-NO measurement and concerning the real biological and clinical meaning of these bioactive species in exhaled air.

Nitric oxide (NO) is a mediator of vasodilation and bronchodilatation. It is synthesized from L-arginine by the class of enzymes known as nitric oxide synthases (NOS) [1–2]. In the respiratory tract, NO is produced endogenously by several types of pulmonary cells, including airway epithelial and endothelial cells and inflammatory cells [3, 4]. Since *in vitro* NO synthase may be induced in bronchial epithelium by proinflammatory cytokines, it has been hypothesized that NO may be relevant to the pathogenesis of inflammatory airway diseases [4, 5].

In the last 5 years, several reports have demonstrated that NO can be recovered in expired air from normal subjects, and that increased levels are present in the expired air of patients with asthma [4, 6–9]. Exhaled NO (e-NO) production may indeed reflect cytokine-mediated inflammation, since its levels are increased during the late-phase reaction that follows allergen inhalation challenge [10]. In addition, consistent with the observation that corticosteroids inhibit the expression of inducible (i)NOS in epithelial cell cultures [4], it has been shown that inhaled steroids are extremely effective in controlling not only airway inflammation and in improving airway obstruction, but also in reducing NO concentrations in exhaled air [9–11]. These results suggest that NO may be a surrogate marker of airway inflammation, and that measurement of e-NO concentrations may be clinically useful in the detection and management of inflammatory lung disorders, such as bronchial asthma [8, 9, 12] – also in the pediatric population [13]. Following the first enthusiastic reports, subsequent studies, however, have raised questions concerning the technical aspects of e-NO measurement [14] and concerning the real biological and clinical meanings of these bioactive species in exhaled air.

Sources of NO in the Airways

In humans, the relative contribution of the different cellular sources to NO levels in exhaled air remains uncertain. NO is formed by at least three isoforms of NOS, including two constitutive forms (i. e., endothelial NOS (eNOS), or type III NOS, and neuronal NOS (nNOS) or type I NOS) and one inducible form (iNOS or type II NOS) [1–3]. The two constitutive isoforms, eNOS and nNOS, are basally expressed in many cells in the airways of normal individuals, including airway epithelium, and may account for the low NO levels measured in exhaled air [3]. In contrast, a variety of observations suggest that exhaled NO in asthma is likely to be derived mainly from iNOS, rather than from constitutive NOS expression. Indeed, iNOS is rapidly induced by proinflammatory cytokines in a variety of cells, including macrophages and airway epithelial cells [8]. In addition, immunohistochemical studies of bronchial biopsies have demonstrated increased iNOS expression in asthmatic patients, as

---

* Divisione di Pneumologia, Istituto G. Gaslini, Genova, Italy
** Valeas Industria Chimica e Farmaceutica, Italy

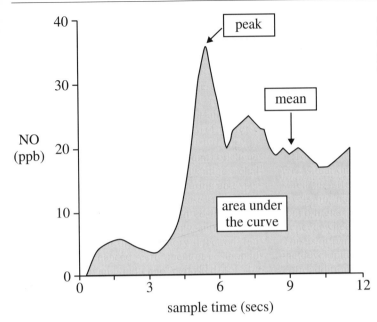

Figure 1. Representative print out of e-NO evaluation in an asthmatic child. The levels of e-NO are expressed on the ordinate and time on the abscissa.

compared to normals [4]. Although we do not know the pathways that link together the inflammatory events characterizing asthma and NO production in the airways, it has been clearly demonstrated that inhalation of aminoguanidine, a selective iNOS inhibitor, decreases exhaled NO in asthmatic subjects, but not in normals [15]. In humans, high concentrations of NO are produced in the upper airways [16, 17], which may contribute to NO in exhaled air in normal and asthmatic individuals if no closure of the soft palate is achieved [18, 19]. However, NO is also derived from the lower respiratory tract, and it can be measured in intubated patients via direct bronchoscopic sampling [20].

Measuring e-NO and Analyzing Data in Children

Quantitative comparisons of e-NO in adults in various studies have been complicated by different experimental setups. Indeed, NO has been measured in mixed inhaled air [6], or by using single breath analyses either during slow vital capacity manoeuvres [5, 7] or during exhalation after breathholding [21].

Measuring e-NO with chemiluminescence analyzers, adapted for online recording of NO concentration, obviates the need for collection in a reservoir, with its variable loss of reactive NO [14]. With these instruments, subjects are asked to perform a slow vital capacity maneuver over 15–20 seconds into wide-bore teflon tubing [5, 6, 11, 22]. NO is sampled continuously at a rate of approximately 50–100 mL/minute with the patient blowing against a positive pressure of 6–8 cm H_2O (exhaled NO-obstructed). This maneuver results in increased oropharyngeal pressure and closure of the soft palate, thereby diminishing the nasal NO component [11].

Different measurement techniques have also been used in pediatric studies, and most authors produced results similar to those described in adults [13, 22–27]. However, while some studies showed correlations between exhaled air NO levels and patient height [24], no relations have been described with body mass index [22] or lung volume and flow [27]. As in adults, in pediatric populations nasal-derived NO may also contribute to NO in exhaled air, if no closure of the soft palate is achieved, thereby producing false-positive results [18, 28]. However, a mixture of nasal and oral NO is unlikely to account for more than a minor component of e-NO when the child is able to perform a slow expiratory maneuver against a resistance [14, 27].

With regard to data analysis, it has been suggested that *"area under the curve," "peak NO levels,"* and *"plateau levels"* can be used, as long as the same analysis is performed in all subjects (Figure 1) [29]. In agreement with the recent recommendation published in the *European Respiratory Journal*, we feel that – at least in pediatric patients – *plateau level* is preferable because the *peak level* is at least partially contaminated by nasal NO and the *area under the curve* measure may be different when the maneuver is terminated prematurely [14, 30].

E-NO, Airway Inflammation, and Bronchial Hyperreactivity

There is convincing evidence that bronchial inflammation is present even in mild asthma, and that mediators released by inflammatory cells may induce acute damage and a progressive loss of respiratory function, even in asymptomatic patients [31–34]. Therefore, since control of airway inflammation is an important therapeutic goal, treatment with inhaled antiinflammatory drugs should be started as early as possible [32]. Since over two-thirds of all patients with asthma have a mild form of the disease, determining the appropriate circumstances for starting antiinflammatory treatment is an issue of major importance, particularly in the pediatric population [27, 32].

In contrast to e-NO levels measurements, which is a noninvasive, simple, and well-tolerated test, induced sputum and bronchoalveolar lavage cannot be performed easily on a routine basis to assess and gauge the intensity of airway inflammation, even in adult patients [14]. e-NO production may indeed reflect cytokine-mediated inflammation in asthma, for three reasons:

1. It is increased during the late phase reaction that follows natural exposure to allergens or experimental allergen-inhalation challenge [10].
2. It correlates with parameters of "inflammation" [27].
3. It is effectively inhibited by treatment with inhaled glucocorticosteroids [9–11] (Figure 2).

In addition to airway inflammation, bronchial hyperresponsiveness is recognized as a major characteristic of bronchial asthma [31–34]. Among methods able to quantify airway responsiveness, inhalation challenge test (more frequently with methacholine than with histamine) has become important in clinical practice, epidemiology, and research, even in the pediatric population [35]. However, these tests are time-consuming and require levels of collaboration not always possible in younger patients. The mechanisms underlying airway hyperresponsiveness and their causal relationships with airway inflammation remain unclear [34–36].

In an evaluation of children with mild to intermittent asthma, we were unable to show correlations between e-NO levels and (a) pulmonary function parameters [27], (b) degree of bronchial responsiveness to methacholine [37], and (c) intensity of methacholine-induced bronchoconstriction [37].

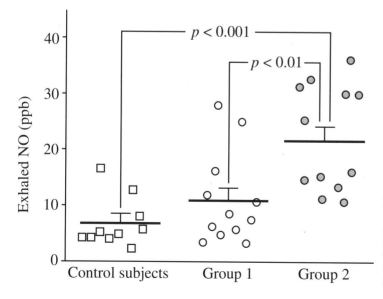

Figure 2. NO levels in orally exhaled air in control subjects and in asthmatic patients treated with inhaled glucocorticosteroids (Group 1) or with inhaled β_2-agonists on an as-necessary basis (Group 2). NO concentration is expressed on the ordinate, as parts per billion (ppb), and the different study groups on the abscissa.

Even if a causal relationship between airway inflammation and hyperresponsiveness is suggested by a variety of studies in allergic asthma [1, 32–34], this concept is questionable because frequent dissociation between airway inflammation and hyperresponsiveness in allergic asthma has been demonstrated [36, 38]. Our data are similar to those reported by Taylor et al., showing no correlations between e-NO levels and airway responsiveness to methacholine in mild asthmatics [39]; but they disagree with the results published by Dupont et al., who found significant correlations between e-NO levels and bronchial reactivity to histamine [40].

Conclusions

Measurement of e-NO levels in orally expired air represents a noninvasive test that would appear to be simple and well tolerated by the vast majority of school-age children. A number of recent observations suggest that this test accurately reflects airway inflammation in allergic children with asthma. Our results suggest that – at least in steroid-naive children with mild to intermittent asthma – e-NO measurements do not correlate with pulmonary function parameters and are poor predictors of the degree of airway responsiveness to methacholine. Further studies are required to determine whether the degree of airway inflammation, reflected by e-NO levels, may be useful for gauging the severity of the disease, for judging therapeutic need and the efficacy of anti-inflammatory treatment, i. e., to evaluate the real relevance of this test in clinical practice.

Acknowledgments

Supported by grants from Valeas S.p.A., Milan-Italy and by "Ricerca Corrente," Ministero della Pubblica Istruzione, Rome, Italy.

Address for correspondence:

Giovanni A Rossi
Divisione di Pneumologia
Istituto G. Gaslini
Largo G. Gaslini, 4
I-16148 Genoa
Italy
Tel. +39 010 563-6547/8
Fax +39 010 377-6590
E-mail giovannirossi@ospedale-gaslini.ge.it

References

1. Moncada S, Palmer RMJ, Higgs EA. Nitric oxide physiology, pathophysiology and pharmacology. Pharm Rev 1991; 43:109.

2. Nathan C, Xie Q-W. Nitric oxide synthase: Roles, tolls, and controls. Cell 1994; 78:915.

3. Kobzik L, Bredt DS, Lowenstein CJ, Drazen J, Gaston B, Sugarbaker D, Stamler JS. Nitric oxide synthase in human and rat lung: Immunocytochemical and histological localization. Am J Respir Cell Mol Biol 1993; 9:371.

4. Hamid Q, Springall DR, Riveros-Moreno V, Chanez P, Howarth P, Redington A, Bousquet J, Godard P, Holgate S, Polak J. Induction of nitric oxide synthase in asthma. Lancet 1993; 342:1510.

5. Kharitonov SA, Wells AU, O'Connor BJ, Cole PJ, Hansell DM, Logan-Sinclair RB, Barnes PJ. Elevated levels of exhaled nitric oxide in bronchiectasis. Am J Respir Crit Care Med 1995; 151:1889.

6. Alving K, Weitzbel E, Lundberg JM. Increased amount of nitric oxide in exhaled air of asthmatics. Eur Respir J 1993; 6:368.

7. Kharitonov SA, Yates D, Robbins RA, Logan-Sinclair R, Shinebourne EA, Barnes PJ. Increased nitric oxide in exhaled air of asthmatic patients. Lancet 1994; 343:133.

8. Barnes PJ, Liew FY. Nitric oxide and asthmatic inflammation. Immunol Today 1995; 16:128.

9. Kharitonov SA, Yates D, Barnes PJ. Inhaled glucocorticoids decrease nitric oxide in exhaled air of asthmatic patients. Am J Respir Crit Care Med 1996; 153:454.

10. Taylor DA, Lim S, Barnes PJ, O'Connor BJ. Exhaled nitric oxide production and increased airway responsiveness in asthma reflects different inflammatory pathways. Eur Respir J 1996; 9:416S.

11. Massaro A, Gaston B, Kita D, Fanta C, Stamler JS, Drazen JM. Expired nitric oxide levels during treatment of acute asthma. Am J Respir Crit Care Med 1995; 152:800.

12. Ten Hacken NHT, Meijer RJ, Kerstjens HAM, van der Mark ThW. Expired nitric oxide in stable asthmatic patients does not relate to parameters of disease severity. Eur Respir J 1996; 9:416S.

13. Dotsch J, Demirakça S, Terbrack HG, Huls G, Rascher G, Kuhl PG. Airway nitric oxide in asthmatic children and patients with cystic fibrosis. Eur Respir J 1996; 9:2537.

14. Kharitonov S, Alving K, Barnes PJ. Exhaled and nasal nitric oxide measurements: Recommendations. Eur Respir J 1997; 10:1683.

15. Yates DH, Kharitonov SA, Worsdell M, Thomas PS, Barnes PJ. Exhaled nitric oxide is decreased after inhalation of a specific inhibitor of inducible nitric

oxide synthase in asthmatic but not in normal subjects. Am J Respir Crit Care Med 1996; 154:247.

16. Zapol WM, Rimar S, Gillis N, Marletta M, Bosken CH. Nitric oxide and the lung. Am J Respir Crit Care Med 1994; 149:1375.

17. Scheding U, Frostell C, Persson MG, Jacobsson J, Andersson G, Gustafsson LE. Contribution from upper and lower airways to exhaled endogenous nitric oxide in humans. Acta Anaesth Scand 1995; 39:327.

18. Kimberly B, Nejadnik B, Giraud CD, Holden WE. Nasal contribution to exhaled nitric oxide at rest and during breathholding in humans. Am J Respir Crit Care Med 1996; 153:829.

19. Gerlach H, Rossaint R, Pappert D, Knorr M, Falke KJ. Autoinhalation of nitric oxide after endogenous synthesis in nasopharynx. Lancet 1994; 343:518.

20. Kharitonov SA, Chung KF, Evans D, O'Connor BJ, Barnes PJ. Increased exhaled nitric oxide in asthma is mainly derived from the lower respiratory tract. Am J Respir Crit Care Med 1996; 153:1773.

21. Persson MG, Viklund NP, Gustafsson LE. Endogenous nitric oxide in single exhalation and the change during exercise. Am Rev Respir Dis 1993;1 48:1210.

22. Artlich A, Hagenah JU, Jonas S, Ahrens P, Gortner L. Exhaled nitric oxide in childhood asthma. Eur J Pediatric 1996; 155:689.

23. Lundberg JM, Nordvall SL, Weitzbel E, Kolberg H, Alving K. Exhaled nitric oxide in pediatric asthma and cystic fibrosis. Arch Dis Child 1996; 75:323.

24. Guerrieri A, Persky V, Sceff P, Ramakrishnan V, Rubinstein I. Exhaled nitric oxide levels in children with mild asthma in inner city Chicago. Am J Respir Crit Care Med 1997; 155:A268.

25. Cailland M, Kaufman C, Fourot-Bauzan, Nguyen L, Bedu M, Dinh-Xuan AT. Exhaled nitric oxide in children with mild asthma. Am J Respir Crit Care Med 1997; 155:A824.

26. Baraldi E, Azzolin NM, Zanconato S, Dario C, Zacchello F. Corticosteroids decrease exhaled nitric oxide in children with acute asthma. J Pediatrics 1997; 131:381.

27. Silvestri M, Spallarossa D, Frangova Youroukova V, Battistini E, Fregonese B, Rossi GA. High proportion of atopic children with mild-intermittent asthma has increased orally exhaled nitric oxide levels which are related to the degree of blood eosinophilia. Eur Respir J 1999; 13:321.

28. Nelson BV, Sear S, Woods J, Ling CY, Hunt J, Clapper LM, Gaston B. Expired nitric oxide as a marker for childhood asthma. J Pediatrics 1997; 130:423.

29. Dinarevic S, Byrnes CA, Bush A, Shinebourne EA. Measurement of expired nitric oxide levels in children. Ped Pulmonol 1996; 22:396.

30. Spallarossa D, Silvestri M, Battistini E, Sacco O, Gianiorio P, Frangova Yourukova V, Fregonese B, Gianiorio P, Rossi GA. How should we evaluate nitric oxide (NO) levels in exhaled air in asthmatic children. Am J Respir Crit Care Med 1998; 157:A469.

31. Kay AB.Asthma and inflammation. J Allergy Clin Immunol 1991; 87:893.

32. Expert panel report 2. Guidelines for the diagnosis and management of asthma. January 1997; NIH publication no. 97-4051.

33. Oddera S, Silvestri M, Balbo A, Jovovich BO, Penna R, Crimi E, Rossi GA. Airway eosinophilic inflammation, epithelial damage and bronchial hyperresponsiveness in patients with mild-moderate stable asthma. Allergy 1996; 51:100.

34. Boushey HA, Holtzman MJ, Sheller JR, Nadel JA. Bronchial hyperactivity. Am Rev Respir Dis 1980; 121:389.

35. Galvez RA, McLaughlin FJ, Levison H. The role of the methacholine challenge in children with chronic cough. J Allergy Clin Immunol 1987; 79:331.

36. Crimi E, Spanevello A, Neri M, Ind PW, Rossi GA, Brusasco V. Dissociation between airway inflammation and airway hyperresponsiveness in allergic asthma. Am J Resp Crit Care Med 1998; 157:4.

37. Silvestri M, Spallarossa D, Battistini E, Brusasco V, Rossi GA. Dissociation between exhaled nitric oxide levels and airway responsiveness to methacholine in atopic children with mild-intermittent asthma. Am J Respir Crit Care Med 1999; 159:912A.

38. Haley KJ, Drazen JM. Inflammation and airway function. What you see is not what you get. Am J Resp Crit Care Med 1998; 157:1.

39. Taylor DA, Lim S, Barnes PJ, O'Connor BJ. Exhaled nitric oxide production and increased airway responsiveness in asthma reflects different inflammatory pathways. Eur Respir J 1996; 9:416S.

40. Dupont LJ, Rochette F, Demedts MG, Verleden GM. Exhaled nitric oxide correlates with airway hyperresponsiveness in steroid-naive patients with mild asthma. Am J Resp Crit Care Med 1998; 157:894.

Asthma in the Tropics: The Importance of Parasitic Infection

Neil R Lynch, Isabel Hagel, Maria C Di Prisco*

Keywords: Asthma, parasites, helminths, IgE, tropics

The characteristics of asthma and other allergic diseases in the tropics can differ from those in more temperate climates, and a major factor in determining this is parasitic infection. Helminthic parasites, which affect the vast majority of the world's population, have a dramatic effect on the IgE response, which can modulate the allergic reactivity of infected individuals. Such infections can result in increased allergic reactivity by two mechanisms: First, the specific IgE response against the parasite antigens can directly produce pulmonary dysfunction; second, helminthic infections induce "bystander" polyclonal activation of IgE synthesis, which in situations of mild infection can potentiate the IgE response against other environmental allergens. In contrast, inhibition of allergic reactivity can occur in situations of intense helminthic infection, as a very strong polyclonal stimulus can cause mast cell blockade and also result in a reduction of specific IgE responses.

The close association between helminthic infection and allergic reactivity has led to the suggestion that the principal activity of the IgE response lies in protecting against parasitic infection. Evidence has been obtained that indicates that persons with an atopic disposition have an increased resistance to helminths. This might have determined the evolutionary development of genes that favor an elevated IgE response, but it may have also resulted in a greater propensity toward allergic reactivity against intrinsically inoffensive environmental antigens. The control of parasitic infection by improvements in sanitary conditions could be an important contributory factor to the elevated prevalence of allergic diseases in industrialized countries.

In the tropical environment, asthma and other allergic diseases can present characteristics that differ from those commonly seen in more temperate climates. For example, in our experience over a period of 20 years in the allergy clinic of a large public hospital in Caracas, Venezuela, allergic reactivity to weed, grass, or tree pollens is relatively uncommon. This is probably because the major means of pollination in the tropics is insect-borne and not airborne. Although it might be expected that molds and the remnants of insect cuticles could be important allergens in the tropics, once again our experience has been that these are not necessarily of great significance on a population basis [1]. Without any doubt, the principal source of airborne allergens for our patients is house dust mite [2].

There is, however, a major factor that differentiates the allergic reactivity in the tropics from that in temperate climates – the occurrence of parasitic infections. Not only does the tropical climate favor the survival of parasite eggs, larvae, and cysts in the environment, but also the adverse socio-economic conditions of most tropical countries has impeded the eradication of these infections – resulting in the majority of the world's population being infected by a wide variety of metazoan and protozoan parasites.

It is an interesting point of reflection that because common airborne allergens are the major causes of allergic disease in temperate, industrially more developed countries, relatively little attention has been paid to the fact that probably the most potent allergens that exist in nature are in fact derived from helminthic parasites [3]. Parasites of many genera, such as *Ascaris*, *Necator*, *Ancylostoma*, *Strongyloides*, *Schistosoma*, *Wunchereria*, *Brugia*, *Onchocerca* (to name only a few) have the capacity to stimulate strong IgE responses in the majority of infected individuals. For example, serum levels of IgE antibody against the common intestinal helminth, *Ascaris lumbricoides*, in persons in an area endemic for this parasite, are far higher than against the most common airborne allergen, house-dust mite [1, 4].

It is well recognized that the IgE response

* Institute of Biomedicine, Faculty of Medicine, Central University of Venezuela, Caracas, Venezuela

against helminths can contribute to the pathology of these infections, and indeed a variety of pulmonary conditions have been associated with parasites that have lung-migratory phases [3]. We have found that the pulmonary function of children infected with *Ascaris* improved after the elimination of the parasite by anthelmintic treatment, even if the child did not present clinical evidence of allergic disease [5]. In addition, in a study of asthmatic patients from an area endemic for *Ascaris*, we showed that the inhalation of extracts of this parasite can cause significant bronchoconstriction [6]. Furthermore, clinical improvement of asthmatic patients from an *Ascaris*-endemic area occurred after anthelmintic treatment [7].

It is of great interest, however, that the influence of helminthic infection on the allergic response may not be due only to the presence of antiparasite IgE. This is because helminthic parasites have the capacity to nonspecifically stimulate an IL-4-dependent polyclonal synthesis of IgE [3, 8]. The result is that helminthic infections of light to moderate intensity, via a "bystander" effect, can potentiate the IgE response against common environmental allergens, thus increasing the prevalence of allergic diseases in tropical populations [9–11]. In addition, it seems that protozoan parasites such as *Giardia*, by causing tissue damage, can increase the permeability of the gut mucosa to macromolecules, thus increasing the allergic reactivity to food allergens [12, 13].

It is important to note, however, that the influence of helminthic infection on allergic reactivity is complex. For example, in situations of high-intensity infection, where the polyclonal stimulation of IgE synthesis is very strong, the total IgE levels are highly elevated and mast cell saturation occurs [11, 14, 15]. The blockade of mast cell function by excess IgE can result in an inhibition of allergic reactivity, and this is probably a major contributory factor to the low prevalences of allergic diseases reported in tropical populations where parasitic infection is highly endemic [11, 16, 17]. We have shown that the total IgE levels of such groups are significantly diminished by anthelmintic treatment [18, 19], and that this is accompanied by a reactivation of mast cell function and a substantial increase in allergic reactivity [19]. In view of these considerations [20], we feel that appropriate action should be taken to attend the risk of an elevated prevalence of allergic diseases occurring as a consequence of programs eradicate parasitic infections in highly endemic areas.

Another finding of considerable importance in the context of the relationship between allergic reactivity and helminthic infection is that when sufficiently strong, the polyclonal stimulation of IgE synthesis induced by the parasites also reduces the specific IgE antibody response to any given antigen, including those of the parasite itself [15]. This is of relevance because there is evidence to indicate that the specific IgE antibody response against helminth antigens is an important component of protective immune mechanisms against these parasites [3, 11]. For example, the local allergic reactions stimulated by intestinal parasites could provide a hostile environment to the worm and facilitate the access of the immune system to these. In addition, eosinophils are chemotactically drawn to sites of allergic reactions, and these cells can exert IgE-mediated cytotoxic activity against parasitic larvae. Because the persistence of parasites in their hosts often depends upon their capacity to evade the protective immune response, it can be hypothesized that the polyclonal IgE response they induce can, via mast cell saturation and the reduction of specific IgE production, result in diminished antiparasite activity [21, 22]. In this respect, we found that the rate of reinfection by *Ascaris* occurring after the anthelmintic treatment of children in an area endemic for this parasite is directly associated with the magnitude of the polyclonal IgE response: Children with the highest total serum IgE levels and the lowest specific antiparasite IgE antibody levels are the most susceptible to reinfection [23].

The findings described above lead to the consideration of an important teleological question concerning the allergic response: would such a complex and sophisticated system have developed in the process of evolution only to cause disease? It can, in fact, be argued that the fundamental role of the allergic response is in the defence against parasitic infections, and that allergic diseases represent a misdirection of the IgE response against intrinsically inoffensive environmental antigens. An extension of this concept is that the substantial increase in the prevalence of asthma and other allergic diseases that has occurred in industrialized countries over the past decades is due, at least in part, to the elimination of parasitic infections by improved sanitary conditions.

Also implicit in the hypothesis of a protective effect of allergic reactions is the possibility that genes that enhance the IgE response would be conserved in evolution because of the advantage they provide in the resistance to parasitic infection. However, these same genes may well result in a predisposition to allergic diseases. We have obtained indirect evidence to support this concept by studying an island population of Venezuela where, possibly due to the operation of a "founder effect," the prevalence of asthma is very high [24]. This atopic island group had an IgE response to the helminthic parasite *Ascaris* that was significantly less polyclonal than that of a nonatopic mainland population with similar socio-economic characteristics. In addition, although the prevalences of infection were similar in the two groups, thus indicating a comparable risk of exposure to the parasite, the *intensities* of infection in the atopic group were significantly lower than in the nonatopics. This indicates that the resistance mechanisms of the asthmatic individuals were more effective than in their nonallergic counterparts, which may be due to a skew toward a more specific, rather than a polyclonal, IgE response to the parasites in the atopic subjects. More direct evidence of the genetic determination of resistance to parasitic infection related to the asthmatic condition has also been found in this island population, where an association has been demonstrated between polymorphisms in the β2-adrenoreceptor and the intensity of *Ascaris* infection [25].

In conclusion, in the tropical situation, parasitic infection is an important factor in the evaluation of asthma and other allergic diseases. In addition, the consideration of the relationship between allergic reactivity and helminthic infection has far-reaching implications in the understanding of allergic conditions, even in countries where these infections occur only rarely.

Acknowledgments

Partially supported by grants: World Bank VEN. 96.002.14, CDCH/UCV 09.35.4055.97

Address for correspondence:

Dr Neil Lynch
Instituto de Biomedicina
Aptdo. 4043
Caracas
Venezuela 1010A
Fax +48 2 8615-530
E-mail nlynch@telcel.net.ve

References

1. Lynch NR, Lopez RI, Di Prisco-Fuenmayor MC, Hagel I, Medouze L, Viana G, Ortega C, Prato G. Allergic reactivity and socio-economic level in a tropical environment. Clin Allergy 1987; 17:199–207.

2. Lynch NR, Puccio FA, Di Prisco MC, Lopez RI, Hazell LA, Smith WA, Thomas WR. Reactivity to recombinant house-dust mite allergens in asthma and rhinitis in a tropical situation. Allergy 1998; 53:808–811.

3. Lynch NR. Immediate hypersensitivity (allergic) reactions to intestinal helminthic infections. In Z Pawlowski Ed) Intestinal helminthic infections. Baillieres Clinical Tropical Medicine and Communicable Diseases Bailliere Tindall/WB Saunders, London 1987; 2:573–593.

4. Lynch NR, Perez M, Lopez RI, Turner KJ. Measurement of anti-Ascaris IgE antibody levels in tropical allergic patients, using modified ELISA. Allergol Immunopath 1987; 15:19–24.

5. Lynch NR, Hagel I, Perez M, Di Prisco MC, Alvarez N, Rojas E. Bronchoconstriction in helminthic infection. Int Archs Allergy Immunol 1992; 98:77–79.

6. Lynch NR, Isturiz G, Sanchez Y, Perez M, Martinez A, Castes M. Bronchial challenge of tropical asthmatics with Ascaris lumbricoides. J Invest Allergol Clin Immunol 1992; 2:97–105.

7. Lynch NR, Palenque M, Hagel I, Di Prisco MC. Clinical improvement of asthma after anthelminthic treatment in a tropical situation. Am J Resp Crit Care Med. 1997; 156:50–54.

8. Lynch NR, Hagel I, Vargas M, Perez M, Lopez RI, Garcia N, Di Prisco MC, Arthur IH. Effect of age and helminthic infection on the IgE levels of slum children. J Invest Allergol Clin Immunol 1993; 3:96–99.

9. Lynch NR, Di Prisco-Fuenmayor MC. High allergic reactivity in a tropical environment. Clin Allergy 1984; 14:233–240.

10. Hagel I, Lynch NR, Di Prisco MC, Lopez RI, Garcia N. Allergic reactivity of children of different socio-economic level in tropical populations. Int Archs Allergy Immunol 1993; 101:209–214.

11. Lynch NR. Influence of socio-economic level on helminthic infection and allergic reactivity in tropical countries. In R Moqbel (Ed), Allergy and immunity to helminthic infection: Common mechanisms or divergent pathways? London: Taylor & Francis 1992, pp. 51–62.

12. Di Prisco MC, Hagel I, Lynch NR, Barrios RM, Alvarez N, Lopez RI. Possible relationship between allergic disease and infection by Giardia lamblia. Ann Allergy 1993; 70:210–215.

13. Di Prisco MC, Hagel I, Lynch NR, Jimenez JC, Rojas R, Gil M, Mata E. Association between giardiasis and

allergy. Ann Allergy Asthma Immunol 1998; 81:261–264.

14. Hagel I, Lynch NR, Perez M, Di Prisco MC, Lopez RI, Rojas E. Relationship between the degree of poverty and the IgE response to Ascaris infection in slum children. Trans Royal Soc Trop Med Hyg 1993; 87:16–18.

15. Hagel I, Lynch NR, Perez M, Di Prisco MC, Lopez IR, Rojas E. Modulation of the allergic reactivity of slum children by helminthic infection. Paras Immunol 1993; 15:311–315.

16. Lynch NR, Lopez RI, Isturiz G, Tenias-Salazar E. Allergic reactivity and helminthic infection in amerindians of the Amazon basin. Int Archs Allergy Appl Immunol 1983; 72:369–372.

17. Lynch NR, Medouze L, Di Prisco-Fuenmayor MC, Verde O, Lopez RI, Malave C. Incidence of atopic disease in a tropical environment: Partial independence from intestinal helminthiasis. J Allergy Clin Immunol 1984; 73:229–233.

18. Lynch NR, Di Prisco-Fuenmayor MC, Soto JM. Diagnosis of atopic conditions in the tropics. Ann Allergy 1983; 51:547–551.

19. Lynch NR, Hagel I, Perez M, Di Prisco MC, Lopez IR, Alvarez N. Effect of anthelmintic treatment on the allergic reactivity of children in a tropical slum. J Allergy Clin Immunol 1993; 2:404–411.

20. Lynch NR, Hagel I, Di Prisco MC, Lopez RI, Garcia N, Perez M. Serum IgE levels, helminthic infection and socio-economic change. Parasitol Today 1992; 8:166–167.

21. Hagel I, Lynch NR, Di Prisco MC, Perez M, Sanchez G. Nutritional status and the IgE response against Ascaris lumbricoides in children from a tropical slum. Trans Royal Soc Trop Med Hyg 1995; 89:562–565.

22. Lynch NR. Allergic reactivity and helminthic infection. In MA Ozcel, MZ Alkan (Eds), Parasitology for the 21st century. Oxon, UK: CAB International 1996, pp. 211–218.

23. Hagel I, Lynch NR, Di Prisco MC, Rojas E, Perez M, Alvarez N. Ascaris reinfection of slum children: Relation with the IgE response. Clin Exp Immunol 1993; 94:80–83.

24. Lynch NR, Hagel IA, Palenque ME, Di Prisco MC, Escudero JE, Corao LA, Sandia JA, Ferreira LJ, Botto C, Perez M, Le Souef PN. Relationship between helminthic infection and IgE response in atopic and non-atopic children in a tropical environment. J Allergy Clin Immunol 1998; 101:217–221.

25. Ramsay C, Hayden C, Tiller K, Burton P, Hagel I, Palenque M, Lynch NR, Goldblatt J, Le Souef P. Association of polymorphisms in the β2-adrenoreceptor gene with higher levels of parasitic infection. Hum Genetics (in press).

Involuntary Smoking and Asthma

Jonathan M Samet*

Keywords: Asthma, passive smoking, epidemiology, tobacco smoke

Passive smoking, the involuntary inhalation of cigarette smoke by nonsmokers, is a cause of morbidity and mortality. It is causally linked in adults to lung cancer and heart disease, and in children to respiratory illnesses and symptoms, reduced lung growth, middle ear disease, and onset and exacerbation of asthma. Various governmental and agency reports contain reviews of this evidence and find causal associations, and the conclusions in these reports have already had a significant impact on public policy and on clinical management of asthma. Controlling children's exposure to passive smoking can best be accomplished by keeping environments where children spend time smoke-free. This involves preventing smoking in such locations, particularly the home, which is usually the dominant locus of exposure for children. Finding effective strategies to reduce children's exposure to ETS is challenging, as parents must be dissuaded from smoking around their children.

Introduction

Worldwide, active cigarette smoking is one of the major preventable causes of morbidity and mortality [1] and tragically, the epidemic of smoking-caused premature deaths is predicted to mount as smoking becomes more prevalent in the developing countries. Passive smoking, the involuntary inhalation of cigarette smoke by nonsmokers, is also a cause of morbidity and mortality [2] and rising active smoking implies rising passive smoking, absent interventions to protect nonsmokers. Three decades of research have shown that passive smoking has diverse adverse effects; it has been causally linked in adults to lung cancer and heart disease, and in children to respiratory illnesses and symptoms, reduced lung growth, middle ear disease, and onset and exacerbation of asthma (Table 1) [3–6].

This review addresses the evidence on passive smoking and asthma, covering the composition and characteristics of environmental tobacco smoke (ETS), the mixture of sidestream smoke and exhaled mainstream smoke to which nonsmokers are

Table 1. Adverse effects from exposure of children to tobacco smoke.

Health Effect	SG 1984	SG 1986	EPA 1992	CalEPA 1997	UK 1998
Increased prevalence of respiratory illnesses	Yes/a	Yes/a	Yes/c	Yes/c	Yes/c
Decrement in pulmonary function	Yes/a	Yes/a	Yes/a	Yes/a	
Increased frequency of bronchitis, pneumonia	Yes/a	Yes/a	Yes/a	Yes/c	
Increase in chronic cough, phlegm		Yes/a		Yes/c	
Increased frequency of middle ear disease		Yes/a	Yes/c	Yes/c	Yes/c
Increased severity of asthma episodes and symptoms			Yes/c	Yes/c	Yes/c
Risk factor for new asthma			Yes/a	Yes/c	
Risk factor for SIDS				Yes/c	Yes/a

Yes/a = association, Yes/c = cause
SG = Reports of the Surgeon General of the United States [3, 14]; EPA = Environmental Protection Agency [11]; CalEPA = California Environmental Protection Agency [5]; UK = Report of the Scientific Committee on Tobacco and Health [6]

---

* School of Hygiene and Public Health, Johns Hopkins University, Baltimore, MD, USA

exposed, and the epidemiologic and experimental findings on the consequences of ETS exposure. While scientific research on ETS and asthma has only been carried out for several decades, clinicians have previously recognized the potential role of ETS exposure in exacerbating asthma. A case report, published in the *Journal of the American Medical Association* in 1950, described an asthmatic child whose clinical condition worsened with exposure to tobacco smoking [7]. Centuries earlier, Sir John Floyer in England, had cautioned against the adverse effect of tobacco smoke on persons with asthma [8]. He commented "During the Fit of the Asthma, the Smoak of Tobacco is so offensive that it very much straitens the Breath . . There are many asthmatics that cannot bear the smell of it . . " Today, clinical practice guidelines recommend that persons with asthma should avoid exposure to ETS [9].

This review summarizes the now extensive literature on exposure to ETS and on ETS and asthma, emphasizing the findings for children and their clinical implications. This evidence has been periodically reviewed in various governmental and agency reports. These reports should be consulted for their summaries of the evidence and comprehensive bibliographies. Some key reports include the 1986 report of the US Surgeon General on smoking and health [10], the 1986 report by the US National Research Council [4], the 1992 report of the US Environmental Protection Agency [11], the 1997 report of the Environmental Protection Agency for the State of California [5], and the 1998 report of the UK Scientific Committee on Tobacco [6]. Conclusions of these reports with regard to asthma and other effects in children are provided in Table 1. These conclusions have already had significant impact on public policy and on clinical management of asthma.

Exposure to ETS

Characteristics of Environmental Tobacco Smoke

Nonsmokers inhale ETS, the combination of the sidestream smoke that is released from the cigarette's burning end and the mainstream smoke exhaled by the active smoker [12]. The inhalation of ETS is generally referred to as passive smoking or involuntary smoking. ETS, like tobacco smoke, is a complex mixture of particulate matter with many different gaseous compounds. The mixture changes after its generation as components undergo chemical modification or adsorb onto materials and the particles age and change in their size distribution. Broad classes of the compounds in ETS would be expected to adversely affect persons with asthma directly through their irritative properties or indirectly by impairing host defenses against inhaled agents, including infectious organisms.

The exposures of involuntary and active smoking differ quantitatively and, to some extent, qualitatively [4, 10, 11, 13–15]. Because of the lower temperature in the burning cone of the smoldering cigarette, most partial pyrolysis products are enriched in sidestream as compared to mainstream smoke. Consequently, at the time of its generation, sidestream smoke has higher concentrations of some toxic and carcinogenic substances than mainstream smoke; however, dilution by room air markedly reduces the concentrations inhaled by the involuntary smoker in comparison to those inhaled by the active smoker. Nevertheless, involuntary smoking is accompanied by exposure to toxic agents generated by tobacco combustion [4, 10, 11, 13, 14].

Environmental Tobacco Smoke Concentrations

Not surprisingly, tobacco smoking in indoor environments increases levels of tobacco smoke components, such as respirable particles, nicotine, polycyclic aromatic hydrocarbons, carbon monoxide (CO), acrolein, nitrogen dioxide (NO_2), and many other substances. Tables 2 and 3 provide a summary of data from a number of recent studies [16]. The extent of the increase in concentrations of these ETS components varies with the number of smokers, the intensity of smoking, the rate of exchange between the indoor air and the outdoor air, and the use of air-cleaning devices. Several components of ETS have been measured in indoor environments as markers of the contribution of tobacco combustion to indoor air pollution. Particles have been measured most often because both sidestream and mainstream smoke contain high concentrations of particles in the respirable size range and measurement techniques are available for particles [4]. Other, more specific markers have also been measured, including nicotine [15], which can be measured with active sampling methods and also using passive diffusion badges [15, 17]. Studies of levels of ETS components have been conducted, largely in public buildings; fewer studies have been conducted in homes and offices [4, 10].

Table 2. Occupational ETS exposures in non-office settings (nonsmokers only).

Company Type	Year sampled	# samples	Mean	Standard deviation	Geometric mean	Concentration of nicotine, μg/m³		
						min.	median	max.
Smoking Allowed								
Specialty chemicals	1991–92	8	0.60	0.91	0.24	<0.05	0.46	2.78
Railroad workers (personal)	1983–84	152	0.80	3.30	0.18	<0.1	0.10	38.10
Tool manufacturing	1991–92	13	1.59	1.05	1.16	0.15	1.85	3.40
Textile finishing B	1991–92	11	1.74	1.69	1.10	0.31	0.93	5.09
Labels & paper products	1991–92	1	2.31				2.31		
Die manufacturer	1991–92	12	2.70	1.27	2.46	1.23	2.41	5.42
Sintering metal	1991–92	12	2.88	2.59	2.11	0.62	2.24	9.72
Newspaper B	1991–92	5	2.96	1.37	2.68	1.23	2.78	4.63
Miscellaneous	<1990	282	4.30	11.80	1.70	<1.6	<1.6	126.00
Textile finishing A	1991–92	11	4.33	8.82	1.77	0.46	1.39	30.71
Flight attendants (personal)	1988	16	4.70	4.00	2.32	0.10	4.20	10.50
Fire fighters A *	1991–92	16	5.39	3.81	4.08	1.20	4.84	13.42
Fire fighters B	1991–92	24	5.83	6.77	3.83	0.71	3.65	27.50
Barber shop (personal)	1986–87	2	8.80			4.00		13.70
Hospital (personal)	1986–87	5	24.80	22.80	16.80	6.30	10.00	53.20
Smoking Restricted								
Work clothing	1991–92	9	0.17	0.32	0.06	<0.05	<0.05	0.93
Filtration products	1991–92	10	0.32	0.87	0.08	<0.05	<0.05	2.78
Film and imaging	1991–92	6	0.82	0.83	0.39	<0.05	0.70	2.16
Fiber optics	1991–92	13	1.34	2.79	0.63	0.20	0.64	10.57
Newspaper A	1991–92	4	4.86	6.65	2.62	0.93	1.85	14.81
Valve manufacturer	1991–92	10	5.80	7.85	3.62	1.16	3.26	27.31
Rubber products	1991–92	2	5.85	5.36	4.18	2.06	5.85	9.64
Smoking Prohibited								
Infrared & imaging systems	1991–92	1	<0.05			<0.05	<0.05	
Hospital products	1991–92	5	0.08	0.17	<0.05	<0.05	<0.05	0.39
Weapons systems	1991–92	12	0.08	0.20	<0.05	<0.05	<0.05	0.63
Aircraft components	1991–92	12	0.20	0.18	0.13	<0.05	0.21	0.61
Radar communications components	1991–92	13	0.31	0.36	0.14	<0.05	0.26	1.08
Computer chip equipment	1991–92	10	0.51	0.33	0.41	0.15	0.39	1.08

From [16]. * Omits one data point, 101 μ/m³

Table 3. Nicotine concentrations in homes.

	Year sampled	# samples	Mean	Standard deviation	Concentration of nicotine, $\mu g/m^3$		
					min.	median	max.
North Carolina homes (weekly)	1988	13	1.50	1.10	1.00	1.40	4.40
Personal (each sampled 3×)	1988	15					
Males (personal) * (16 hours)	1993–94	86	2.13			1.29	>8.08
New York homes (weekly)	1986	47	2.20		0.10	1.00	9.40
Females (personal) * (16 hours)	1993–94	220	2.93			1.14	>7.81
North Carolina homes 14 hours (5 pm – 7 am)	1986	13	3.74			c. 3.3	6.5
Minnesota homes (weekly)	c. 1989–	25	5.80		0.10	3.00	28.60

* 16 hour ave.; "away from work," ** 95th percentile, as given in paper, ***assumed 16-hour exposure. From [16]

The contribution of various environments to personal exposure to tobacco smoke varies with the time-activity pattern, i. e., the distribution of time spent in different locations. Time-activity patterns may strongly influence lung airway exposures in particular environments for persons with asthma. For children, the home is generally the dominant locus of exposure while the workplace may contribute significantly for adults. The contribution of smoking in the home to indoor air pollution has been demonstrated by studies using personal monitoring and monitoring of homes for respirable particles. In one of the early studies, Spengler et al. [18] monitored homes in six US cities for respirable particle concentrations and found that a smoker of one pack of cigarettes daily contributed about 20 mg/m³ to 24-hour indoor particle concentrations. Because cigarettes are not smoked uniformly over the day, higher peak concentrations must occur when cigarettes are actually smoked.

For children, exposures would further depend on the coupling of their time-activity patterns to those of the smoking adults. In several studies, small numbers of homes have been monitored for nicotine, which is a vapor-phase constituent of ETS. In a study of ETS exposure of daycare children, the average nicotine concentration during the time that the ETS-exposed children were at home was 3.7 µg/m³; in homes without smoking, the average was 0.3 µg/m³ [19]. Coultas and colleagues [20] measured 24-hour nicotine and respirable particle concentrations in the air of 10 homes on alternate days for a week and then on five more days during alternate weeks. The mean levels of nicotine were around 2–4 µg/m³ but some 24-hour values were as high as 20 µg/m³.

The Total Exposure Assessment Methodology (TEAM) Study, conducted by the US Environmental Protection Agency, provided extensive data on concentrations of 20 volatile organic compounds, many generated by cigarette smoking, in a sample of homes in several communities [21]. Indoor monitoring showed higher concentrations of benzene, xylenes, ethylbenzene, and styrene in homes with smokers compared to homes without smokers. These volatile organic compounds are present in tobacco smoke.

More extensive information is available on levels of ETS components in public buildings and workplaces of various types, locations that are generally not relevant to children [15, 16] (Tables 2 and 3). Monitoring in locations where smoking may be intense, such as bars and restaurants, has generally shown substantial elevations of particles and other markers of smoke pollution where smoking is taking place [4, 10]. Transportation environments may also be polluted by cigarette smoking and children may receive substantial exposures in vehicles when smoking is taking place.

Biological Markers of Exposure

Biological markers of exposure are indicators of the presence of an agent in biological materials, such as blood, tissue, or saliva. Biological markers can be used to describe the prevalence of exposure to environmental tobacco smoke, to investigate the dosimetry of involuntary smoking, and to validate questionnaire-based measures of exposure. In both active and involuntary smokers, the detection of tobacco smoke components or their metabolites in body fluids or alveolar air provides evidence of exposure to tobacco smoke, and levels of these markers can be used to gauge the intensity of exposure and of the dose of materials actually taken into the nonsmoker. At present, the most sensitive and specific markers for tobacco smoke exposure are nicotine and its metabolite, cotinine [4, 22, 23]. Neither nicotine nor cotinine is usually present in body fluids in the absence of exposure to tobacco smoke; consequently, both are highly specific markers. Cotinine, formed by oxidation of nicotine by cytochrome P-450, is one of several primary metabolites of nicotine [23]. Cotinine itself is extensively metabolized, and only about 17% of cotinine is excreted unchanged in the urine.

Because the circulating half-life of nicotine is generally shorter than 2 h [24], nicotine concentrations in body fluids reflect more recent exposures. In contrast, cotinine has a half-life in the blood or plasma of nonsmokers of around 20 hours [23, 25]; hence, cotinine levels provide information about more chronic exposure to tobacco smoke in involuntary smokers. Whether cotinine has the same half-lives in plasma, saliva, and urine has been uncertain, as is the choice of the optimal body fluid for measuring cotinine for research purposes [26–28]. Cotinine levels have been measured in adult nonsmokers and in children [25]. In the studies of adult nonsmokers, exposures at home, in the workplace, and in other settings determined cotinine concentrations in urine and saliva. The cotinine levels in involuntary smokers ranged from less than 1% to about 8% of cotinine levels measured in active smokers.

Cotinine levels have been measured in children in a number of studies (Table 4). Smoking by parents is the predominant determinant of cotinine levels in their children. Coultas et al. [29] examined determinants of a detectable level of cotinine in the saliva of children in a community sample. A multivariable statistical model showed that the major determinants of a detectable level were mother's smoking, associated with a three-fold increased risk, father's smoking, associated with a two-fold increased risk, and smoking by other household members, associated with a four-fold increased risk. In a study in North Carolina, Greenberg et al. [30] found significantly higher concentrations of cotinine in the urine and saliva of infants exposed to cigarette smoke in their homes than in unexposed controls. Urinary cotinine levels in the infants increased with the number of cigarettes smoked during the previous 24 h by the mother. In a study of school children in England, salivary cotinine levels rose with the number of smoking parents in the home [31]. In a study of a national sample of participants in the Third National Health and Nutrition Examination Survey (NHANES), 1988–1991, 88% of nonsmokers had a detectable level of serum cotinine using liquid chromatography-mass spectrometry as the assay method [32]. Cotinine levels in this national sample increased with the number of smokers in the household and the hours exposed in the workplace. In children ages 4–16 years, cotinine levels were approximately ten-fold higher for those with home ETS exposure and the number of smokers in the home was a significant predictor of cotinine level. These studies document the key role of exposures in the home and the need to target the smoking of parents as a predominant source of children's exposure to ETS.

ETS and Childhood Asthma

Wheezing in Children

Data from numerous surveys demonstrate a greater frequency of the most common respiratory symptoms: cough, phlegm, and wheeze in the children of smokers [5, 10, 33]. In these studies the subjects have generally been school children, and the effects of parental smoking have been examined. Many studies have demonstrated increased wheezing in ETS-exposed children, compared to nonexposed children. While a report of the symptom of wheezing does not correspond to a diagnosis of asthma, the findings on ETS and wheezing have general relevance to asthma.

For the symptom of chronic wheeze, the preponderance of the early evidence indicated an excess associated with involuntary smoking. In a survey of 650 school children in Boston, one of the first studies on this association, persistent wheezing, was the most frequent symptom [34]; the prevalence of persistent wheezing increased significantly, comparing children with no smoking parents, one smoking parent, and two smoking parents. In a large study of children in six US communities, the prevalence of persistent wheezing during the previous year was significantly increased if the mother smoked [35].

Cook and Strachan [33] have recently conducted a quantitative summary of studies on passive smoking and respiratory symptoms in children, including 41 on the symptom of wheeze. Overall, the pooled analyses indicated an increased risk for wheezing of approximately 20% associated with parental smoking.

Table 4. Cotinine concentration in children (selected studies).

Study (ref. no.)	Year	No. of subjects	Smoking status	Exposure level	Analytical method	Plasma or serum cotinine (ng/ml)	Salivary cotinine (ng/ml)
Jarvis et al. [61]	1985	269	Nonsmokers, children	Neither parent smoked	GC		0.4 (median 0.2)
		96	Nonsmokers, children	Father smoked	GC		1.3 (median 1.0)
		76	Nonsmokers, children	Mother smoked	GC		2.0 (median 1.7)
		128	Nonsmokers, children	Both parents smoked	GC		3.4 (median 2.4)
Coultas et al. [29]	1987	68	Nonsmokers aged < 5 years	No smoker in home	RIA		1.7 (median 0)
		41	Nonsmokers aged < 5 years	1 smoker in home	RIA		4.1 (median 3.8)
		21	Nonsmokers aged < 5 years	2/+ smokers in home	RIA		5.6 (median 5.4)
		200	Nonsmokers aged 5–17 years	No smoker in home	RIA		1.3 (median 0)
		96	Nonsmokers aged 5–17 years	1 smoker in home	RIA		2.4 (median 1.8)
		25	Nonsmokers aged 5–17 years	2/+ smokers in home	RIA		5.6 (median 5.3)
Strachan et al. [62]	1989	405	Nonsmoker, age 7 years	No smoker in home	GC		1.1 nM/liter
		241	Nonsmoker, age 7 years	1 smoker in home	GC		10.2 nM/liter
		124	Nonsmoker, age 7 years	2/+ smokers in home	GC		37.5 nM/liter
Cook et al. [63]	1994	1260	Nonsmokers age 5–7 years	No smokers in home	GC		0.29 (GM) (95% CI 0.28–0.31)
		293	Nonsmokers age 5–7 years	Mother smoker	GC		2.2 (GM) (95% CI 1.9–2.5)
		521	Nonsmokers age 5–7 years	Father smoker	GC		1.2 (GM) (95% CI 1.1–1.3)
		553	Nonsmokers age 5–7 years	Both parents smokers	GC		4.0 (GM) (95% CI 3.7–4.4)
Pirkle et al. [32]	1996	1071	Nonsmokers age 4–11 years	No home ETS exposure	LC-MS	0.12 (GM) (95% CI 0.10–0.14)	
		713	Nonsmokers age 4–11 years	Home ETS exposure only	LC-MS	1.14 (GM) (95% CI 0.98–1.34)	
		379	Nonsmokers age 12–16 years	No home ETS exposure	LC-MS	0.11 (GM) (95% CI 0.10–0.15)	
		268	Nonsmokers age 12–16 years	Home ETS exposure only	LC-MS	0.81 (GM) (95% CI 0.62–1.04)	

Abbreviations: GC, gas chromatography; RIA, radioimmunoassay; CI, confidence interval; GM, geometric mean; LC-MS, liquid chromatography-mass spectrometry.

Childhood Asthma

Although involuntary exposure to tobacco smoke has been associated with the symptom of wheeze, evidence for association of involuntary smoking with childhood asthma was initially conflicting. Exposure to ETS might cause asthma as a long-term consequence of the increased occurrence of lower respiratory infection in early childhood or through other pathophysiological mechanisms including inflammation of the respiratory epithelium [36, 37]. The effect of ETS may also reflect, in part, the consequences of *in utero* exposure. Children whose mothers smoke during pregnancy are invariably exposed to ETS after birth as the mother continues to smoke. Assessment of airways responsiveness shortly after birth has shown that infants whose mothers smoke during pregnancy have increased airways responsiveness compared with those whose mothers do not smoke [38]. Maternal smoking during pregnancy also reduced ventilatory function measured shortly after birth [39]. These observations suggest that *in utero* exposures from maternal smoking may affect lung development, perhaps reducing relative airways size. This reduction in airways size would increase the risk for wheezing, particularly in the presence of lower respiratory infections.

Lower respiratory illnesses in early childhood have long been postulated to increase risk for later development of airways disease, including asthma (see [36] for a review). Exposure to ETS, by increasing risk for lower respiratory infections, might increase risk for subsequent asthma. This postulated causal pathway has not been directly tested, however, and a number of studies show an inverse relationship between viral infections and asthma occurrence [40]. One current hypothesis concerning pathogenesis posits that viral infections maintain an immunologic phenotype with Th1-like T cells and lower risk for allergic disease.

While the underlying mechanisms remain to be identified, the epidemiologic evidence linking ETS exposure and childhood asthma is mounting [5, 33]. The quantitative synthesis by Cook and Strachan [33] shows a significant excess of childhood asthma if both parents or the mother smoke (Table 5). This meta-analysis draws on the findings of numerous case-control and cohort studies.

The epidemiologic evidence indicates that ETS exposure increases risk for both incidence (onset of new asthma) and for worsening of childhood asthma. Data on incidence derive from cohort (follow-up) and cross-sectional (surveys) studies. A particularly informative study of the case-control design was conducted in Montreal, Canada. Infante-Rivard [41] compared family characteristics and environmental exposures of 3- and 4-year old children with incident asthma to those of control children without asthma. Mother's smoking increased risk for asthma with an odds ratio of 2.77 (95% confidence limits 1.35–5.66) if the mother smoked 20 or more cigarettes per day compared with no smoking by the mother. The presence of other smokers in the home approximately doubled the risk, although the increase was not statistically significant.

This evidence has been interpreted in the California Environmental Protection Agency report as indicating that ETS exposure increases asthma risk in children [5]. The United Kingdom's Scientific Committee on Tobacco and Health emphasized the role of parental smoking in exacerbating asthma, considering this triggering as the explanation for the association of ETS exposure with asthma onset in cohort studies [6].

The studies reported to date more definitively indicate that involuntary smoking worsens the status of those with asthma. The possibility that ETS

Table 5. Summary of pooled random effects odds ratios with 95% confidence intervals (number of studies in parentheses).

	Asthma			Wheeze#		
	OR	(95% CI)	[n]	OR	(95% CI)	[n]
Either parent smokes	1.21	(1.10 to 1.34)	[21][a]	1.24	(1.17 to 1.31)	[30][a]
One parent smokes	1.04	(0.78 to 1.38)	[6]	1.18	(1.08 to 1.29)	[21]
Both parents smoke	1.50	(1.29 to 1.73)	[8]	1.47	(1.14 to 1.90)	[11]
Mother only smokes	1.36	(1.20 to 1.55)	[11]	1.28	(1.19 to 1.38)	[18][b]
Father only smokes	1.07	(0.92 to 1.24)	[9]	1.14	(1.06 to 1.23)	[10]

#Excluding EC study, in which the pooled odds ratio was 1.20. * Data for phlegm and breathlessness restricted as several comparisons are based on fewer than five studies. [a]Two age groups from reference [64] included as separate studies. [b]Reference [65] included as three separate studies. From [33]

adversely affects children with asthma was described as early as 1950 in a case report entitled "Bronchial asthma due to allergy to tobacco smoke in an infant" [7]. More recently, Murray and Morrison [42, 43] evaluated asthmatic children followed in a clinic. Level of lung function, symptom frequency, and responsiveness to inhaled histamines were adversely affected by maternal smoking. Population studies have also shown increased airways responsiveness for ETS-exposed children with asthma [44, 45]. The increased level of airway responsiveness associated with ETS exposure would be expected to increase the clinical severity of asthma. In a clinic-based study of children in Maine, both reported exposure and urine cotinine levels were associated with measures of morbidity: number of exacerbations and lung function level [46]. In this regard, exposure to smoking in the home has been shown to increase the number of emergency room visits made by asthmatic children [47]. Asthmatic children with smoking mothers are more likely to use asthma medications [48], a finding that confirms the clinically significant effects of ETS on children with asthma. This extensive evidence has uniformly been interpreted as showing that ETS exposure exacerbates childhood asthma.

ETS and Asthma in Adults

Neither epidemiological nor experimental studies have definitively established the role of ETS in exacerbating asthma in adults. The acute responses of asthmatics to ETS have been assessed by exposing persons with asthma to tobacco smoke in a chamber. This experimental approach cannot be readily controlled because of the impossibility of blinding subjects to exposure to ETS. However, suggestibility does not appear to underlie physiological responses of asthmatics to ETS [49]. Of three studies involving exposure of unselected asthmatics to ETS, only one showed a definite adverse effect [50–53]. Stankus et al. [54] recruited 21 asthmatics who reported exacerbation with exposure to ETS. With challenge in an exposure chamber at concentrations much greater than typically encountered in indoor environments, seven of the subjects experienced a more than 20% decline in FEV_1.

The epidemiologic evidence is extremely limited, but suggests that ETS can exacerbate asthma in adults [55]. In a prospective cohort study of adults with asthma in Switzerland, self-reported ETS exposure was associated with wheezing and a report of physician-diagnosed asthma [56]. In a prospective cohort study of 451 adult asthmatics in California, self-reported ETS exposure was associated with greater severity, lower quality of life, and increased health care utilization [57]. The findings of a cross-sectional study in India were similar [58]. A small cross-sectional study in Sweden showed a small and nonsignificant association between prevalent asthma and passive exposure to tobacco smoking in the workplace [59].

Conclusions

In many countries worldwide, ETS is ubiquitous and children may be unable to avoid exposure from the smoking of their parents at home and in vehicles. The mounting evidence on ETS and childhood asthma establishes passive smoking both as a cause and exacerbating factor for asthma. Exposure control can best be accomplished by keeping environments where children spend time smoke-free. This involves not smoking in places where children spend time, particularly the home. Finally, effective strategies to reduce children's exposure to ETS will be challenging, as parents must be dissuaded from smoking around their children [60].

Address for correspondence:

Jonathan M Samet, MD, MS
School of Hygiene and Public Health
Johns Hopkins University
615 North Wolfe Street, Suite W6041
Baltimore, Maryland 21205-2179
Tel. +1 410 955-3286
Fax +1 410 955-0863
E-mail jsamet@jhsph.edu

References

1. Murray CJL, Lopez AD. Evidence-based health policy – Lessons from the global burden of disease study. Science 1996; 274:740–743.

2. Samet JM, Wang SS. Environmental tobacco smoke (in press). In Lippmann M (Ed), Environmental toxicants: Human exposures and their health effects (2nd

ed., Chapter 11). New York: Van Nostrand Reinhold 1999.

3. US Department of Health and Human Services (USDHHS). US Public Health Services: The health consequences of involuntary smoking. Report of the Surgeon General. Public Health Service, Office of the Assistant Secretary of Health, Office of Smoking and Health 1986. DHHS Pub No. (PHS) 87–8398.

4. National Research Council (NRC), Committee on Passive Smoking. Environmental tobacco smoke: Measuring exposures and assessing health effects. Washington, DC: National Academy Press 1986.

5. California Environmental Protection Agency (Cal EPA), Office of Environmental Health Hazard Assessment. Health effects of exposure to environmental tobacco smoke. California Environmental Protection Agency 1997.

6. Scientific Committee on Tobacco and Health, HSMO. Report of the Scientific Committee on Tobacco and Health. The Stationary Office 1998. Report No. 011322124x.

7. Rosen FL, Levy A. Bronchial asthma due to allergy to tobacco smoke in an infant: A case report. JAMA 1950; 144(8):620–621.

8. Sakula A. Sir John Floyer's A Treatise of the Asthma (1698). Thorax 1983; 39:248–254.

9. US Department of Health and Human Services (USDHHS), Public Health Service, National Institute of Health, National Heart Lung and Blood Institute. Practical guide for the diagnosis and management of asthma. NIH 1997. Publication No. 97–4053.

10. US Department of Health and Human Services (USDHHS). The health consequences of involuntary smoking: A report of the Surgeon General. Washington, DC: US Government Printing Office 1986. DHHS Publication No. (CDC) 87–8398.

11. US Environmental Protection Agency (EPA). Respiratory health effects of passive smoking: Lung cancer and other disorders. Washington, DC: US Government Printing Office 1992. Report No.EPA/600/006F.

12. First MW. Constituents of sidestream and mainstream tobacco and markers to quantify exposure to them. In Gammage RB (Ed), Indoor air and human health. Chelsea, MI: Lewis Publishers 1985.

13. National Research Council (NRC), Committee on Indoor Pollutants. Indoor pollutants. Washington, DC: National Academy Press 1981.

14. US Department of Health and Human Services (USDHHS). The health consequences of smoking — chronic obstructive lung disease. A report of the Surgeon General. Washington, DC: US Government Printing Office 1984.

15. Guerin MR, Jenkins RA, Tomkins BA. The chemistry of environmental tobacco smoke: Composition and measurement. Center for Indoor Air Research (Eds). Chelsea, MI: Lewis Publishers 1992.

16. Hammond SK. Exposure of US workers to environmental tobacco smoke. Environ Health Perspect 1999; 107:329–340.

17. Leaderer BP, Hammond SK. Evaluation of vapor-phase nicotine and respirable suspended particle mass as markers for environmental tobacco smoke. Environ Sci Technol 1991; 25:770–777.

18. Spengler JD, Dockery DW, Turner WA, Wolfson JM, Ferris BG, Jr. Long-term measurements of respirable sulfates and particles inside and outside homes. Atmos Environ 1981; 15:23–30.

19. Henderson FW, Reid HF, Morris R, Wang OL, Hu PC, Helms RW, Forehand L, Mumford J, Lewtas J, Haley NJ, Hammond SK. Home air nicotine levels and urinary cotinine excretion in preschool children. Am Rev Respir Dis 1989; 140:197–201.

20. Coultas DB, Samet JM, McCarthy JF, Spengler JD. Variability of measures of exposure to environmental tobacco smoke in the home. Am Rev Respir Dis 1990; 142:602–606.

21. Wallace LA, Pellizzari ED. Personal air exposures and breath concentrations of benzene and other volatile hydrocarbons for smokers and nonsmokers. Toxicol Lett 1987; 35(1):113–116.

22. Jarvis MJ, Russell MA. Measurement and estimation of smoke dosage to nonsmokers from environmental tobacco smoke. Eur J Respir Dis Suppl 1984; 133:68–75.

23. US Department of Health and Human Services (USDHHS). The health consequences of smoking: Nicotine addiction. A report of the Surgeon General. Washington, DC: US Government Printing Office 1988.

24. Rosenberg J, Benowitz NL, Jacob P, Wilson KM. Disposition kinetics and effects of intravenous nicotine. Clin Pharmacol Ther 1980; 28:517–522.

25. Benowitz NL. Cotinine as a biomarker of environmental tobacco smoke exposure. Epidemiol Rev 1996; 18(2):188–204.

26. Jarvis MJ, Russell MAH, Benowitz NL, Feyerabend C. Elimination of cotinine from body fluids: Implications for noninvasive measurement of tobacco smoke exposure. Am J Public Health 1988; 78:696–698.

27. Wall MA, Johnson J, Jacob P, Benowitz NL. Cotinine in the serum, saliva and urine of nonsmokers, passive smokers, and active smokers. Am J Public Health 1988; 78:699–701.

28. Haley NJ, Colosimo SG, Axelrod CM, Hanis R, Sepkovic DW. Biochemical validation of self-reported exposure to environmental tobacco smoke. Environ Res 1989; 49:127–135.

29. Coultas DB, Howard CA, Peake GT, Skipper BJ, Samet JM. Salivary cotinine levels and involuntary tobacco smoke exposure in children and adults in New Mexico. Am Rev Respir Dis 1987; 136(2):305–309.

30. Greenberg RA, Haley NJ, Etzel RA, Loda FA. Measuring the exposure of infants to tobacco smoke: Nicotine and cotinine in urine and saliva. N Engl J Med 1984; 310:1075–1078.

31. Jarvis MJ, Russell MA, Feyerabend C, Eiser JR, Morgan M, Gammage P, Gray EM. Passive exposure to tobacco smoke: Saliva cotinine concentrations in a representative population sample of nonsmoking school children. Br Med J 1985; 291:927–929.

32. Pirkle JL, Flegal KM, Bernert JT, Brody DJ, Etzel RA, Maurer KR. Exposure of the US population to environmental tobacco smoke. The Third National Health and Nutrition Examination Survey, 1988 to 1991. JAMA 1996; 275(16):1233–1240.

33. Cook DG, Strachan DP. Parental smoking and prevalence of respiratory symptoms and asthma in school age children. Thorax 1997; 52(12):1081–1094.

34. Weiss ST, Tager IB, Speizer FE, Rosner B. Persistent wheeze: its relation to respiratory illness, cigarette smoking, and level of pulmonary function in a population sample of children. Am Rev Respir Dis 1980; 122:697–707.

35. Ware JH, Dockery DW, Spiro A, III. Passive smoking, gas cooking, and respiratory health of children living in six cities. Am Rev Respir Dis 1984; 129:366–374.

36. Samet JM, Tager IB, Speizer FE. The relationship between respiratory illness in childhood and chronic airflow obstruction in adulthood. Am Rev Respir Dis 1983; 127:508–523.

37. Tager IB. Passive smoking-bronchial responsiveness and atopy. Am Rev Respir Dis 1988; 138:507–509.

38. Young S, Le Souef PN, Geelhoed GC, Stick SM, Turner KJ, Landau LI. The influence of a family history of asthma and parental smoking on airway responsiveness in early infancy. N Engl J Med 1991; 324(17):1168–1173.

39. Hanrahan JP, Tager IB, Segal MR, Tosteson TD, Castile RG, Van Vunakis H, Weiss ST, Speizer FE. The effect of maternal smoking during pregnancy on early infant lung function. Am Rev Respir Dis 1992; 145:1129–1135.

40. Von Mutius E, Martinez FD. Epidemiology of childhood asthma. In Murphy S, Kelly HW (Eds), Pediatric asthma (Vol. 126). New York: Marcel Dekker 1999, pp. 1–39.

41. Infante-Rivard C. Childhood asthma and indoor environmental risk factors. Am J Epidemiol 1993; 137(8): 834–844.

42. Murray AB, Morrison BJ. The effect of cigarette smoke from the mother on bronchial responsiveness and severity of symptoms in children with asthma. J Allergy Clin Immunol 1986; 77(4):575–581.

43. Murray AB, Morrison BJ. Passive smoking by asthmatics: its greater effect on boys than on girls and on older than on younger children. Pediatrics 1989; 84(3):451–459.

44. O'Connor GT, Weiss ST, Tager IB, Speizer FE. The effect of passive smoking on pulmonary function and nonspecific bronchial responsiveness in a population-based sample of children and young adults. Am Rev Respir Dis 1987; 135:800–804.

45. Martinez FD, Antognoni G, Macri F, Bonci E, Midulla F, DeCastro G, Ronchetti R. Parental smoking enhances bronchial responsiveness in nine-year-old children. Am Rev Respir Dis 1988; 138:518–523.

46. Chilmonczyk BA, Salmun LM, Megathlin KN, Neveux LM, Palomaki GE, Knight GJ, Pulkkinen AJ, Haddow JE. Association between exposure to environmental tobacco smoke and exacerbations of asthma in children. New Engl J Med 1993; 328(23):1665–1669.

47. Evans D, Levison MJ, Feldman CH, Clark NM, Wasilewski Y, Levin B, Mellins RB. The impact of passive smoking on emergency room visits of urban children with asthma. Am Rev Respir Dis 1987; 135:567–572.

48. Weitzman M, Gortmaker S, Walker DK, Sobol A. Maternal smoking and childhood asthma. Pediatrics 1990; 85(4):505–511.

49. Urch RB, Silverman F, Corey P, Shephard RJ, Cole P, Goldsmith LJ. Does suggestibility modify acute reactions to passive cigarette smoke exposure? Environ Res 1988; 47:34–47.

50. Shephard RJ, Collins R, Silverman F. "Passive" exposure of asthmatic subjects to cigarette smoke. Environ Res 1979; 20(2):392–402.

51. Coultas DB, Samet JM. Respiratory disease prevention. In Wallace RB, Doebbeling BN, Last JM (Eds), Public Health & Preventive Medicine. Stanford: Appleton & Lange 1998, pp. 981–990.

52. Dahms TE, Bolin JF, Slavin RG. Passive smoking: effect on bronchial asthma. Chest 1981; 80(5):530–534.

53. Murray AB, Morrison BJ. The effect of cigarette smoke from the mother on bronchial responsiveness and severity of symptoms in children with asthma. J Allergy Clin Immunol 1986; 77(4):575–581.

54. Stankus RP, Menan PK, Rando RJ, Glindmeyer H, Salvaggio JE, Lehrer SB. Cigarette smoke-sensitive asthma: Challenge studies. J Allergy Clin Immunol 1988; 82:331–338.

55. Leaderer BP, Samet JM. Passive smoking and adults: New evidence for adverse effects. Am J Resp Crit Care Med 1994; 150:1216–1218.

56. Leuenberger P, Schwartz J, Ackermann-Liebrich U, Blaser K, Bolognini G, Bongard JP, Brandli O, Braun P, Bron C, Brutsche M, Domenighetti G, Elsasser S, Guldimann P, Hollenstein C, Hufschmid P, Karrer W, Keller R, Keller-Wossidlo H, Kunzli N, Luthi JC, Martin BW, Medici T, Perruchoud AP, Radaelli A, Schindler C, Schoeni MH, Solari G, Tschopp JM, Villiger B, Wuthrich B, Zellweger JP, Zemp E. Passive

smoking exposure in adults and chronic respiratory symptoms (SAPALDIA Study). Am J Resp Crit Care Med 1994; 150:1222–1228.

57. Eisner MD, Yelin EH, Henke J, Shiboski SC, Blanc PD. Environmental tobacco smoke and adult asthma. The impact of changing exposure status on health outcomes. Am J Resp Crit Care Med 1998; 158:170–175.

58. Jindal SK, Gupta D, Singh A. Indices of morbidity and control of asthma in adult patients exposed to environmental tobacco smoke. Chest 1994; 106:746–749.

59. Flodin U, Jönsson P, Ziegler J, Axelson O. An epidemiologic study of bronchial asthma and smoking. Epidemiol 1995; 6:503–505.

60. Samet JM, Lewitt EM, Warner KE. Involuntary Smoking and Children's Health. Critical Health Issues for Children and Youth 1994; 4(3):94–114.

61. Jarvis MJ, Russell MA, Feyerabend C, Eiser JR, Morgan M, Gammage P, Gray EM. Passive exposure to tobacco smoke: saliva cotinine concentrations in a representative population sample of nonsmoking schoolchildren. Br Med J (Clin Res Ed) 1985; 85:927–929.

62. Strachan DP, Jarvis MJ, Feyerabend C. Passive smoking, salivary cotinine concentrations, and middle ear effusion in 7 year old children. Br Med J 1989; 298(6687):1549–1552.

63. Cook DG, Whincup PH, Jarvis MJ, Strachan DP, Papacosta O, Bryant A. Passive exposure to tobacco smoke in children aged 5–7 years: Individual, family, and community factors. Br Med J 1994; 308:384–389.

64. Comstock GW, Lundin FE. Parental smoking and perinatal mortality. Am J Obstet Gynecol 1967; 98(5):708–718.

65. Lindbohm ML, Sallmen M, Hemminki K, Taskinen H. Paternal occupational lead exposure and spontaneous abortion. Scand J Work Environ Health 1991; 17:95–103.

Major Risk Factors According to Age: The Relevance of Indoor Allergens to the Increase in Asthma

Thomas AE Platts-Mills*

Keywords: Asthma, risk factors, children, dust mites, cats, cockroach, RSV, rhinovirus

It has been clear for the last 20 years that sensitization to dust mite allergens is a major risk factor for asthma. More recently, evidence that animal dander and the German cockroach are also important sources of allergens has come from several parts of the world. The strength of these associations suggests that there must be a causal relationship between these allergens and asthma. However, there is a real question whether the change has been an increase in allergy of which increasing asthma is a part – or an increase in the percentage of allergic individuals who wheeze. Analyses of the causes of the increase need to consider not only those factors that could have increased the expression of the atopic response, i. e., Th2 and IgE, but also the range of lifestyle changes that could have increased the expression of asthma among allergic individuals.

Introduction

Over the last 40 years of the 20th century, some remarkable changes have occurred in the prevalence and severity of allergic disease [1]. Under-standing the reasons for the increases is important both in terms of management but also in understanding the etiology of the diseases. In the UK and Germany the published studies suggest that the increase in asthma is part of an overall increase in skin test reactivity [2] or of allergic disease [3]. By contrast, in the USA there is little evidence for an increase in hayfever over the last 30 years, and it appears that there has been a selective rise in asthma (Table 1) [4, 5]. Similarly, in comparing Guang Chou in Southern China with Hong Kong, Leung and his colleagues found very similar prevalence of skin test reactivity, but a much higher (and increasing) prevalence of asthma in Hong Kong [6]. A general rise in allergic disease could be explained by an increase in immune responses of the Th2 type. By contrast, a selective rise in asthma would best be explained by either an increase in an exposure that selectively effects the lungs or by a progressive loss of some factor that protects the lungs from wheezing.

When Coca first coined the term "atopic" he included those diseases in which a family history and positive skin tests were common, i. e., atopic

Table 1. The prevalence of allergic rhinitis in the United States: When did the increase occur?

Date	Authors	Site	Allergic Dis. Prevalence	Rhinitis
1924	Spain and Cooke	New York	3.3%	
1930–34	Jimenez	Michigan	12.0%	
1937	Rowe	California	10–13%	
1932–50	Ratner & Silberman	New York	10–13%	
1954	Tips	Indiana	18.7%	
1959	Van Arsdale	Washington	16.7%	
1960	Mathews	Michigan	19.2%	(16.6%)
1962	Nagy & Settipane	Rhode Island	25%	(21.1%)
1997	Nathan et al.	USA	–	18.4%

Courtesy of Dr. Harold Nelson, who concluded: "There is no clear evidence of an increase in the last 30–40 years in the prevalence of allergic rhinitis in the US."

* Asthma & Allergic Diseases Center, University of Virginia, Charlottesville, VA, USA

Table 2. Sensitization as a risk factor for asthma (symptomatic BHR).

Country	Study	Dominant Allergen	Odds ratio	Pollen	Author
UK	Prospective	Mite (cat)	19.7**	n.s.	Sporik et al.[1]
NZ	Prospective	Mite (Asp.)	6.6**	n.s.	Sears et al.[2]
Sweden	Population	Cat, dog	3.9**	Birch*	Ronmark et al.[3]
Australia	School(s)	Mite	≥10**	n.s.	Peat et al.[4]
USA:					
Virginia	School(s)	Mite (cat, CR)	6.6**	n.s.	Squillace et al.[5]
Atlanta	Acute (ER)	Mite, CR	8.2**	n.s.	Call et al.[6]
Arizona	Prospective	Alternaria	**	n.s.	Halonen et al.[7]
NM	School	Cat, dog	6.2*	n.s.	Sporik et al.[8]

[1]N Engl J Med 1990; 323:502; [2]Clin Exp Allergy 1989; 19:419; [3]Respir Med 1998; 92:316; [4]AJRCCM 1996; 153:141; [5]AJRCCM 1997; 156:170; [6]J Peds 1992; 121:862; [7]AJRCCM 1997; 155:1356; [8]AJRCCM 1995; 151:1388
** p < 0.001

dermatitis, hayfever and extrinsic asthma. The allergens that are relevant to these diseases are now well defined. It is also clear that the different allergic diseases are associated with different groups of allergens. Seasonal rhinitis or hayfever is strongly associated with positive skin tests to allergens derived from pollens and outdoor fungi. By contrast in most studies the dominant allergens associated with asthma are present in the environment all year. In general, this means indoor allergens, e. g., dust mite, animal dander, cockroach; however, in several areas of the world the fungus *Alternaria* is also significantly associated with asthma (Table 2) [7–15]. Thus, the important characteristic of the allergens associated with asthma may be exposure for many months of the year rather than the site of exposure. Multiple different proteins and glycoproteins are involved including molecules which have diverse biological roles, and not surprisingly, many of the defined allergens have extensive homology with known enzymes [16]. While it is possible that enzymic activity plays a role in the immunogenicity of these proteins, there are several reasons for doubting this role. In general the putative enzymes have not been shown to have enzymic activity under the circumstances prevailing in the respiratory tract [17]. Most studies have not found any evidence that allergens have an effect on non-allergic individuals. At least two allergens, which are very important in asthma, have no homology with known enzymes: the Group 2 mite allergens (Der p 2 and Der f 2) and Fel d 1 from the cat. At this time the idea that enzymatic activity of allergens plays an important role in immunogeneity should be regarded as a hypothesis which still lacks direct support [18, 19]. The main characteristics of

an allergen are that they are immunologically foreign, freely soluble, and are inhaled repeatedly.

The Immune Response to Inhalant Allergens

In 1935 Cooke and his colleagues established that the serum of allergic individuals had two different kinds of antibodies, skin sensitizing antibodies and blocking antibodies. Subsequent studies established that the response includes IgG and IgA antibodies, as well as the IgE antibodies which bind to the high affinity receptor on mast cells and basophils. Once it became possible to study specific T cell responses, it was found that allergic individuals gave proliferative responses to purified allergens while most nonallergic individuals did not [20, 21]. Subsequent studies established that the allergen specific T cells were predominantly CD4+ and produced cytokines characteristic of Th2 cells [22, 23, 24]. In some cases it has been possible to clone allergen specific T cells from nonallergic individuals, and these were found to have a different cytokine profile [24]. This evidence has been taken as support for the view that the normal or nonallergic response to allergens is a Th1 response. Indeed, this argument has been taken further to argue that allergy represents an abnormal persistence of the neonatal Th2 response [25]. There are however major problems with accepting the view that normal individuals have made a Th1 response. First, inhalant allergens are not associated with delayed hypersensitivity skin test responses. Second, the *in vitro* T cell responses of nonallergic individuals to mite or cockroach allergen are generally very small (i. e., S.I. < 3) and are not comparable to those found with Th1 responses to tetanus, Trichophyton, Candida or PPD [26]. Third, there are no examples of the major indoor allergens (e. g., mite, cat or cockroach) giving rise to lung disease such as hypersensitivity pneumonitis that could be associated with a Th1 response. Finally, the antibody response in nonallergic individuals is not typical of a Th1 response; high titer IgG1 antibodies are unusual; precipitins to common allergens very rare; and many of the sera that have IgG antibodies also have IgG4 antibodies [27, 28]. The presence of IgG4 is significant because this isotype is dependent on Th2 cytokines. Vercelli and her colleagues have demonstrated that the expression of IgG4 is dependent on IL-4 [29]. An immune response that includes IgG4, with or without IgE, is probably dependent on a Th2 response. Although there may be T cells with a Th1 phenotype in some nonallergic individuals, these cells are not sufficient to give proliferative responses in most patients; and there are no DH skin responses, no precipitins and no disease typical of Th1. The correct conclusion is that in most cases the nonallergic state is either a nonresponse or a modified Th2 response.

Determinants of an Early Response

The human fetus is capable of making immune responses from the beginning of the third trimester. Indeed, there is clear evidence that some infants are allergic to food antigens when they are born or become allergic during the first few months of life. It is also possible that a response to inhalant allergens occurs in utero or infancy. However, the quantities of an inhalant allergen such as dust mite reaching the fetus must be very low indeed, and there is no consistent evidence to support the hypothesis. The most widely quoted phenomena is the proliferation of cord blood T cells in response to mite allergens in vitro [30, 31, 32]. While the exact significance of this response is not clear, the evidence available does not support the idea that this proliferation represents an immune response. Firstly, the response is transient and is not found at 6 months. Secondly, other groups find that the response is less common than originally described and that it has no predictive significance [33, 34]. Finally, the response

does not appear to be influenced by exposure of the mother. Thus, in Sweden mothers who are exposed to less than 1 fg Der p 1/g dust still have babies whose cord blood T cells divide when exposed to mite extract [31]. Some groups have reported evidence of antibody production to common inhalant allergens in early life. These results have been obtained using ELISA which is susceptible to nonspecific binding, and tends to over detect low affinity antibody [35]. Using radio immunoprecipitation assays there is no nonspecific binding from IgG, and because radiolabeled antigen is bound in the fluid phase it requires high affinity antibody [27, 36]. These assays can be modified to measure other isotypes including IgE and IgG4 [27]. In a prospective study in England most of the children had no detectable antibody before age 4 years. At age 2 years we could only identify one quarter of the infants who subsequently became allergic. After age 2 years the children who were going to become allergic developed IgG, IgG4, and IgE antibodies to Der p 1 in parallel [7, 27]. At present the hard evidence about the immune response to inhalant allergens does not support an event in utero or in early infancy and it is much more likely that the response occurs over the first 4 years. It is patently absurd to refer to universal sensitization to dust mite antigens in utero on the basis of the currently available evidence [37].

Sensitization of infants in utero would have to be influenced by the immune status of the mother, because passage of allergen across the placenta would inevitably be influenced by maternal antibody. In support of this concept it has been reported that the mother's history has more influence over the development of asthma in early childhood, than the father's history of asthma. However, this influence of the mother is only over early wheezing and not over allergic responses or asthma developing after age 4 years. At age 10–13 the parents have equal genetic influence over allergy and asthma.

Factors Influencing the Clinical Outcome

Given the strength of the epidemiological association between immediate hypersensitivity to indoor allergens and asthma, it is logical to assume that allergen exposure plays a role in the disease. In fact, there is a wide range of experimental evidence supporting the view that inhaled antigen is a contributor to the inflammation and symptoms of asthma, if not a primary cause of the disease [38]. The evidence can be focused in three areas:

- The association with sensitization to indoor allergens is very strong; has been consistently found in many parts of the world; and generally reflects the allergens found in the average house in the community [39].
- Bronchial provocation with allergen can produce immediate and late responses in the lung. Indeed, provocation of the lung with a relevant allergen is the best established method for recruiting eosinophils into the lung and producing a prolonged increase in BHR [40, 41].
- Moving patients with asthma away from their homes to sanitoria or hospital rooms has consistently resulted in decreases in symptoms and decreases in BHR [39, 42]. In addition, the controlled trials of avoidance that have achieved prolonged decreases in dust mite exposure in patients have also resulted in significant decreases in BHR [39, 43].

Although the evidence that allergens play a role in asthma is very convincing, it is an entirely different question whether increased exposure can explain increases in asthma occurring over a 40-year period. Increases in asthma have been associated with sensitization to dust mite, cat, cockroach and *Alternaria* allergens in different communities and in different parts of the world [7–15]. Changes in lifestyle have increased the amount of time spent indoors. In addition there have been many changes in houses that could have increased exposure to allergens, e. g., warmer, lower ventilation, increased furnishings. However, in order to explain the increase in asthma simply by increased exposure one would have to propose that multiple different allergens had increased in parallel. It seems unlikely that changes in mite, cat and cockroach allergens could have occurred in parallel, or that the changes have been sufficient to explain the scale of the changes in asthma.

The question then is what other changes in Western lifestyle could have increased allergic disease. At this point it becomes important to decide whether the increase in asthma has been part of an overall increase in allergic disease. An increase in allergic disease could be explained by a change in immunity. The possible explanations include: changes in diet; the introduction of broad spectrum antibiotics; increased vaccination in early childhood; decreased

infections overall; or decreased viral infections in early childhood. There are epidemiological studies supporting each of these possibilities, however none of them are supported by direct evidence that the changes can cause the disease. Furthermore, the odds ratios associated with these effects, i. e., 1.1–1.3, are not comparable to the odds ratios associated with sensitization to indoor allergens [44].

If, as we have argued earlier, the evidence is for an increase in wheezing among allergic individuals then the arguments are different. Increased wheezing could occur because of a selective insult to the lungs or because of the progressive loss of a factor that under normal circumstances protects the lungs from wheezing. The association between indoor exposure and asthma is well established. What is less well recognized is that indoor exposure is very uncommon as a cause of conjunctivitis. Thus, an increase in asthma with a decline in conjunctivitis might have occurred simply on the basis of spending more time indoors. Figures available from managed care organizations in the USA show that a large number of asthmatics are also being treated for rhinitis. However, it is not clear whether rhinitis has increased since 16% of the population reported rhinitis as early as 1960 (see Table 1).

The possibility that sedentary lifestyle is harmful to the lungs has received very little attention until recently [45]. Children today are spending as much as three hours per day in front of video screens, televisions and computers [46]. The evidence in the Surgeon General's report about increasing obesity in the USA is also best explained by decreased physical activity [47]. Luder et al. reported in 1998 that asthmatic children in New York are heavier than their counterparts in that city [48]. Thus, it appears that the decline in physical activity is at least as severe among those children who have asthma as it is in the community in general. Sedentary lifestyle could influence the lungs in several ways. It has long been recognized that full expansion of the lungs can decrease lung resistance, and that patients with spinal cord injuries have BHR. Skloot et al. have demonstrated that relatively short periods of time spent without taking a deep breath can make the lungs of a normal individual hyper-reactive to methacholine [49]. Recently, Fredburg and his colleagues in Boston have provided a mechanism for the bronchodilator effects of full lung expansion. They have shown that without regular extension smooth muscle will start to contract at a shorter length. They went further to speculate that a decline in spontaneous sigh rates would give rise to BHR

Table 3. Increase in asthma/allergic disease: Three hypotheses (from [17]).

- *Changes in housing and lifestyle* – including increased time indoors – have increased exposure to perennial allergens that are most likely to cause chronic inflammation in the lung.
- *Changes in Western society* – including antibiotic use, diet, and immunization – have altered immune responsiveness such that more individuals develop immediate hypersensitivity.
- *Changes in lifestyle over the past 40 years,* including the decline in physical activity have, not only influenced immune responsiveness and exposure to indoor allergens, but also lowered the threshold for wheezing.

---

[50]. Prolonged periods spent in any sedentary activity will decrease full expansion of the lungs. However, we have recently shown that spontaneous sigh rates are significantly lower while watching a screen compared to reading [51]. Thus, some passive visual activities might decrease sigh rates below a critical level. The alternative hypothesis would be that prolonged physical activity (such as children's play) is beneficial to the lungs either physiologically or via an effect such as accelerated healing of allergen-induced inflammation [17]. Clearly direct experiments on the effects of exercise on the lungs of asthmatics are needed.

Conclusion

In some Western countries the increase in asthma is such that as many as three quarters of the children who are currently presenting for treatment would not have had symptoms in 1950. Given these figures it is clearly very important to identify the causes of the increase. The main theories can be divided into three types which may well overlap (Table 3). The most striking fact about the epidemiology is that sensitization to indoor allergens remains as strong a risk factor for asthma today as it was in 1970 when increases were first reported. Thus, it is obvious that the increase is primarily among allergic individuals. Nonetheless, increase in allergen exposure is not a convincing explanation of the progressive rise in asthma associated with so many different allergens. For this reason several theories have been developed about factors that could have increased immune responses or decreased the threshold for wheezing among allergic individuals.

In the United States asthma has increased as judged by treatment, national surveys, hospital admissions and mortality rates. The "epidemic" in the USA is striking because it is worst among individuals living in poverty, and particularly African Americans living in poverty [14, 15, 52]. In most other countries in the Western World asthma is not associated with poverty. In fact many of the theories proposed to explain the increase in wheezing in Europe and Australasia cannot explain what has happened in the American cities. Thus crowded and very poor housing remain common in the big cities; furthermore, vaccination rates are generally lower and infection rates are generally higher. The rise in obesity among children which is appearing in many countries, is most marked among poor children in the US. Thus, decline in physical activity has to be considered as a possible factor contributing to the severity of asthma in American cities. As we have seen this may interact with high exposure to allergens such as dust mite and cockroach and high levels of sensitization. While it is possible that risk factors for asthma in the USA are different from those in other countries, it seems more likely that the progressive increase in asthma that has occurred over the period 1960–1995 in so many communities has common causal elements.

Acknowledgments

This research was supported by NIH Grants AI-20565 and U19 NIEHS/NIAID-34607.

Address for correspondence:

Thomas AE Platts-Mills, MD, PhD
Asthma & Allergic Diseases Center
Box 225 HSC, University of Virginia
Charlottesville, VA 22908
USA
Tel. +1 804 924-5917
Fax +1 804 924-5779
E-mail NKM8T@virginia.edu

References

1. Woolcock AJ, Peat JK. Evidence for the increase in asthma worldwide. In Ciba Foundation (Ed), The rising trends in asthma. Chichester: Wiley 1997, pp. 122–139.
2. von Mutius E, Martinez FD, Fritzsch C, Nicolai T,

Roell C, Thiemann HH. Prevalence of asthma and atopy in two areas of West and East Germany. Am J Respir Crit Care Med 1994; 149:358–364.

3. Butland BK, Strachan DP, Lewis S, Bynner J, Butler N, Britton J. Investigation into the increase in hay fever and eczema at age 16 observed between the 1958 and 1970 British birth cohorts. Br Med J 1997; 315:717–721.

4. Broder I, Higgins NW, Mathews KP, Keller JB. Epidemiology of asthma and allergic rhinitis in a total community. Tecumseh Michigan. IV. Natural History. J Allergy 1974; 54:100.

5. Nathan RA, Meltzer EO, Selner JC, Storms W. Prevalence of allergic rhinitis in the United States. J Allergy Clin Immunol 1997; 99:5808.

6. Leung R, Ho P. Asthma and atopy in three southeast Asian populations. Thorax 1994; 49:1205–1210.

7. Sporik RB, Holgate ST, Platts-Mills TAE, Cogswell J. Exposure to house dust mite allergen (Der p I) and the development of asthma in childhood: A prospective study. N Engl J Med 1990; 323:502–507.

8. Peat JK, Tovey E, Toelle BG, Haby MM, Gray EJ, Mahmic A, Woolcock AJ. House dust mite allergens. A major risk factor for childhood asthma in Australia. Am J Respir Crit Care Med 1996; 153:141–146.

9. Sporik R, Ingram JM, Price W, Sussman JH, Honsinger RW, Platts-Mills TAE. Association of asthma with serum IgE and skin-test reactivity to allergens among children living at high altitude: Tickling the dragon's breath. Am J Res Crit Care Med 1995; 151:1388–1392.

10. Halonen M, Stern DA, Wright AL, Taussig LM, Martinez FD. *Alternaria* as a major allergen in children raised in a desert environment. Am J Resp Crit Care Med 1997; 155:1356–1361.

11. Perzanowski MS, Sporik R, Squillace SP, Gelber LE, Call R, Carter MC, Platts-Mills TAE. Association of sensitization to *Alternaria* allergens with asthma among school age children. J Allergy Clin Immunol 1998; 101:626–632.

12. Ronmark E, Lundback B, Jonsson E, Platts-Mills TAE. Asthma, type-1 allergy and related conditions in 7- and 8-year-old children in Northern Sweden: Prevalence rates and risk factor patterns. Resp Med 1998; 92:316–324.

13. Sears MR, Hervison GP, Holdaway MD, Hewitt CJ, Flannery EM, Silva PA. The relative risks of sensitivity to grass pollen, house dust mite, and cat dander in the development of childhood asthma. Clin Exp Allergy 1989; 19:419–424.

14. Call RS, Smith TF, Morris E, Chapman MD, Platts-Mills TAE. Risk factors for asthma in inner city children. J Pediatr 1992; 121:862–866.

15. Rosenstreich DL, Eggleston P, Kattan M, Baker D, Slavin RG, Gergen P, Mitchell H, McNiff-Mortimer K, Lynn H, Ownby D, Malveaux F. The role of cockroach allergy and exposure to cockroach allergen in causing morbidity among inner-city children with asthma. N Engl J Med 1997; 336:1356–1363.

16. Stewart GA, Thompson PJ. The biochemistry of common aeroallergens. Clin Exp Allergy 1996; 26:1020–1044.

17. Platts-Mills TAE, Wheatley LM, Aalberse RC. Indoor versus outdoor allergens in allergic respiratory disease. Curr Op Immunol 1998; 10:634–639.

18. Hewitt CRA, Brown AP, Hart GD, Pritchard DI. A major house dust cleaving CD23. J Exp Med 1995; 182:1537–1544.

19. Schultz O, Sewell HF, Shakib F. Proteolytic cleavage of CD-25 by Der p 1, a major mite allergen with cysteine protease activity. J Exp Med 1998; 187:271–275.

20. Black PL, Marsh DG. Correlation between lymphocyte responses and immediate hypersensitivity to purified allergens. J Allergy Clin Immunol 1980; 66:394–401.

21. Rawle FC, Mitchell EB, Platts-Mills TAE. T cell responses to the major allergen from the house dust mite *Dermatophagoides pteronyssinus*, Antigen P1: comparison of patients with asthma, atopic dermatitis, and perennial rhinitis. J Immunol 1984; 133:195–201.

22. O'Hehir RE, Garman RD, Greenstein JL, Lamb JR. The specificity and regulation of T-cell responsiveness to allergens. Ann Rev Immunol 1991; 9:67–95.

23. Romagnani S. Regulation of the development of type 2 T-helper cells in allergy. Curr Opin Immunol 1994; 6:838–846.

24. Wierenga EA, Snoek M, DeGroot C, Chretien I, Bos JD, Jansen HM, Kapsenberg ML. Evidence for compartmentalization of functional subsets of $CD4^+$ lymphocytes in atopic patients. J Immunol 1990; 144:4651–4656.

25. Holt PG, Sly PD, Bjorksten B. Atopic versus infectious diseases in childhood: A question of balance. Pediat Allergy Immunol 1997; 8:53–58.

26. Slunt JB, Taketomi EA, Woodfolk JA, Hayden ML, Platts-Mills TAE. The immune response to Trichophyton tonsurans: distinct T cell cytokine profiles to a single protein among subjects with immediate and delayed hypersensitivity. J Immunol 1996; 157:5192–5197.

27. Rowntree S, Platts-Mills TAE, Cogswell JJ, Mitchell EB. A subclass IgG4-specific antigen-binding radioimmunoassay (RIA). J Allergy Clin Immunol 1987; 80:622–630.

28. Blumenthal KB, Hochmair MJ, Gold D, Platts-Mills TAE. Monitoring of isotype specific antibodies in mothers and children from Boston, Massachusetts. J Allergy Clin Immunol 1999; 103:S244.

29. Vercelli D, De Monte L, Monticelli S, Di Bartolo C, Agresti A. To E or not to E: Can an IL-4-induced B

cell choose between IgE and IgG4? Int Arch Allergy Immunol 1998; 116:1–4.

30. Miles EA, Warner JA, Jones AC, Colwell BM, Bryant TN, Warner JO. Peripheral blood mononuclear cell proliferative responses in the first year of life in babies born to allergic parents. Clin Exp Allergy 1996; 26:780–788.

31. Bjorksten B, Holt BJ, Baron-Hay MJ, Munir AKM, Holt PG. Low level exposure to house dust mites stimulates T cell responses in early childhood independant of atopy. Clin Exp Allergy 1996; 26:775–779.

32. Prescott SL, Macaubas C, Holt BJ, Smallacombe TB, Loh, R, Sly PD, Holt PG. Transplacental priming of the human immune system to environmental allergens: universal skewing of initial T-cell responses toward the Th-2 cytokine profile. J Immunol 1998; 160:4730–4737.

33. Becker AB. Personal communication.

34. Smillie FI, Elderfield AJ, Cain G, Patel FY, Tavernier G, Brutsche M, Simpson B, Simpson A, Custovic A, Woodcock AA. Cord blood lymphoproliferative responses in neonates with defined atopic risk and maternal indoor allergen exposure. J Allergy Clin Immunol 1999; 103:S109.

35. Mariani R, Price JF, Kemeny DM. The IgG subclass antibody response to an inhalant antigen *(Dermatophagoides pteronyssinus)* during the first year of life. Clin Exp Allergy 1992; 22:29–33.

36. Platts-Mills TAE. Local production of IgG, IgA and IgE antibodies in grass pollen hay fever. J Immunol 1979; 122:2218–2225.

37. Prescott SL, Macaubas C, Smallacombe T, Holt BJ, Sly PD, Loh R, Holt PG. Reciprocal age-related patterns of allergen-specific T-cell immunity in normal vs atopic infants. Clin Exp Allergy 1998; 28:39–49.

38. Sporik RB, Chapman MD, Platts-Mills TAE. House dust mite exposure as a cause of asthma (Editorial). Clin Exp Allergy 1992; 22:897–906.

39. Platts-Mills TAE, Vervloet D, Thomas WR, Aalberse RC, Chapman MD (Co-chairmen). Indoor allergens and asthma. Third International Workshop. Cuenca Spain. J Allergy Clin Immunol 1997;100:S1–S24.

40. Calhoun WJ, Dick EC, Schwartz LB, Busse WW. A common cold virus, rhinovirus 16, potentiates airway inflammation after segmental antigen bronchoprovo-

cation in allergic subjects. J Clin Invest 1994; 94:2200–2208.

41. Cockcroft DW, Ruffin RE, Dolovich J, Hargreave FE. Allergen-induced increase in nonallergic bronchial reactivity. Clin Allergy 1977; 7:503–513.

42. Platts-Mills TAE, Tovey ER, Mitchell EB, Moszoro H, Nock P, Wilkins SR. Reduction of bronchial hyperreactivity during prolonged allergen avoidance. Lancet 1982; 2:675–678.

43. Platts-Mills TAE, Chapman MD, Wheatley LM. Control of house dust mite in managing asthma: Conclusions of meta-analysis were wrong (Letter to Editor). Br Med J 1999; in press.

44. Peak JK. Can asthma be prevented? Evidence from epidemiological studies of children in Australia and New Zealand in the last decade. Clin Exp Allergy 1998; 28:261–265.

45. Platts-Mills TAE, Sporik RB, Chapman MD, Heymann PW. The role of domestic allergens. In Chadwick DJ, Cardew G (Eds), Rising trends in allergy. Chichester, UK: Wiley 1997, pp. 173–189.

46. Gortmacher SL, Must A, Sobol AM, Peterson K, Colditz GA, Dietz WH. Television viewing as a cause of increasing obesity among children in the United States. Arch Ped Adol Med 1996; 150:356–362.

47. Digest of Educaiton Statistics, Washington-US Department of Education, National Center for Education Statistics; 1996. NOES 96–133. [US Government Printing Office]; 64.

48. Luder E, Melink TA, DiMaio M. Association of being overweight with Hispanic children. J Pediat 1998; 132:699–703.

49. Skloot G, Permutt S, Togias A. Airway hyperresponsiveness in asthma. J Clin Invest 1995; 96:2393–2403.

50. Fredberg JJ, Inouye DS, Mijailovich SM, Butler JP. Perturbed equilibrium of myosin binding in airway smooth muscle and its implications in bronchospasm. AJRCCM 1999; in press.

51. Hark WT, Thompson WM, McLaughlin T, Platts-Mills TAE. The influence of behavior on resting sigh and respiratory rates in normal and asthmatic subjects. J Allergy Clin Immunol 1998; 101:S183.

52. Lang DM, Polansky M. Patterns of asthma mortality in Philadelphia from 1969 to 1991. N Engl J Med 1994; 331:1542–1546.

Sinusitis in Children

Charles K Naspitz*

Keywords: Sinusitis, rhinitis, asthma, bronchial hyperresponsiveness, antibiotics

Physicians caring for children must recognize that children do indeed develop acute and chronic infections of their sinuses with signs and symptoms that may be quite different from those of adults. The lack of classical signs and symptoms of sinusitis in children, particularly in the very young, is well recognized. Acute sinusitis occurs as a complication of approximately 0.5% of common colds. If one considers that children have an average of six to eight colds a year, sinusitis may be regarded as a frequently encountered disease. The paranasal sinuses appear radiologically at different age periods in children, and it is important to note that there is much variation in the shape and size of the sinuses at all ages. The pathogenesis of sinusitis usually involves blockage of the ostia, which can be initiated by infection, allergy, structural abnormalities, or any edema of the nasal mucosa. The most commonly found pathogens of sinusitis in children are similar to those found in adults. The diagnosis of sinusitis is based on a clinical history, physical examination, laboratory results, and imaging studies. Standard radiographs are still the most frequently used radiologic modality for evaluating sinus disease. However, computed tomography is the gold standard for the precise delineation of inflammatory sinus disease. Sinusitis in children is associated with allergic rhinitis and/or asthma. In asthmatic children, there is an improvement of asthmatic symptoms and pulmonary function following diagnosis and optimal treatment of concomitant sinusitis.

Without question, symptoms related to the upper respiratory tract are the most frequent ones affecting children. Children all over the world experience the common cold, allergy, and infections of the ears, nose, throat, or sinuses and regularly seek medical attention for these conditions. In most cases the symptoms are treated without firm determination of the etiology of the problem. In chronic or recurrent cases more attention should be given to making the diagnosis with respect to the causative agent in order that more effective and (hopefully) long-lasting results can be attained.

The influence of the developing child on the pathophysiology of the upper airway has more than simply academic interest; it is the essence of establishing a patient-specific diagnostic and management plan for a variety of disorders that affect children. In order to gain a better perspective on the interaction of the dynamics of a growing child and the presentation of many of these disorders, it is necessary to clearly establish the growth and development patterns of the anatomy and physiology of the normal child and to delve from there into the questions of the pathophysiological state.

Acute sinusitis occurs as a complication of approximately 0.5% of all common colds. If one considers that children on average have six to eight colds per year, sinusitis may be considered a frequently encountered disease. It is a disease associated with infection of the paranasal sinuses, occlusion of the sinus ostia, and inflammation of the sinus and nasal mucosa. Symptoms such as purulent rhinorrhea and nasal congestion overlap with those of various forms of rhinitis or occur in conjunction with rhinitis. However, the lack of signs and symptoms of sinusitis in children, particularly in the very young, is well recognized [1].

The true prevalence of sinusitis in children is unknown, but it closely parallels the incidence of acute infections of the upper respiratory tract. However, sinusitis has also been described in association with allergic rhinitis as well as asthma; the possibility of a recurrent or persistent sinusitis associated with perennial allergic rhinitis should also be considered [2]. In the United States, sinusitis develops in approximately 31 million individuals each year. An average of 4 days are lost from work each year because of acute sinusitis [3]. Overall health-care expenditures attributable to sinusitis in the United States in 1996 were estimated at $5.8 billion, of which $1.8 billion (31%) was for

* Division of Allergy, Clinical Immunology and Rheumatology, Department of Pediatrics, Federal University of São Paulo, Brazil

children 12 years or younger. This economic burden is quite significant and may in fact lie too low [4].

There is no universally accepted classification of asthma, but commonly used terminology is:

- *Acute sinusitis* – Symptoms lasting for 3 to 4 weeks consisting of some or all of the following: persistent symptoms of an upper respiratory infection, purulent rhinorrhea, postnasal drainage, anosmia, nasal congestion, facial pain, headache, fever, and cough.
- *Chronic sinusitis* – Symptoms lasting for 3 to 8 weeks or longer of varying severity consisting of the same symptoms as seen in acute sinusitis.
- *Recurrent sinusitis* – three or more episodes of acute sinusitis per year. Patients with recurrent sinusitis may be infected by different organisms at different times [3].

The paranasal sinuses encompass the paired air-containing cranial cavities that develop as outpouchings of the nasal mucosa. The ethmoid and maxilary sinuses first appear radiologically as air-filled spaces between the 3rd and 12th months of life. The frontal bone is not pneumatized until the first or second year of life, assuming its definitive shape by the third year and become radiologically visible between years 3 and 6. The sphenoids, which form about the third year of life, do not appear radiographically until the ninth year. It is important to note that there is much variation in the shape and size of the sinuses at all ages. The normal physiology of the sinuses resembles that of the adjacent nasal respiratory structures (pseudostratified ciliated columnar cells interspersed with goblet cells). Secretions are a mixture of viscid mucus from the seromucous gland and watery secretions from the anterior serous glands. The adhesive properties of mucus and the strength and constant beating of the cilia are such that bacteria usually cannot penetrate to the epithelium. However, the protective mucous layer is less effective against viruses. Lactoferrin, interferon, and secretory IgA are present in the mucosal secretions and form an important part of the local mechanisms of defence [2]. The role of cytokines in infectious sinusitis helps in the understanding the pathomechanics of inflammation, especially in chronic sinusitis and nasal polyposis, which is crucial for further success in disease treatment [5].

The pathogenesis of sinusitis usually involves blockage of the ostia. The blockage of the ostia can be initiated by infection, allergy, structural abnor-

malities, or any edema of the nasal mucosa, which impede ventilation and appropriate drainage of the sinuses and lead to mucous impaction and decreased oxygenation in the sinus cavities. Regeneration of the mucosa is usually prompt and the outcome is benign. However, when acute sinusitis is not resolved but becomes chronic, the epithelial lining may be irreversibly damaged. This may lead to thickening of the mucosa and the development of mucoceles or polyps [2, 3].

In acute sinus disease, viral upper respiratory infections (rhinovirus, adenovirus, influenza type A, and parainfluenza virus) frequently precede bacterial superinfection. The most commonly found pathogens of sinusitis in children are similar to those found in adults. The predominant organisms in two-thirds of acute sinusitis infections are *Streptococcus pneumoniae, Haemophilus influenzae*, and *Moraxella catarrhalis*. In addition to the organisms mentioned above, the most common organisms in chronic sinusitis are *Pseudomonas aeruginosa*, Group A streptococcus, and *Staphylococcus aureus*, as well anerobes such as *Bacteroides* spp. and *Fusobacteria*. In children, there are reports of fungal sinusitis caused by *Aspergillus, Mucor, Candida*, or other species [1, 2, 3, 6].

The diagnosis of sinusitis is based on a combination of clinical history with physical examination, and laboratory and imaging studies. A differential diagnosis [7] must be considered to other conditions associated with chronic sinusitis: allergic rhinitis (often associated with asthma), anatomical abnormalities of the ostiomeatal complex, nasal anatomic variations, cystic fibrosis, immunodeficiencies, and, less commonly, ciliary dyskinesia and Kartagener's syndrome. Children may exhibit nasal congestion, purulent rhinorrhea, postnasal drainage, increased irritability, vomiting (mucus), and a prolonged cough, frequently with a more severe nocturnal component. In our experience, the history of asthma, presence of nasal purulent secretion, elevated blood eosinophils, and elevated serum IgE had a significant correlation with the presence of sinusitis [1].

Standard radiographs are still the most frequently used radiologic imaging means for evaluating sinus disease. There are many controversies in the interpretation of sinus x-rays in children, particularly regarding the relationship between radiologic abnormalities and bacterial infection. We evaluated children with chronic tonsillitis and/or adenoid enlargement without previous diagnosis of sinusitis. The maxillary sinus was punctured at adenoidectomy and/or tonsillectomy, and the aspirates were cultured. On the same day of the surgery, a radiograph was taken of the sinuses. *Streptococcus pneumoniae* was isolated from 67% of the patients whose x-rays showed complete opacified maxillary sinuses. Based on these results and the fact that sinusitis was not diagnosed either by the primary physician or by the ENT specialist, children with complete radiologic opacification of maxillary sinuses are treated with antibiotics, regardless of their clinical symptoms, in an effort to prevent the harmful complications of sinusitis in the pediatric group [1].

Computed tomography (CT) is the modality of choice in the preoperative evaluation of the nose and paranasal sinuses and is the gold standard for precise delineation of inflammatory sinus disease secondary to obstruction of the ostiomeatal complex, by revealing disease that does not appear on routine x-ray films [3]. However, because of the high cost of CT, in developing countries standard radiographs still remain the main imaging diagnostic tool.

Fiberoptic rhinoscopy permits more detailed examination of the anterior and posterior nasopharyngeal structures, such as sinus ostia, sphenoetmoidal recess, and eustachian tube ostia.

Laboratory evaluation is mainly used for differential diagnosis of recurrent sinusitis, including nasal cytology, quantitative sweat chloride determination, tests for immunodeficiency and ciliary tests.

Sinusitis in children can also be associated with allergic rhinitis, which commonly precedes the development of chronic or recurrent sinusitis. This IgE-mediated hypersensitivity disorder of the nasal mucous membrane causes edema, increased production of seromucous secretions, and interruption of normal mucociliary clearance leading to retention of mucopurulent secretions within the sinus cavities. The prevalence of allergic rhinitis is around 30% in the pediatric population [8]. Evidence of allergic rhinitis has been found in 25% to 70% of young patients with chronic sinusitis [9]. Because of the close relationship between allergic rhinitis and sinusitis, especially patients with chronic or recurrent sinusitis should have an allergy evaluation. Once the atopic state and allergen(s) have been defined, the management of allergic rhinitis includes environmental control, pharmacologic treatment, and, if necessary, immunotherapy. The reduction of the inflammation and swelling that compromises the sinus ostia may help in the control

of the concomitant sinusitis [10]. Recently, the role of allergy in sinus disease was extensively reviewed [11].

For many years the association between sinusitis and asthma has been described. At the beginning of this century, several studies described the incidence of sinusitis in asthmatic patients as varying between 12% and 90%. Later it was believed that sinusitis reflected only broader changes of the respiratory tract, so that management of sinusitis would have little effect on the course of lower respiratory tract disease [9, 12]. Children with asthma showed remarkable improvement of asthmatic symptoms and pulmonary function after the diagnosis and treatment of concomitant sinusitis [2]. Sinus surgery in patients with asthma has also been shown to bring about improvement in lower airway disease [9]. On the other hand, it can be said that sinusitis and asthma merely coexist and represent different end products of the same inflammation occurring in different organ systems. The most common mechanisms proposed to explain the relationship between asthma and sinusitis are sinonasobronchial reflex; inhalation of cold, dry air; aspiration of nasal secretions; cellular and soluble mediators; and diminished β-agonist responsiveness [2]. However, no direct causal factor has yet been found.

To help to decipher whether sinusitis and asthma are independent manifestations of the same disease, we studied the effect of clinical therapy for sinusitis in atopic children with concomitant rhinitis and/or asthma. (Sinusitis was defined as a complete radiological opacification of the maxillary sinuses.) Methacholine PC_{20} was determined before and 30 days after clinical treatment. Sinus radiographs were also repeated. The improvement of bronchial hyperresponsiveness was observed only in patients with rhinitis and asthma with opacified maxillary sinuses at entry and who had normal sinus radiographs at 30 days. In asthmatic patients, infection/inflammation in the maxillary sinuses may contribute to heightened bronchial hyperresponsiveness, and the appropriate clinical treatment of the sinusitis is important. This might be true only for asthmatic patients, since there were no changes in the hyperresponsiveness of rhinitic patients with sinusitis but without asthma. On the basis of these results, we recommend that the presence of sinusitis be considered in children with asthma that is difficult to control despite optimal appropriate therapy, and who have associated significant upper airway symptoms. The presence of complete opacification of one or two maxillary sinuses justifies aggressive pharmacologic intervention, resulting in improvement in symptoms and bronchial hyperresponsiveness [12]. In a recent study of a group of asthmatics presenting to the emergency department with marked spirometric abnormalities and significantly elevated nitric oxide levels, it was shown that 42% had CT evidence of severe sinusitis that had gone unrecognized by the treating ED physician. This study demonstrates the need to consider examining all severe asthmatics for sinusitis and to consider additional therapy based on the results [13]. Another recent study showed that the mean total asthma costs during a 1-year follow-up were $415 for patients with a history of sinusitis vs. $316 for those without. These findings underscore both the high prevalence of sinusitis in patients with asthma and the importance of jointly managing diseases of the upper and lower airways [14].

Antibiotics are the primary therapy for bacterial sinusitis in the management of sinusitis. In acute or chronic sinus disease, the most common bacteria observed are polysaccharide-encapsulated organisms. In patients with uncomplicated disease, amoxicillin alone or associated with clavulanate is a reasonable choice. Another excellent drug for initial therapy is sulfamethoxazole-trimethoprim (SMX-TMP), especially in developing countries. The drug has an adequate antimicrobial spectrum and is inexpensive. Second- and third-generation cephalosporins, erythromycin analogs, such as azithromycin and clarithromycin, are also available as suspensions and easily used in young children [3]. The choice of an antibiotic for the treatment of sinusitis depends on the physician's experience and the microorganisms predominant in the region. The duration of treatment is not well defined. Treatment for 14 days is usually adequate for most children with acute sinusitis. Chronic sinusitis generally requires prolonged antibiotic treatment (3 to 6 weeks). In children with chronic sinusitis and allergic rhinitis, the administration of an oral second-generation antihistamine associated to a decongestant might help in the management of sinusitis. Topical nasal steroids, as an adjunct to antibiotical therapy, are beneficial in treating both acute and chronic sinusitis. At times, a short course of oral prednisolone (3–4 days) may be useful to further promote decrease in nasal mucosal edema and encourage sinus drainage.

Recently, investigations on sinusitis suggest the involvement of leukotrienes in chronic sinusitis. Four patients with chronic sinusitis unresponsive to conventional therapy were treated successfully with leukotriene pathway modifiers. While these drugs are currently targeted for the treatment of mild to moderate asthma and possibly rhinitis, they may also play a role in the treatment of chronic sinusitis. Further randomized controlled trials are necessary [15].

The complex interaction of children with their environment, the interplay of allergens, irritants and infectious agents is clearly seen in childhood sinusitis and rhinitis. Physicians caring for children must recognize that children do indeed develop acute and chronic infections of their sinuses with signs and symptoms that may be quite different from those of adults.

Address for correspondence:

Prof. Charles K Naspitz
Rua Sergipe 634–13^A
01243-000 São Paulo, SP
Brazil
Tel. +55 11 256-8186
Fax +55 11 257-3738
E-mail cnaspitz@mandic.com.br

References

1. Arruda LK, Mimica IM, Sole D, Weckx LLM, Schoettler J, Heiner DC, Naspitz CK. Abnormal maxillary sinus radiographs in children: Do they represent bacterial infection? Pediatrics 1990; 85:553–558.

2. Friday GA, Fireman P, Sukanich A, Steinberg ML. In Naspitz CK, Tinkelman DG (Eds), Childhood rhinitis and sinusitis. New York: Marcel Dekker 1990, pp. 193–215.

3. Parameters for the diagnosis and management of sinusitis. J Allergy Clin Immunol 1998; 102:S107–S144.

4. Ray NF, Baraniuk JN, Thamer M, Rinehart CS, Gergen PJ, Kaliner M, Josephs S, Pung YH. Healthcare expenditures for sinusitis in 1996: Contributions of asthma, rhinitis and other airway disorders. J Allergy Clin Immunol 1999; 103:404–414.

5. Bachert C, Wagenmann M, Rudack C, Hopken K, Hillebrandt M, Wang D, van Cauwenberge P. The role of cytokines in infectious sinusitis and nasal polyposis. Allergy 1998; 53:2–13.

6. Gwaltney, JM. Microbiology of sinusitis. In Druce HM (Ed), Sinusitis – pathophysiology and treatment. New York: Marcel Dekker 1994, pp. 41–56.

7. Kaliner M. Medical management of sinusitis. Am J Med Sci 1998; 316:21–28.

8. Worlwide variations in prevalence of symptoms of asthma, allergic rhinoconjunctivitis, and atopic eczema. The International Study of Asthma and Allergies in Childhood (ISAAC). Lancet 1998; 351:1225–1232.

9. Slavin RG. Complications of allergic rhinitis: Implications for sinusitis and asthma. J Allergy Clin Immunol 1998; 101:S357–S360.

10. Dykewicz MS, Fineman, S. Diagnosis and manangement of rhinitis: Parameter documents of the Joint Task Force on practice parameters in allergy, asthma and immunology. Ann Allergy Asthma Immunol 1998; 81:512–513.

11. Pelikan Z. The role of allergy in sinus disease. Clin Rev Allergy Immunol 1998; 16:55–156.

12. Oliveira CAA, Sole D, Naspitz CK, Rachelefsky GS. Improvement of bronchial hyperresponsiveness in asthmatic children treated for concomitant sinusitis. Ann Allergy Asthma Immunol 1997; 79:70–74.

13. Peters EJ, Crater SE, Philipps CD, Murphy AE, Platts-Mills TAE. Occult sinusitis in patients with an acute exacerbation of asthma. J Allergy Clin Immunol 1998; 101:S253.

14. Huse DM, Russell NW, Kuriyama N. Weiss ST, Hartzl SC. Asthma treatment costs are increased in patients with sinusitis. Eur Resp J 1998; 12:49S.

15. Kukhta AL, Bratton DL, Chan KH, Wood RP, Langmack EL, Westcott JY, Wenzel SL, Liu AH. Leukotrienes pathway modifiers: Are they the newest line of therapy for chronic sinusitis? J Allergy Clin Immunol 1998; 101:S252.

Bronchopulmonary Dysplasia

Oliviero Sacco, Bruno Fregonese, Andrea Boscarini, Laura Fregonese, Donata Girosi, Emilio Pallecchi, Giovanni A Rossi*

Keywords: Lung damage, oxygen toxicity, pulmonary fibrosis, infants

Bronchopulmonary dysplasia (BDP), the most common chronic lung disease in infancy, is the result of lung injury and inadequate lung repair in infants who have experienced mechanical ventilation and oxygen therapy for respiratory failure at birth. The main pathogenetic events of BDP are oxygen-induced injury and inflammation, which increases lung microvascular permeability and reduces surfactant production and ciliary motility. The development of BDP is facilitated by immature defense systems against reactive oxygen species and low production of factors promoting lung differentiation. The most common radiologic findings in BPD are diffuse, fine infiltrates with or without emphysema. Physiologic abnormalities include increased total respiratory resistance, airways flow limitation, and reduced dynamic lung compliance, which in the most severe cases lead to ventilation-perfusion mismatching and hypoxia with or without hypercapnia.

The therapy of BDP is based mainly on respiratory management. Maintaining an adequate oxygenation can promote normal somatic and neurologic growth and avoid the development of permanent damage. Management of BDP with (a) diuretic drugs, (b) bronchodilators, (c) corticosteroids, and (d) vasoactive drugs has proved to be effective in some cases of BDP, even if no drug can be considered completely effective because of the complex nature of the disease.

Introduction

Bronchopulmonary dysplasia (BPD) is a syndrome characterized by oxygen dependence, radiographic abnormalities, and symptoms that persist beyond the fourth week of life in infants with respiratory failure at birth [1–3]. This disorder represents the most common chronic lung disease in infants and is thought to be the result of three interacting factors: lung immaturity, lung injury caused by oxygen

Table 1. Risk and pathogenetic factors leading to bronchopulmonary dysplasia.

– Lung immaturity
– Lung injury caused by oxygen radicals and mechanical ventilation
– Inadequate repair of the initial lung injury
– Immature defence mechanisms toward reactive oxygen metabolites
– Low production of factors promoting lung differentiation.

therapy and mechanical ventilation, and inadequate repair of the initial lung injury [2–4]. Facilitating factors aggravating the development of BDP include immature defense mechanisms toward reactive oxygen metabolites, and low production of factors promoting lung differentiation (Table 1).

Advances in neonatal-perinatal medicine have made it possible to lower the incidence of BPD in moderately premature babies (of 30–32 weeks of gestation); however, despite surfactant replacement therapy in premature infants with respiratory distress syndrome, BPD continues to be an important sequela of mechanical ventilation [5, 6]. In addition, since there has been an increase in the survival rates of premature infants of 25 to 28 weeks of gestation, more than 75% of patients with BPD belong to this very low birthweight group. Indeed, in these immature infants, even minimal exposure to oxygen and mechanical ventilation can lead to BDP [6].

Risk and Pathogenetic Factors

The key risk factor for the development of BPD is respiratory failure at birth, caused by any variety of factors, including lung immaturity and perinatal lung disorders. Because most infants with immature

* Divisione di Pneumologia, Istituto G. Gaslini, Genova, Italy

lungs have very low birthweights, the most important single predictive factor for the development of BPD is in fact birthweight [2–4].

Although the term "lung immaturity" is usually associated with incomplete development of the alveolar structures and with reduced functional activity of the surfactant system in type II cells, all components of the immature respiratory system can be underdeveloped at birth, and all may contribute to respiratory failure. Immature infants have a flail chest wall, incompletely developed respiratory control system, lower tone, and lack of coordination of respiratory muscles [7]. In addition, at 22 to 26 weeks of gestation, most of the lung capillaries are still embedded in mesenchymal tissue and show increased permeability to water and proteins. This can lead to pulmonary edema soon after birth, when pulmonary blood flow increases. This would explain why BPD continue to occur even in infants whose type II cells development has been accelerated by maternal corticosteroid treatment or in infants treated with surfactant replacement therapy [8].

In addition to lung immaturity, a second key pathogenetic factor in BDP is lung injury due to oxygen therapy and mechanical ventilation. It is nearly impossible to define a safe level or duration of oxygen exposure for infants with immature lungs. Indeed, even 21% oxygen (PAO2 ~ 110 mmHg) is relatively hyperoxic for the premature infant, whose *in utero* alveolar O_2 tension was less than 40 mmHg.

Although high concentrations of oxygen can be toxic for all lung cellular components (Table 2), the endothelial cells appear to be particularly vulnerable to oxygen-induced injury. Because intracellular oxidant production is markedly accelerated and antioxidant defenses are inadequate, oxygen-induced toxicity markedly increases lung microvascular permeability and the development of pulmonary edema [3]. In addition, the oxidant stress of acute oxygen exposure can disrupt normal lung development, interfere with surfactant production and ciliary motility, and cause oxidative inactivation of cellular antioxidants [4–6].

Long-term exposure to high concentrations of oxygen has other detrimental effects as well, including recruitment and activation of polymorphonuclear leukocytes, necrosis of bronchiolar epithelium and of type I cells, hyperplasia of type II cells and marked proliferation of fibroblasts and myofibroblasts in the lung interstitium. All of these pathologic features are present in infants with BPD [9].

Table 2. Oxygen-induced toxicity in bronchopulmonary dysplasia.

- Cytotoxicity to all lung parenchymal cells
- Increased lung microvascular permeability
- Development of pulmonary edema
- Decreased surfactant production
- Impaired ciliary motility
- Inactivation of cellular antioxidants and interstitial antiproteases
- Recruitment and activation of polymorphonuclear leukocytes

Finally, positive airway pressure of even a mild degree can augment oxygen toxicity by increasing PAO2 in previously unventilated alveolar units with low compliance. The immature lung can also be directly injured by the mechanical effects of positive-pressure ventilation and high tidal volume ventilation can increase lung microvascular permeability and edema formation [9, 10].

Airway Inflammation and Lung Damage and Repair

The intubated infant with respiratory failure is exposed to a variety of irritants that can induce an inflammatory reaction and alter the balance between inflammatory and antiinflammatory mechanisms within the lung. Neutrophil- and macrophage-derived inflammatory mediators have been proposed as prominent risk factors for the development of BPD. Neutrophils can produce and release oxygen species toxic to lung cells and proteases able to derange the intercellular matrix [11]. Bronchoalveolar lavage fluid from infants who will develop BPD contains elevated levels of neutrophil-derived proteases, reduced or inactivated antiprotease defenses [12] and high concentrations of proinflammatory cytokines and of vasoactive and bronchoactive metabolites [5, 12]. Leukotriene B4, the anaphylatoxin C5a, and interleukin-8, all important chemoattractants for neutrophils, have been detected in BAL fluid of such infants [13], and the expression of intercellular adhesion molecule-1 (ICAM-1) appears to be increased in airway secretion of premature infants who later develop BDP [14]. In addition, other proinflammatory mediators and substances with known effects on microvascular permeability can be detected within the airways of infant with BDP. These include IL-6, leukotrienes, prostacyclin, and platelet-activating factor (PAF) [13–16]. It has recently shown that elevation of IL-6 and IL-8 in tracheal aspirate precedes neutrophil influx in preterm infants who develop BDP, suggesting that these cytokines initiate the inflammatory cascade in the lungs [17]. Finally, in BDP lungs there are increased numbers of pulmonary neuroendocrine cells and neuroepithelial bodies, cells containing a variety of bioactive peptides, including bombesin-like-peptides (BLP). Since BLP exert mitogenic effects on epithelial cells and fibroblast and may play a role in lung growth and maturation, the involvement of these peptides in the pathogenesis of BDP has been suggested [18].

Morphologic Changes and Their Clinical Manifestations

On the basis of morphologic changes, BDP may be classified into four stages, as a function of post-injury days:
– Stage I, acute (2–4 days);
– Stage II, regenerative (4–8 days);
– Stage III, transitional (8–16 days);
– Stage IV, chronic (after 16 days) [2, 19].

Pathologic changes of the chronic stage include obliterative airway disease and interstitial fibrosis. Hyperexpanded units are present alongside fibrotic units and granulomatous nodules, concentric fibrosis, and polyps may cause tracheal or bronchial obstruction. In addition, muscular hyperplasia around pulmonary arteries and especially around bronchioles can be identified. However, all these abnormalities may be focal, and normal broncho-vascular anatomy may be seen in many lung regions [2, 19].

Cardiac involvement has been demonstrated in most infants with severe BPD. There may be evidence of myocardial ischemia or myocardial infarction, of left-sided and biventricular hypertrophy; myocardial fibrosis may also be present.

Clinically, tachypnea, dyspnea, and wheezing may be intermittently or chronically present. Inspiratory stridor due to subglottic stenosis or intratracheal scars may be present in infants who have been intubated for long periods. The chest wall may appear hyperinflated or flat, and digital clubbing is seen in the most severe cases. The most common

Table 3. Physiologic abnormalities in bronchopulmonary dysplasia.

– Increased in total respiratory resistance
– Severe flow limitation (especially at low lung volumes)
– Reduction in dynamic lung compliance
– Ventilation-perfusion mismatching
– Pulmonary vascular hypertension.

radiologic abnormalities seen in patients with BDP are diffuse, fine infiltrates with or without appreciable emphysema.

The major physiologic abnormalities are related to focal small airway narrowing due to edema, fibrosis, and muscle hypertrophy; they include increased total respiratory resistance, severe flow limitation (especially at low lung volumes) and reduced dynamic lung compliance (Table 3) [11]. The reduction in compliance results not only from small airway narrowing, but also from interstitial fibrosis, edema, and actelectasis. These abnormalities lead to an increase in the work of breathing and to ventilation-perfusion mismatching. Pulmonary vascular hypertension may also be present in infants with BPD: It is characterized pathologically by structural remodeling of pulmonary arterioles and by altered vasoreactivity. As a result of these abnormalities, hypoxia with or without hypercapnia is often present.

Most infants with BPD show improvement of pulmonary function with time, so that lung function is in the normal range by 2 to 3 years of age in a consistent proportion of patients. Whether this improvement represents repair of damaged lung or growth of new lung (or both) is not clear.

Therapy

The goals of respiratory management of infants with BPD are to maintain normal oxygenation avoiding the interventions that may increase the risk of further pulmonary damage or delay lung repair. Maintenance of adequate oxygenation is mandatory to promoting normal somatic growth and neurologic development, and to preventing the development of pulmonary vascular disease and right ventricular hypertrophy.

Positive-pression ventilation via endotracheal tube should be discontinued as soon as possible. Because of the difficulties involved in home care, risks of recurrent infections, accidental decannulation, and airway obstruction due to tracheal distortion, the decision to perform a tracheostomy in infants with severe BPD should be undertaken only for clear-cut indications. The value of chest physiotherapy in either ventilated or spontaneously breathing infants, although unproved, is probably useful. Despite meticulous care, approximately 10–30% of infants with BPD at 28 days of life die before discharge. The cause of death may be intercurrent respiratory infection or unexpected sudden death.

Because of the complex nature of the disease, there is no drug regimen that is likely to be effective in all infants with BPD. In addition, there is no simple relationship between improvement in lung mechanics and improvement in gas exchange. Pharmacotherapy in infants with BPD include the use of

- Drugs with diuretic properties,
- Bronchodilators,
- Corticosteroids,
- Vasoactive drugs.

Drugs with diuretic properties have been shown to reduce pulmonary edema and to improve gas exchange [20]. Diuretic therapy is used intermittently when symptoms of acute fluid intolerance occur and increased respiratory symptoms or oxygen requirements that cannot be explained by infection.

The rationale for bronchodilator therapy is based on short-term clinical trials showing that inhaled or parenteral β2-adrenoreceptor agonists and methylxanthines improve lung mechanics and gas exchange [21]. These drugs may also reduce lung edema, enhance mucociliary transport, and improve pulmonary blood flow. However, the physician should be mindful of their short duration of action, their cardiac side effects, and the possibility of rebound bronchospasm.

Corticosteroid therapy is perhaps the most controversial area of BPD care. Early reports have suggested improvement in pulmonary function, but they also show that incidence of bacterial sepsis and hypertension was higher than expected and long-term benefits could not be demonstrated [22]. The role of inhaled corticosteroid therapy has yet to be evaluated.

There has been an increased interest in the role of vasoactive drugs, such as nifedipine captopril and hydralazine, for the treatment of abnormal circulatory dynamics and gas exchange in infants with BPD. These drugs have been reported to be effective in some patients [23].

Acknowledgment

Supported by Grant "Ricerca Corrente" from Ministero della Sanità, Rome, Italy.

Address for correspondence:

Giovanni A Rossi, MD
Pulmonary Division
G. Gaslini Institute
Largo G Gaslini 5
I-16147 Genoa
Italy
Tel. +39 010 563-6547
Fax +39 010 377-6590
E-mail giovannirossi@ospedale-gaslini.ge.it

References

1. Shepard F, Gray J, Stahlman MT. Occurrence of pulmonary fibrosis in children who had idiopathic respiratory distress syndrome. J Pediatr 1964; 65:1078.
2. Stahlman MT. Medical complications in premature infants. N Engl J Med 1989; 1551:320.
3. Hazinski TA. Bronchopulmonary dysplasia. In Chernick V, Kendig EL (Eds), Disorders of the respiratory tract in children. Philadelphia: W. B. Saunders 1990, p. 300.
4. Taghizadeh A, Reynolds EOR. Pathogenesis of bronchopulmonary dysplasia following hyaline membrane disease. Am J Pathol 1976; 82:241.
5. Groneck P, Speer CP. Pulmonary inflammation in the pathogenesis of bronchopulmonary dysplasia. Pediatr Pulmonol 1997; Suppl 16:29.
6. Rojas MA, Gonzalez A, Banclari E, Claure N, Poole C, Silva-Neto G. Changing trends in the epidemiology and pathogenesis of neonatal lung diseases. J Pediatr 1995; 126:605.
7. Chang KN, Noble-Jamieson CM, Elliman A, Bryan EM, Silverman M. Lung function in children with low birthweight. Arch Dis Child 1989; 64:1284.
8. Wang JY, Yeh TF, Lin YJ, Chen WY, Lin CH. Early postnatal dexamethasone therapy may lessen lung inflammation in premature infants with respiratory distress syndrome on mechanical ventilation. Pediatr Pulmonol 1997; 23:193.
9. De Lemos RA, Coalson JJ, Gerstmann DR. Oxygen toxicity in the premature baboon with hyaline membrane disease. Am Rev Respir Dis 1987; 136:677.
10. Sadeghi H, Lowenthal DB, Dozor AJ. Inspiratory flow limitation in children with bronchopulmonary dysplasia. Pediatr Pulmonol 1998; 26:177.

11. Weiss SJ. Tissue destruction by neutrophils. N Engl J Med 1989; 320:365.

12. Merritt TA, Cochrane cG, Holcomg K, Bohl B, Hallman M, Strayer D. Elastase and a1-proteinase inhibitor activity in tracheal aspirate during respiratory distress syndrome. J Cin Invest 1983; 72:656.

13. Groneck P, Gotze-Speer B, Oppermann M, Eiffert H, Speer CP. Association of pulmonary inflammation and increased microvascular permeability during the development of bronchopulmonary dysplasia: A sequential analysis of inflammatory mediators in respiratory fluids of high risk preterm infant. Pediatrics 1994; 93:712.

14. Kotecha S, Chan B, Azam N, Silverman M, Shaw RJ. Increase in interleukin-8 and soluble intercellular adhesion molecule in bronchoalveolar lavage fluid from premature infants who develop chronic lung disease. Arch Dis Child 1995; 72:90.

15. Bagchi A, Viscardi RM, Tacia KV, Ensor JE, McCrea KA, Hesday JD. Increased interleukin-6 but not tumor necrosis-α in lung lavage of premature infants is associated with the development of bronchopulmonary dysplasia. Pediatr Res 1994; 36:244.

16. Stenmark KR, Voelkei NF. In Bancalari E, Stocker JT (Eds). Potential role of inflammation and lipid mediators in the pathogenesis and pathophysiology of bronchopulmonary dysplasia. Bronchopulmonary dysplasia (p. 59). Washington, DC: Hemisphere Publishing Corp. 1988.

17. Munshi UK, Niu JO, Siddiq MM, Parton LA. Elevation of interleukin-8 and interleukin-6 precedes the influx of neutrophils in tracheal aspirates from preterm infants who develop bronchopulmonary dysplasia. Pediatr Pulmonol 1998; 24:331.

18. Scher H, Miller YE, Aguayo SM, Johnson KJ, Miller JE, McCray PB Jr. Urinary bombesin-like peptide levels in infants and children with bronchopulmonary dysplasia and cystic fibrosis. Pediatr Pulmonol 1998; 26:326.

19. Toti P, Buonocore G, Tanganelli P, Catella AM, Palmeri MLD, Vatti R, Seemayer TA. Bronchopulmonary dysplasia of the premature baby: an immunohistochemical study. Pediatr Pulmonol 1997; 24:22.

20. Engelhardt BE, Elliott S, Hazinski TA. Short- and long-term effects of furosemide on lung function in infants with bronchopulmonary dysplasia. J Pediatr 1986; 109:1034.

21. Gappa M, Gartner M, Poets CF, von der Hardt H. Effects of salbutamol delivered from a metered dose inhaler versus jet nebulizer on dynamic lung mechanics in very preterm infants with chronic lung diseases. Pediatr Pulmonol 1997; 23:442.

22. Mammel MC, Green TP, Johson DE, Thompson TR. Controlled clinical trials of dexamethasone therapy in infants with bronchopulmonary dysplasia. Lancet 1983; 6:1356.

23. Brownlee JR, Beejman RH and Rosental A. Acute hemodynamic effects of nifedipine in infants with bronchopulmonary dysplasia and pulmonary hypertension. Pediatr Res 1988; 24:186.

Respiratory Manifestations in Children with Primary Immunodeficiencies

Magda MS Carneiro-Sampaio*, Dirceu Solé**

Keywords: Primary immunodeficiency, recurrent infections, asthma

The authors describe their clinical experience on recurrent respiratory infections in children with primary immunodeficiency diseases. They also discuss asthma as a manifestation of primary immunodeficiency and present some patients with asthma associated with humoral immunodeficiencies. The frequency of IgA deficiency (IgAD) among severe asthmatic children was 1:50 – that is 20 times higher than the frequency of IgAD among the general Brazilian population, according to the authors' data.

Upper and lower respiratory tract infections are the major clinical manifestations presented by children with primary and secondary immunodeficiencies. Patients with these diseases are usually recognized because they have (1) increased frequency of infections, sometimes without symptom-free intervals, (2) increased severity of infections, with unexpected complications, and/or (3) longer duration of infections.

Main Etiological Agents of Pulmonary Infections

Etiologic agents of pulmonary infections differ according to type of immunodeficiency (Table 1). In patients with antibody deficiencies, the most common agents are encapsulated bacteria such as *S. pneumoniae* and *H. influenzae*. These patients usually present with recurrent infections, which in most cases can be completely cured by treatment. Among patients with cellular or combined immunodeficiency syndromes, *P. carinii* and fungi are the microorganisms most frequently isolated from the lungs. Infections in these patients have a protracted course and may be resistant to the antibiotics commonly used in pediatric practice. In patients with neutropenias or functional phagocyte disorders, *S. aureus* is the major etiological agent of pneumonias, which may progress to pulmonary abscesses, pleural effusions, or pneumatoceles (Figures 1 and 2).

Table 1. Main etiological agents isolated from pulmonary lesions according to the type of primary immunodeficiency.

	Type of primary immunodeficiency			
	Predominantly antibody deficiencies	Cellular deficiencies	Neutropenias/ granulocyte dysfunctions	Complement deficiencies
Bacteria	*S. pneumoniae* *H. influenzae* *K. pneumoniae* *Pseudomonas* sp. *E. coli*	*M. tuberculosis* Atypical micobacteria BCG	*S. aureus* *S. marcescens* *Pseudomonas* sp. *E. coli* BCG	Capsulated bacteria
Virus	rare	Varicella-zoster CMV	rare	rare
Fungi	rare	*Candida* sp. *Aspergillus* sp. *H. capsulatum*	*Aspergillus* sp. *Nocardia*	rare
Protozoa	rare	*P. carinii*	rare	rare

* Department of Immunology, University of São Paulo (USP), Brazil
** Department of Pediatrics, Federal University of São Paulo (UNIFESP), Brazil

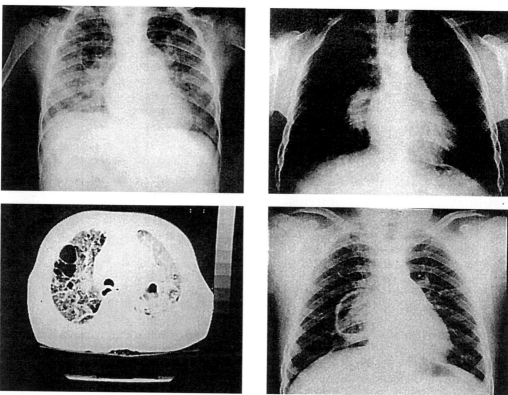

Figure 1. Chest X-ray (antero-posterior view) (top) and computed tomography (bottom) showing area of consolidation and pneumatoceles in a patient with chronic granulomatous disease.

Figure 2. Chest X-ray (antero-posterior view) of a patient with hyper IgE syndrome and pulmonary abscess before (top) and after (bottom) coughing up abundant amount of purulent secretion.

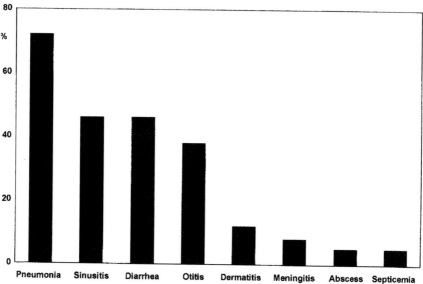

Figure 3. Frequency of infectious illnesses in 138 patients with primary immunodeficiencies followed at a referral center.

The images seen on chest X-rays or computed tomography may be helpful in selecting appropriate antibiotic treatment, if suggestive of a particular etiologic agent. However, in patients with severe infections, particularly those with a protracted course or with significant complications, one should attempt to identify the specific agent, even if invasive procedures need to be carried out, in order to guide adequate antibiotic choice.

Respiratory Manifestations of Primary Immunodeficiencies

Since the establishment of our center, we have diagnosed 161 patients with primary immunodeficiencies. In almost all of these patients, the reason for referral was the presence of recurrent or severe infections. Figure 3 shows the main clinical manifestations of infections reported by 138 patients; the respiratory manifestations were the most common, followed closely by gastrointestinal manifestations. Recurrent pneumonias were reported by 72% of the patients, sinusitis by 46%, otitis by 35%,

and chronic diarrhea by 46%. Manifestations of skin and other organs as well as very severe infections were present in a lower percentage of the patients. In keeping with what others have reported, our results could be explained by the fact that the most prevalent types of immunodeficiency in our series were the predominantly humoral deficiencies.

A detailed analysis of infectious respiratory illnesses associated with the primary immunodeficiencies we have diagnosed revealed that pneumonias were the most frequent. Among patients with familiar cyclic neutropenia, oral ulcers were the most frequent complaint, with pneumonias second in frequency, though less frequent than in other kinds of immunodeficiencies (Figure 4).

Deficiency of Antipolysaccharide Antibody Synthesis

In the last 4 years, we had the opportunity to follow 10 children 3–8 years of age, diagnosed with the syndrome of deficiency of antipolysaccharide anti-

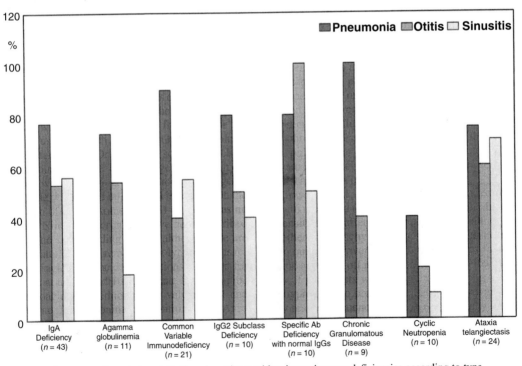

Figure 4. Frequency of respiratory infections in patients with primary immunodeficiencies according to type.

Table 2. Main recurrent infections observed in 10 patients with deficiency of antipolysaccharide antibody synthesis.

Recurrent infections	No. patients
Otitis media	10
Pneumonias	8
Sinusitis	5
Meningitis*	1

* 8-year-old boy presented 3 meningitis (*S. pneumoniae* was isolated twice and *H. influenzae* once)

Table 3. Serum levels of antipolysaccharide (PS) antibodies (mg/ml), against 6 pneumococcus serotypes, pre- and postvaccination, in a 4-year-old boy presenting with a history of numerous otitis media and two pneumonias in the year prior to diagnosis.

PS	1	3	5	6B	9V	14
Pre	0.3	0.1	0.2	0.3	0.1	0.2
Post	1.5	0.2	0.1	0.2	0.2	0.2

body synthesis with normal immunoglobulin levels. The diagnosis of these patients was based on the following criteria, adapted from Ochs and Winkelstein [1]:

1. Abnormal susceptibility to infections, as shown on Table 2, with predominance of manifestations of recurrent respiratory infections, mainly otitis media, seen in all cases [2] (Figure 4).
2. Normal serum levels of IgG, IgM, IgA, and IgG subclasses, compared to normal values for the Brazilian population.
3. Clearly demonstrated deficiency of antibody synthesis, based on the criteria recently proposed by Sorensen to define deficient synthesis of antibody to pneumococcal 23-valent polysaccharide vaccine. Adequate response to a given polysaccharide was considered to have occurred when there was at least a four-fold increase in post-vaccine antibody levels, measured 4 to 6 weeks after vaccination, in relation to prevaccine levels and/or when postvaccine antibody concentrations were equal or greater than 1.3 mg/ml [3]. Since this is a polyvalent vaccine, it is necessary to evaluate the response to each component as well as to the combined antigens. In children 2 to 5 years of age, we consider normal (according to the above criteria) a positive response to at least 50% of the antigens tested. Normal children 6 years and older should have a positive response to at least 70% of the polysaccharides tested. Response to six *S. pneumo-*

niae serotypes (1, 3, 5, 6B, 9V, and 14) in one of the patients is shown on Table 3.

Preliminary results from a survey of 120 clinically healthy children 6 to 144 months old who received the antipneumococcal polyvalent vaccine (Pasteur-Mérieux) revealed that the above criteria are suitable to distinguish a normal from an abnormal response.

Bronchial Asthma as a Manifestation of Immunodeficiency

Some conditions are frequently associated with immunodeficiencies, including autoimmune diseases and asthma. Regarding asthma, we found a frequency of 67.4% (29/43) among patients with IgA deficiency. In patients with common variable immunodeficiency, deficiency of antipolysaccharide specific antibody synthesis and IgG2 deficiency, asthma frequency approaches 20%, which is similar to the frequency in the general population (Figure 5).

The identification of this association is important because frequently the control of asthma can be achieved only after treatment of the associated immunodeficiency. As examples, we had three patients with primary immunodeficiencies (combined IgA and IgG2 deficiencies, common variable immunodeficiency and deficiency of antipolysaccharide specific antibody synthesis) who also had severe corticosteroid-dependent asthma. These patients could not control their asthma despite antiasthma therapy. Replacement treatment with IV immunoglobulin-promoted control of asthma, with total withdrawal of corticosteroids in two of the patients, as well as reduction in the number of infections.

Analysis of serum levels of IgG, IgM, and IgA in a group of 203 children with moderate to severe asthma revealed 4 patients with IgA deficiency, corresponding to a frequency of 1:50 (Figure 5) [9].

In the evaluation of patients with recurrent pneumonias (two or more episodes within the previous year), primary immunodeficiencies were found in up to one-third of the population studied. Some factors have been linked to the variations in prevalence, including age of the patients, inclusion

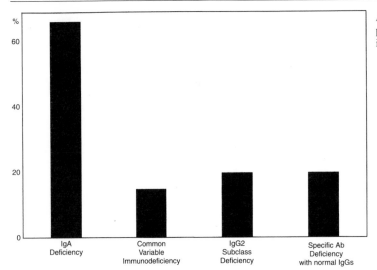

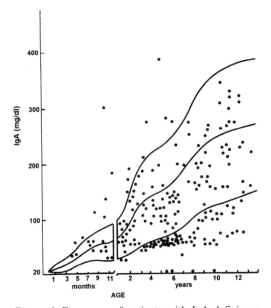

Figure 6. Frequency of patients with IgA deficiency among patients with moderate to severe asthma.

criteria, associated diseases, methods for laboratory investigation, and extent of diagnostic testing. Since the establishment of our center, 402 patients have been referred for investigation of recurrent infections, of whom 170 presented with two or more episodes of bacterial pneumonia. After appropriate immunologic work-up, primary immunodeficiencies were diagnosed in 93 of these patients (54.7%),

of whom 49 also presented with asthma (52.7%). On the other hand, among the 170 patients with recurrent pneumonia, 61.2% (104/170) had asthma, of whom 47% also had a diagnosis of primary immunodeficiency. Although asthma has been associated with primary immunodeficiencies, the evidence suggests that asthma has played an important role in the episodes of recurrent pneumonia. After appropriate asthma treatment, there was a better control of symptoms and a decrease in pulmonary infections. In our series, asthma was the most frequent cause of erroneous patient referral for evaluation of the immune system.

Are asthmatic patients more prone to developing recurrent infectious pulmonary illnesses than the normal population? In a case-control study of children with a mean age of 23.5 months, recurrent wheezing was documented as risk factor for the development of recurrent pneumonias [4]. In a prospective, longitudinal study in the UK that evaluated individuals from birth to 33 years of age, investigators assessed the incidence and prognosis of wheezing illness. The results demonstrated the association of asthma, wheezing illness, and pneumonia in children up to 7 years of age [5]. Other researchers have suggested that the decline of pulmonary function at adult age is a consequence of episodes of pneumonia during the first seven years of life – independent of personal history of wheezing. It is difficult to establish whether preexisting lower pulmonary function could play a role, being a cause instead of a consequence, of pulmonary infections in this case [6].

Viral infections are important triggers of acute exacerbations of asthma. Patients usually have elevations of body temperature, which prompts physicians to obtain a chest X-ray. The underlying inflammatory process associated with infection often determines production of thick mucoid secretion, which may become impacted in the bronchi and may be misinterpreted as pneumonia, leading to hospital admission of these patients [7]. In keeping with other authors' observations, we found a high frequency of patients with pneumonia diagnosed by the attending physician, among patients with acute attacks of asthma. These patients were kept under observation and only one of them required hospital admission for the treatment of infectious pulmonary illness [8].

We believe that further controlled studies will be necessary to conclusively establish the causal relationship between asthma and recurrent infectious pulmonary illnesses.

Address for correspondence:

Magda MS Carneiro-Sampaio
Department of Immunology
Instituto de Ciências Biomédicas da USP
Av. Prof. Lineu Prestes, 2415
05508-900 São Paulo, SP
Brazil
Tel./fax +55 11 818-7438
E-mail icbsedir@icb.usp.br

References

1. Ochs HD, Winkelstein J. Disorders of the B-cell system. In Stiehm ER (Ed) Immunologic disorders in infants and children (4th ed.). Philadelphia: W. B. Saunders Co. 1995, pp. 296–338.

2. Barros-Nunes P, Carneiro-Sampaio MMS, Costa-Carvalho BT, Naspitz CK, Solé D, Leiva L, Sörensen RU. Responses to pneumococcal immunization in patients with recurrent infections. J Allergy Clin Immunol 1997; 99(suppl):20.

3. Sörensen RU. Antigen specific antibody deficiency: Fact or fiction? American Academy of Allergy, Asthma and Immunology, 54th Annual Meeting, Washington 1998.

4. Pereira JCR, Escuder MM. Susceptibility of asthmatic children to respiratory infection. Rev Saude Publica 1997; 31:441–447.

5. Strachan DP, Butland BK, Anderson HR. Incidence and prognosis of asthma and wheezing illness from early childhood to age 33 in a national British cohort. BMJ 1996; 312:1195–1199.

6. Johnston IAD, Strachan DP, Anderson HR. Effect of pneumonia and whooping cough in childhood on adult lung function. N Engl J Med 1998; 338:581–587.

7. Roback MG, Dreitlein DA. Chest radiographs in the evaluation of first time wheezing episodes: Review of current clinical practice and efficacy. Ped Emerg Care 1998; 14:181–184.

8. Soares FJP, Solé D, Naspitz CK. Radiologia do torax em crianças com asma aguda. Rev Bras Alergia Imunopatol 1988; 11:4–9.

9. Solé, D, Carneiro-Sampaio, MMS, Naspitz CK. Níveis séricos de imunoglobulinas (G, A, M e E) em pacientes com alergia respiratória. Rev Assoc Med Bras 1985; 31:236–240.

Diagnosis and Treatment of Exercise-Induced Asthma

Kai-Håkon Carlsen*

Keywords: Exercise-induced asthma, children, sports, diagnosis, treatment

Exercise-induced asthma (EIA) is a frequent presentation in asthma and represents a major obstacle to normal daily activities in many asthmatic children. Mastering EIA is an important part of mastering asthma. Proper diagnosis is a requisite for correct treatment of EIA. There are several differential diagnoses that do not respond to the usual treatment for EIA. EIA is best diagnosed using a standardized exercise test with sufficiently high and precisely standardized exercise load. Cold air inhalation together with exercise may also increase the sensitivity of the test. Following up the patient and assessing the effect of prescribed treatment is also part of the diagnostic process. Exercise tests may also be used to monitor the effect of asthma treatment.

EIA is frequently seen in athletes, especially endurance athletes. Because there are reasons to believe that heavy training may increase airways inflammation and bronchial hyperresponsiveness, special considerations apply for treating EIA in athletes.

Optimal treatment of asthma usually represents proper treatment of EIA. Inhaled steroids improve EIA, but additional treatment before exercise is often needed. Inhaled short- and long-acting β_2-agonists are often the treatment of choice, but chromones have also been used with good effect, and now leukotriene antagonists may prove to be a useful choice. The efficacy of the prescribed treatment for EIA should be controlled by follow-up consultations and the treatment modified if needed.

Exercise-induced asthma (EIA) is a common presentation of asthma in children and adolescents, and is found in 70–80% of all asthmatic children and adults without antiinflammatory treatment [1]. EIA represents an impediment for asthmatic children in their daily play and activities, and it may reduce their self-confidence and self-esteem as children largely measure themselves by their success in physical activity and sports. A national American study reported that 30% of children with asthma suffered from limitations in their physical activity versus 4.5% in the overall pediatric population [2].

One main aim stated in the International Consensus for the treatment of asthma in children is the mastering of EIA [3]. EIA may also be considered a measure of bronchial hyperresponsiveness (BHR). The reduction in forced expiratory volume in one second (FEV_1) after a standardized exercise test may be employed as a measure of "indirect BHR" [4] – indirect because the exercise stimulus causes a release of mediators leading to bronchoconstriction. The reduction in FEV_1 after exercise may be used as a measure of the severity and activity of asthma.

The other connection between physical activity, BHR, and asthma is the frequent occurrence of EIA and BHR among elite athletes, reported especially in endurance sports [5]. Reports have focused especially on cross-country skiing [6, 7], but also among swimmers [8–10] and long-distance runners [11] has an increased occurrence of EIA and BHR been reported. It has been demonstrated that high-intensity training may increase BHR as measured by histamine inhalation [8]; Heir et al. [12] reported that BHR increased in young skiers during the competitive season in January and February. A relationship between BHR and training intensity was also demonstrated [13], as was the aggravating effect upon BHR by respiratory infections while training [14]. Frequently repeated high-intensity training may provoke asthma, especially when performed under unfortunate environmental conditions such as cold-air inhalation (cross-country skiing), chlorine inhalation (swimmers) [10].

Diagnosis of EIA

Good therapy must be based upon a well-conducted examination and diagnosis. Several differential diagnoses for EIA can be mentioned, including exercise-induced laryngeal stridor [15, 16] or

* Voksentoppen Children's Center and Research Institute of Asthma and Allergy, Oslo, Norway

hyperventilation. A diagnosis of EIA ought to be made before starting treatment. An exact clinical history, examination with lung function measurements before and after inhalation of a β_2-agonist, before and after a standardized exercise test such as treadmill run and/or a cold-air inhalation test and measurement of BHR by metacholine inhalation are all parts of the diagnostic process. The extent of diagnostic procedures employed varies from case to case, but one important part of any diagnostic process is to follow up on the patient to evaluate the treatment effect.

Exercise-induced bronchoconstriction may be diagnosed in different ways and by employing different sorts of exercise. In order to compare the results of testing between different individuals, and to compare results from the same individual at different times, it is paramount to standardize the test. Both tests with free running, step-tests, cycling, and running on a motor-driven treadmill have been standardized and used in the diagnosis of exercise-induced bronchoconstriction. Running provokes exercise-induced bronchoconstriction in children more easily than does cycling, because in most children the muscles used during running are usually better trained than the muscles used during cycling. Experience has shown that running on a motor-driven treadmill is particularly useful and easy to standardize. In our laboratory we use running on a motor-driven treadmill with submaximum load. The treadmill has an inclination of 5.5%, and during running the speed of the treadmill is gradually increased until a steady state heart rate of at least 170 beats per minute is reached. However, increased sensitivity of the exercise test was demonstrated by increasing the exercise load to a heart rate of at least 95% of the calculated maximum heart rate [17]. Maximum heart rate is calculated as follows: 220 – patient's age in years. The heart

rate can be measured electronically by devices such as the Sport-Tester PE 3000®. The child then runs for 6 minutes at this steady state. The running is performed with a room temperature of approximately 20°C and a relative humidity of ambient air of approximately 40% Lung function is measured before running, immediately after cessation of running, after 3 minutes, 6 minutes, 10 minutes, 15 minutes, and 20 minutes. FEV_1 is usually the lung function parameter employed, and a fall of 15% is most often used as a sign of exercise-induced bronchoconstriction. Some authors also use 10% reduction in FEV_1 from before and after exercise as a criterion of exercise-induced bronchoconstriction [18, 19]. The degree of bronchoconstriction after exercise may also bee assessed in other ways than by measuring the maximum fall in FEV_1 after exercise. Instead of calculating the maximum reduction in percent of baseline, the reduction in percent of predicted lung function may be assessed, thus taking into account also the baseline lung function. In addition, calculating the area under the curve when drawing the curve of lung function from before to after exercise may assess the bronchoconstriction, and also time to recovery [20]

In addition to diagnosing EIA, the reduction in FEV_1 after standardized exercise may be considered as a measure of nonspecific bronchial reactivity and used to evaluate the severity of asthma, as well as the effects of therapy. This measure of nonspecific bronchial reactivity is an indirect measure [4], as it is thought to work through the release of mediators [1]. It has been shown to correlate well to direct measures of bronchial reactivity, such as histamine or metacholine bronchial provocation [21]. Furthermore, it is a useful physiologic measure, as it reflects the effect of daily activities upon the asthmatic child.

Studies have shown that this test has a very high

Table 1. Comparison of sensitivity, specificity, positive and negative likelihood ratio (LR+ and LR–) in discriminating between asthma and other chronic lung diseases by bronchial responsiveness as measured by metacholine inhalation (PD_{20-M}), standardized exercise test by treadmill run (EIB), and combination of treadmill run and cold-air inhalation (EIB + CA). For metacholine responsiveness PD_{20}, values of 2 and 4 µmol are used as breaking points, for EIB and EIB + CA a reduction after exerise of 10% is used. Results are calculated from [24].

	Sensitivity	Specificity	LR+	LR–
PD_{20-M}				
(2 µmol):	47%	65%	1.34	0.82
(4 µmol):	82%	42%	1.41	0.43
EIB (ΔFEV_1: –10%)	48%	88%	4.0	0.60
EIB + CA (ΔFEV_1: –10%)	72%	72%	25.7	0.38

specificity for the diagnosis of asthma, but a rather low sensitivity when compared to histamine or metacholine bronchial provocation [22, 23]. If one adds an extra stimulus to the exercise test by combining running on a treadmill with the inhalation of dry cold air of –20°C, high specificity is maintained, and sensitivity is markedly increased [24]. By use of sensitivity, specificity, and positive and negative likelihood ratios (LR+ and LR–) it is possible to evaluate the usefulness of a diagnostic test. Table 1 shows how different measures of direct and indirect bronchial responsiveness are of different usefulness in discriminating between bronchial asthma and other chronic lung diseases in a group of children [24]. A LR+ above 10 is of almost certain diagnostic value, whereas values between 2 and 10 provide information about the overall condition. LR+ < 2 provide no important information. From Table 1 one can seen that a LR+ of 25.7 in the exercise cold-air inhalation test is diagnostically conclusive, whereas the exercise test has an LR+ of 4.0, giving important but not diagnostically conclusive information. On the other hand, PD_{20} metacholine gives us no diagnostic information in this aspect.

In many circumstances the availability of treadmills and other equipment used may be limited. A tentative diagnosis based upon case history and physical examination may be done without using exercise or cold-air provocation tests. When prescribing treatment, it is important to follow up on the patient and assess the effectiveness of the treatment. This has also diagnostic value.

General Therapeutic Measures

Both environmental measures, efforts related to training, as well as drug treatment belongs to the treatment strategies. Physical warming-up is among the general efforts related to training procedures. This is an important way of preventing EIA. Protection against cold-air inhalation is also important. Different equipment may be used, employing the principle of warm exchange. The expired air of 37°C warms up the inspired air. In common use in the Nordic countries are Jonaset®, Jonaset Sport®, and Lungplus®. In order to protect themselves from developing BHR, athletes should not perform endurance training or participate in competition

during ongoing viral respiratory infections or during cold-air temperatures.

Drug Treatment of Exercise-Induced Asthma

The medical drug treatment of EIA consists of premedication shortly before physical activity or training and prophylactic treatment. Prophylactic treatment consists mainly of antiinflammatory treatment. Furthermore, symptoms occurring through exercise must be treated.

Prophylactic Antiinflammatory Treatment

In order to master physical activity, the asthmatic disorder should be treated optimally to improve bronchial hyperresponsiveness and to maintain good control of disease activity. The usual guidelines for treating asthma should be followed. Antiinflammatory treatment is presently the cornerstone in treating asthma and is crucial in mastering EIA. Inhaled steroids are the most important treatment. Even after one week's treatment with inhaled steroids (budesonide) a marked reduction in EIA was observed in asthmatic well-trained athletes, as measured by the fall in FEV_1 after a standardized treadmill run [25]. The same was observed in asthmatic children 15 years ago [26], but in order to obtain a significant reduction of the fall in MEF_{25-75} (a measure of peripheral bronchial obstruction), further treatment of 3 to 4 weeks was necessary. It is also demonstrated that a more rapidly occurring effect by inhaled steroids is observed with EIA than with BHR, as measured by metacholine bronchial provocation. After 2–3 months' treatment with inhaled steroids, the anticipated improvement of EIA to be obtained is reached [19]. On the other hand, improvement of BHR, as measured by metacholine provocation, has been observed for up to 22 months [27].

Another treatment principle that is presently being introduced is the use of oral leukotriene antagonists. There are two main groups of leukotriene antagonists, leukotriene synthesis antagonists and leukotriene receptor antagonists. These drugs may reduce EIA. Following a single dose, leukotriene antagonists are significantly better than placebo against EIA [28]. The leukotriene antagonists have both an antiinflammatory and a bronchodilating

Table 2. Treatment principles of exercise induced asthma.

1) Environmental measures and advice on training etc.
2) Medical treatment
   a) Prophylactic (antiinflammatory) treatment
     i)   Inhaled steroids
     ii) Leukotriene-antagonists
     iii) Disodium cromoglycate (?)
   b) Pretreatment (before exercise)
     i)   Inhaled β_2-agonists
       (1) Short-acting
       (2) Long-acting
     ii) Disodium cromoglycate
     iii) Leukotriene antagonists
     iv) Ipratropium-bromide

effect. They have been shown to protect against exercise-induced asthma both in adults [20] and children [29] after use for several weeks. It is not clear how much the antiinflammatory aspect of leukotriene antagonists effect EIA and how much of a direct bronchodilating effect there is.

Another antiinflammatory asthma drug that has been used for many years is disodium cromoglycate (DSCG) as well the related, more recently introduced nedocromile sodium. Some studies report an improvement of BHR after the use of DSCG, whereas other studies do not confirm this finding [30]. The most often reported effect of DSCG and nedocromile sodium upon EIA is obtained when the drugs are taken before exercise [31].

Treatment Before Exercise

A number of different drugs may be taken before exercise to protect against EIA. The effect of these drugs should be evaluated by performing an exercise test or by a control consultation. If there is no effect, treatment should be adjusted or, especially if the diagnosis of EIA is based upon history alone, the diagnosis should be reconsidered. The therapeutic drugs mostly employed before exercise are inhaled β_2-agonists, DSCG, or nedocromile sodium and the more rarely inhaled ipratropium bromide [32].

Both DSCG and nedocromile sodium have been demonstrated to be useful in the pretreatment of EIA [31, 33, 34]. Taken within 15 minutes before physical activity, they reduce the decrease in lung function provoked by the activity. It has been demonstrated that DSCG, in addition to protecting against EIA, also reduces ventilation and energy

consumption during running. Maximum oxygen uptake was significantly lower when compared to placebo when the children inhaled DSCG or the β_2-agonist salbutamol before running or before engaging in physical activity [35]. It has also been shown that DSCG reduces the ventilatory work in children suffering from EIA, but not in healthy children [36]. This suggests that energy consumption during exercise is higher in untreated than in treated asthmatic children, and that pretreatment with DSCG or an inhaled β_2-agonist enables asthmatic children, adolescents, and athletes to participate in sports and physical activity on an equal level with healthy children, adolescents, and athletes.

Both DSCG and the inhaled β_2-agonist terbutaline have been found to protect against EIA for up to 2 hours, whereas the combination of DSCG and terbutaline protected for up to 4 hours [37]. It has been maintained that an inhaled β_2-agonist is preferable when there is baseline bronchial constriction, whereas DSCG should be used when the subject does not demonstrate signs of bronchial constriction prior to physical activity [32]. It is important that DSCG be taken in adequately high doses; 20 mg is to be preferred. This makes treatment impractical, so that inhaled β_2-agonists are often preferred.

Inhaled β_2-agonists are often preferred as protective treatment prior to physical activity. The protective effect against EIA is usually very good, both when bronchial constriction is present before exercise and not [32]. The short-acting inhaled β_2-agonists, salbutamol and terbutaline, are usually preferred. Inhaled β_2-agonists have a better effect than when the drugs are taken orally. The recommended dose of inhaled salbutamol is 0.2–0.4 mg, corresponding to an inhaled dose of 0.25–0.5 mg terbutaline.

The long-acting β_2-agonists for inhalation, salmeterol and formoterol, were recently introduced. Both have been demonstrated to have a good protective effect against EIA [38–40]. Children with EIA will benefit from such long-acting protective drugs as they usually do not plan their activity beforehand. In athletes performing endurance sports, a long-acting β_2-agonist may be of benefit as the usual β_2-agonists may not last long enough. In addition, the use of a long-acting β_2-agonist may improve symptom control and quality of life both in the asthmatic athlete and in asthmatic children and adolescents [41, 42].

Ipratropium bromide may be effective in protecting against EIA in some patients, but they are less useful than inhaled β_2-agonists [32, 43]. However, ipratropium bromide should be tried in certain subjects. Sometimes an additional protective effect may be obtained when ipratropium bromide is added to an inhaled β_2-agonist [44]. This underlines the importance of trying out the effect of the prescribed drugs.

Lately, the protective effect of inhaled furosemide [45] and inhaled heparin [46] upon EIA has been described. This is of considerable theoretical interest, though these drugs do not represent a therapeutic alternative to the other treatments.

The Relationship to Doping

The frequent occurrence of EIA in participants in endurance sports has led to a high consumption of asthma drugs within these branches of athletics [7]. Thus, it has been discussed whether inhaled β_2-agonists in particular could improve performance, especially endurance performance. In animals it has been demonstrated that oral β_2-agonists (clenbuterol) in high doses may cause an increase in muscle mass. This has entailed restrictions in the international doping regulations. Both inhaled steroids and inhaled β_2-agonists are allowed for use in sports in asthmatic athletes. Systemic β_2-agonists and systemic steroids, however, are not allowed. Since 1993 only the inhaled β_2-agonists salbutamol and terbutaline are allowed for asthmatics for use in sports, but after studies demonstrating that both salbutamol, terbutaline, and salmeterol do not improve performance [47–50], salmeterol, too, has been allowed for use in sports (since February 1, 1996). The other long-acting inhaled β_2-agonist, formoterol, is presently not allowed for use in sports.

Conclusions

The asthmatic condition should be treated optimally in athletes suffering from EIA. This often includes the use of inhaled steroids, which reduce BHR and EIA considerably. However, additional protective medication before exercise is frequently needed. Inhaled β_2-agonists, usually short-acting, are most often used. EIA is usually well mastered by combining inhaled steroids and inhaled β_2-agon-

ists. Long-acting inhaled β_2-agonists may be necessary, especially in severe asthma, but also in children, who do not plan their physical activity in the same way as athletes do. Leukotriene antagonists, recently introduced, may also be a useful alternative in the treatment of EIA. The use of asthma drugs is restricted in sports, and it is the athlete's own responsibility to know the doping rules. However, the physician should also know these rules and avoid prescribing drugs not permitted for the use in sports. For the individual patients and the individual athletes it is important that the effectiveness of the prescribed treatment be controlled.

In addition to the medical treatment, certain preventive measures should be ensured in order to help the athlete avoid the dangers of heavy endurance training and competition. Endurance training and competition should not be performed during a respiratory tract infection nor in cold temperatures (below $-10°C$) without cold-protection equipment; in indoor swimming pools, adequate ventilation should be ensured in order not to expose the swimmers to high levels of chlorine in inhaled air.

Address for correspondence:

Prof. Kai-Håkon Carlsen
Voksentoppen Children's Center and Research
Institute of Asthma and Allergy
Ullveien 14
N-0791 Oslo
Norway
Tel. +47 22 136500
Fax +47 22 136505
E-mail kaic@usit-div.uio.no

References

1. Lee TH, Anderson SD. Heterogeneity of mechanisms in exercise-induced asthma. Thorax 1985; 40:481–487.
2. Taylor WR, Newacheck PW. Impact of childhood asthma upon health. Pediatrics 1992; 90:657–662.
3. International Paediatric Consensus Group on Asthma. Asthma: A follow up statement from an international paediatric asthma consensus group. Arch Dis Child 1992; 67(2):240–248.
4. Pauwels R, Joos G, Van der Straten M. Bronchial responsiveness is not bronchial responsiveness is not asthma. Clin Allergy 1988; 18:317–321.

5. Carlsen KH. Bronchial hyperreactivity in athletes. Nord Med 1994; 109:16–18.

6. Larsson K, Ohlsen P, Larsson L, Malmberg P, Rydstrom PO, Ulriksen H. High prevalence of asthma in cross country skiers. BMJ 1993; 307(6915):1326–1329.

7. Heir T, Oseid S. Self-reported asthma and exercise-induced asthma symptoms in high-level competitive cross-country skiers. Scand J Med Sci Sports 1994; 4:128–133.

8. Carlsen KH, Oseid S, Odden H, et al. The response to heavy swimming exercise in children with and without bronchial asthma. In Oseid S, Carlsen KH (Eds), Children and exercise XIII. Champaign, IL: Human Kinetics Publishers, Inc. 1989, pp. 351–360.

9. Fjellbirkeland L, Gulsvik A, Walloe A. Swimming-induced asthma [in Norwegian]. Tidsskr Nor Laegeforen 1995; 115(17):2051–2053.

10. Drobnic F, Freixa A, Casan P, Sanchis J, Guardino X. Assessment of chlorine exposure in swimmers during training. Med Sci Sports Exerc 1996; 28(2):271–274.

11. Helenius IJ, Tikkanen HO, Haahtela T. Association between type of training and risk of asthma in elite athletes.

12. Heir T. Longitudinal variations in bronchial responsiveness in cross-country skiers and control subjects. Scand J Med Sci Sports 1994; 4:134–139.

13. Heir T, Larsen S. The influence of training intensity, airway infections and environmental conditions on seasonal variations in bronchial responsiveness in cross-country skiers. Scand J Med Sci Sports 1995; 5:152–159.

14. Heir T, Aanestad G, Carlsen KH, Larsen S. Respiratory tract infection and bronchial responsiveness in elite athletes and sedentary control subjects. Scand J Med Sci Sports 1995; 5:94–99.

15. Landwehr LP, Wood RP, Blager FB, Milgrom H. Vocal cord dysfunction mimicking exercise-induced bronchospasm in adolescents. Pediatrics 1996; 98(5): 971–974.

16. McFadden ER, Jr., Zawadski DK. Vocal cord dysfunction masquerading as exercise-induced asthma. A physiologic cause for "choking" during athletic activities. Am J Respir Crit Care Med 1996; 153(3):942–947.

17. Engh G, Mørk M, Carlsen KH. Exercise-induced bronchoconstriction depends on exercise load. Am J Respir Crit Care Med 1998; 157(3):A621.

18. Backer V, Ulrik CS. Bronchial responsiveness to exercise in a random sample of 494 children and adolescents from Copenhagen. Clin Exp Allergy 1992; 22:741–747.

19. Waalkens HJ, van Essen-Zandvliet EE, Gerritsen J, Duiverman EJKK, Knol K. The effect of an inhaled corticosteroid (budesonide) on exercise-induced asthma in children. Dutch CNSLD Study Group [see comments]. Eur Respir J 1993; 6:652–656.

20. Leff JA, Busse WW, Pearlman D, Bronsky E, Kemp J, Hendeles L, Dockhorn R, Kundu S, Zhangn J, Seidenberg BC, et al. Montelukast, a leukotriene-receptor antagonist, for the treatment of mild asthma and exercise-induced bronchoconstriction. N Engl J Med 1998; 339:147–152.

21. Carlsen KH, Bech R, Oseid S, et al. Bronchial reactivity measured by exercise-induced asthma test and PC-20-histamine: A comparison of two methods. In Morehouse CA (Ed), Children and exercise XII. Champaign, IL: Human Kinetics Publishers Inc. 1986, pp. 295–300.

22. Godfrey S, Springer C, Noviski N, Maayan Ch, Avital A. Exercise but not metacholine differentiates asthma from chronic lung disease in children. Thorax 1991; 46:488–492.

23. Avital A, Springer C, Bar Yishay E, Godfrey S. Adenosine, methacholine, and exercise challenges in children with asthma or paediatric chronic obstructive pulmonary disease. Thorax 1995; 50(5):511–516.

24. Carlsen KH, Engh G, Mørk M, Schrøder E. Cold air inhalation and exercise-induced bronchoconstriction in relationship to metacholine bronchial responsiveness. Different patterns in asthmatic children and children with other chronic lung diseases. Respir Med 1998; 92(2):308–315.

25. Papalia, S.M. Aspects of inhaled budesonide use in asthma and exercise. Department of Human Movement, University of Western Australia 1996.

26. Henriksen JM, Dahl R. Effects of inhaled budesonide alone and in combination with low-dose terbutaline in children with exercise-induced asthma. Am Rev Respir Dis 1983; 128(6):993–997.

27. van Essen-Zandvliet EE, Hughes MD, Waalkens HJ, Duiverman EJ, Pocock SJ, Kerrebijn KF, The Dutch CNSLD Study Group. Effects of 22 months of treatment with inhaled corticosteroids and/or β2-agonists on lung function, airway responsiveness, and symptoms in children with asthma. Am Rev Respir Dis 1992; 146:547–554.

28. Robuschi M, Riva E, Fuccella LM, Vida E, Barnabe R, Rossi M, Gambaro G, Spagnotto S, Bianco S. Prevention of exercise-induced bronchoconstriction by a new leukotriene antagonist (SK&F 104353). A double-blind study versus disodium cromoglycate and placebo. Am Rev Respir Dis 1992; 145:1285–1288.

29. Kemp JP, Dockhorn RJ, Shapiro GG, Nguyen HH, Reiss TF, Seidenberg BC, Knorr B. Montelukast once daily inhibits exercise-induced bronchoconstriction in 6- to 14-year-old children with asthma. J Pediatr 1998; 133(3):424–428.

30. Hoag JE, McFadden ERJr. Long-term effect of cromolyn sodium on nonspecific bronchial hyperresponsiveness: A review. Ann Allergy 1991; 66:53–63.

31. Benedictis FM, Tuteri G, Bertotto A, Bruni L, Vaccaro R. Comparison of the protective effects of cromolyn sodium and nedocromil sodium in the treatment of exercise-induced asthma in children. J Allergy Clin Immunol 1994; 94:684–688.

32. Anderson SD. Drugs and the control of exercise-induced asthma. Eur Respir J 1993; 6:1090–1092.

33. Comis A, Valletta EA, Sette L, Andreoli A, Boner AL. Comparison of nedocromil sodium and sodium cromoglycate administered by pressurized aerosol, with and without a spacer device in exercise-induced asthma in children. Eur Respir J 1993; 6:523–526.

34. Oseid S, Mellbye E, Hem E. Effect of nedocromil sodium on exercise-induced bronchoconstriction exacerbated by inhalation of cold air. Scand J Med Sci Sports 1995; 5(2):88–93.

35. Zanconato S, Baraldi E, Santuz P, Magagnin G, Zacchello F. Effect of inhaled disodium cromoglycate and albuterol on energy cost of running in asthmatic children. Pediatr Pulmonol 1990; 8(4):240–244.

36. Baraldi E, Santuz P, Magagnin G, Filippone M, Zacchello F. Effect of disodium cromoglycate on ventilation and gas exchange during exercise in asthmatic children with a postexertion FEV_1 fall less than 15% Chest 1994; 106(4):1083–1088.

37. Woolley M, Anderson SD, Quigley BM. Duration of protective effect of terbutaline sulfate and cromolyn sodium alone and in combination on exercise-induced asthma. Chest 1990; 97:39–45.

38. Green CP, Price JF. Prevention of exercise-induced asthma by inhaled salmeterol xinafoate. Arch Dis Child 1992; 67:1014–1017.

39. Carlsen KH, Røksund O, Olsholt K, Njå F, Leegaard J, Bratten G. Overnight protection by inhaled salmeterol on exercise-induced asthma in children. Eur Respir J 1995; 8(11):1852–1855.

40. Boner AL, Spezia E, Piovesan P, Chiocca E, Maiocchi G. Inhaled formoterol in the prevention of exercise-induced bronchoconstriction in asthmatic children. Am J Respir Crit Care Med 1994; 149:935–939.

41. Steffensen I, Faurschou P, Riska H, Rostrup J, Wegener T. Inhaled formoterol dry powder in the treatment of patients with reversible obstructive airway disease. A 3-month, placebo- controlled comparison of the efficacy and safety of formoterol and salbutamol, followed by a 12-month trial with formoterol. Allergy 1995; 50(8):657–663.

42. Juniper EF, Johnston PR, Borkhoff CM, Guyatt GH, Boulet LP, Haukioja A. Quality of life in asthma clinical trials: Comparison of salmeterol and salbutamol. Am J Respir Crit Care Med 1995; 151(1):66–70.

43. Finnerty JP, Holgate ST. The contribution of histamine release and vagal reflexes, alone and in combination, to exercise-induced asthma [see comments]. Eur Respir J 1993; 6:1132–1137.

44. Greenough A, Yuksel B, Everett L, Price JF. Inhaled ipratropium bromide and terbutaline in asthmatic children. Respir Med 1993; 87(2):111–114.

45. Bianco S, Vaghi A, Robuschi M, Pasargiklian M. Prevention of exercise-induced bronchoconstriction by inhaled frusemide. Lancet 1988; 2:252–255.

46. Garrigo J, Danta I, Ahmed T. Time course of the protective effect of inhaled heparin on exercise-induced asthma. Am J Respir Crit Care Med 1996; 153(5): 1702–1707.

47. Meeuwisse WH, McKenzie DC, Hopkins S, Road JD, Hopkins SR. The effect of salbutamol on performance in nonasthmatic athletes. Med Sci Sports Exerc 1992; 24:1161–1166.

48. Morton AR, Papalia SM, Fitch KD. Is salbutamol ergogenic? The effects of salbutamol on physical performance in the high-performance nonasthmatic athletes. Clin J Sport Med 1992; 2:93–97.

49. Carlsen KH, Ingjer F, Thyness B, Kirkegaard H. The effect of inhaled salbutamol and salmeterol on lung function and endurance performance in healthy well-trained athletes. Scand J Med Sci Sports 1997; 7:160–165.

50. Heir T, Stemshaug H. Sabutamol and high-intensity treadmill running in nonasthmatic highly conditioned athletes. Scand J Med Sci Sports 1995; 5:231–236.

118

Environmental Control

Thomas AE Platts-Mills, Judith A Woodfolk*

Keywords: Mites, cockroach, cat, dog, allergen avoidance, asthma

Allergens found inside domestic houses are well recognized as an important contribution to the symptoms of asthma. In keeping with this, controlling exposure to these allergens is a logical part of the treatment. Reducing exposure requires understanding the biology of the source and the ways in which the allergen is distributed. At present, there is good evidence for the efficacy of dust mite avoidance and the methods that should be recommended are well defined. For domestic animals, it is well established that removing cats from the house is an effective method of reducing exposure. By contrast, there are many questions about whether it is possible to control exposure with the animal in the house. For cockroach allergens, the situation is even less satisfactory because it remains unclear whether it is possible to control these insects in low income housing. Overall, it is clear that avoidance should be part of the treatment of allergic disease, but further research is needed into techniques and methods of persuading patients to comply.

In 1929 Storm Van Leuven published his results on treatment of asthma using a "climate chamber." His design of a room included maintaining low dust levels and a supply of clean air. This experiment was based on the observation that many asthmatics improved when they spent time in the high altitude clinics in Switzerland [1]. It was also well known 50 years ago that patients with asthma improved when they were admitted to hospital. Indeed Rackemann included failure to improve in hospital as one of the characteristics of intrinsic asthma [2]. Skin testing with house dust extracts was routine in allergy clinics as early as 1935. However, advice on avoidance of house dust was hampered because the nature of the house dust "atopen" was not known. In 1962, Spieksma saw live mites in house dust and she and her colleagues rapidly developed clear evidence that mites were a major source of allergens in dust [3]. Research relevant to allergen avoidance as a treatment for asthma can now be separated into four areas of interest:

– Biology of dust mites, cockroaches and other living organisms that contribute to the allergen content of houses.
– Immunochemistry of indoor allergens and the development of assays for allergens in dust.
– Analysis of the reasons why patients with asthma improve when they are moved to sanatoria or hospital rooms.
– Detailed studies on techniques for controlling allergens in inhabited houses.

Biology of the Indoor Arthropods: Mites and Cockroaches

Some aspects of mite biology are now well known, i. e., that they live best in warm humid conditions, that they require a "nest" to protect against short term fluctuations in humidity, and that they are photophobic. In addition, it is clear that they can eat human skin scales or fungi but will also thrive on many different complex food sources. The aspects of mite biology that are much less well understood include controlling population size and dispersal within houses [4]. Although it is clear from cultures that breeding can be accelerated by optimizing conditions it is not clear how that translates into growth characteristics within a house. Thus, there are still major differences in individual houses which are not explained. Furthermore although it is known that different species of mites will compete in cultures, the relevance of this to mite growth in houses is not clear.

Among the many different insects that inhabit houses, cockroaches are best recognized as a source of allergens. Cockroaches are tropical in origin and thrive in houses that are continuously warm. Thus, cockroach infestation was extremely rare in

---

* Asthma & Allergic Diseases Center, University of Virginia, Charlottesville, VA, USA

England prior to the introduction of central heating. In addition, cockroaches require food sources and thrive in houses where food or garbage remains open. However, unlike mites, cockroaches are not dependent on ambient humidity and show great talent in finding water sources within a building. Cockroaches can flourish in overheated multistory buildings in New York or Chicago during winters that are very dry. These insects also flourish throughout the South in any house where food is available and the building is not regularly treated. The sources of allergen from cockroaches are not well defined; cockroaches produce fecal particles which look like ground pepper but these are probably too large to become airborne. They also "lick" trails around a house and thus saliva may also be an important source of allergens. Although it is certain that the number of cockroaches in houses can reach very large numbers, no methods currently exist for accurate measurement and the relationship between roach numbers and allergen levels either in floor dust or airborne is not well established.

Immunochemistry

The purification, characterization, and molecular biology of indoor allergens is now as advanced as it is for pollens. In particular, the allergens of dust mites, cats, and the German cockroach are very well defined (Table 1) [5–8]. Not surprisingly, these organisms produce many different proteins (some of which are enzymes) and allergic individuals can

Table 1. Nomenclature and characteristics of indoor allergens.

Source	Allergen[1]	MW	Homology/Function	Sequence[2]
House dust mite:				
Dermatophagoides spp.	Group 1	25 kD	Cysteine protease	cDNA
	Group 2	14 kD	Epididymal protein	cDNA
	Group 3	28–30 kD	Serine protease	cDNA/protein
	Der p 4	60 kD	Amylase	Protein
	Group 5	14 kD	Unknown	cDNA
	Der p 6	25 kD	Chymotrypsin	Protein
	Group 7	22 kD	Unknown	cDNA
	Der p 8	26 kD	Glutathione-S transferase	cDNA
	Der p 9	30 kD	Serine protease	cDNA
	Group 10	36 kD	Tropomyosin	cDNA
Euroglyphus maynei	Eur m 1	25 kD	Cysteine protease	PCR
Blomia tropicalis	Blo t 5	14 kD	Unknown	cDNA
Lepidoglyphus destructor	Lep d 1	14 kD	Unknown	None
Mammals:				
Felis domesticus	Fel d 1	36 kD	Uteroglobin	PCR
Canis familiaris	Can f 1	25 kD	Unknown	cDNA
Mus musculus	Mus m 1	19 kD	Calycins, pheromone	cDNA
Rattus norvegicus	Rat n 1	19 kD	Binding proteins	cDNA
Cockroach:				
Blattella germanica	Bla g 1	20–25 kD	Unknown	cDNA
	Bla g 2	36 kD	Aspartic protease	cDNA/protein
	Bla g 4	21 kD	Calycin	cDNA
	Bla g 5	23 kD	Glutathione-S transferase	cDNA/protein
	Bla g 6	18 kD	Troponin C	cDNA
Fungi:				
Aspergillus fumigatis	Asp f 1	18 kD	Cytotoxin (mitogillin)	cDNA

[1]New nomenclature proposed by WHO/IUIS sub-committee, [2]Method given for full sequence determination where available. Amino acid sequence obtained by sequencing the natural protein is incomplete; N-terminal or internal peptide sequences have been determined.

produce IgE antibodies to a large number of these allergens. The use of a single protein to measure sensitization will underestimate the number of allergic individuals. On the other hand, measurement of a single allergen in house dust may be an adequate index of exposure. Clearly, this depends on several assumptions:

1. That the protein or major allergen measured is always produced by the organism. This may not be true if the protein is an inducible enzyme only expressed under certain circumstances, or if there is a closely related organism in which the relevant protein is antigenically distinct.

2. That the proteins produced by different sources become airborne in the same form. It is clear that cat allergens remain airborne (unlike mite or cockroach allergens). However, it is assumed that all allergens derived from cats behave in the same way. For the dust mite allergens there is considerable evidence that the Group 2 allergen (Der p 2 and Der f 2) are airborne on different particles to the Group 1 proteins [9]. However, the overall behavior of allergens of the two groups is very similar. Preliminary evidence from two groups suggests that cockroach allergens become airborne during domestic disturbance but are not measurable in undisturbed rooms [10, 11]. Thus, cockroach allergens appear to have similar airborne characteristics to mite allergens, which is in keeping with the fact that most cockroach allergic patients are *not* aware of a rapid onset of symptoms in an infested house.

Effects of Moving Allergic Patients out of Their Houses

Although families in the United States move repeatedly they generally take their furniture with them and maintain the "new" house in the same condition as the old. On the other hand, real change may occur when families move from a wet climate to a dry climate. There are many apocryphal stories of patients with asthma improving when they move, but no controlled trials. On the other hand there have been extensive studies on children who are moved from their houses to sanatoria. The most important conclusion is that children kept in these allergen free conditions have decreased bronchial reactivity as well as decreased symptoms of asth-

ma. Results of that kind have been reported from three high altitude sanatoria in Davos, Briancon, and Misurina. Similar results have also been shown with young adults admitted to a hospital "allergen-free" unit [12, 13, 14, 15].

Dr. Boner and his colleagues in Verona have reported detailed studies on the immunological events that occur during periods of time at a sanatorium [14, 16, 17]. They demonstrated decreases in serum and nasal antibodies, but more significantly they found decreased numbers of eosinophils in induced sputum. It was suggested that decreased numbers of eosinophils in sputum correlated with decreased nonspecific bronchial reactivity. The effects of moving to the sanatorium reversed when children went home and studies demonstrated that these effects were reproducible [14–18]. These findings strongly support the view that symptoms and bronchial hyperreactivity (BHR) in children with asthma are maintained by continued exposure to antigens in the home. However, it is very important to recognize what the sanatoria and hospital units represent. In addition to having very low levels of mite allergens these units have no carpets, no animals, very low mold spores, good ventilation and in many cases an exercise program. Thus, although the dominant skin sensitivity of the children in each of these studies was to dust mites, it would be simplistic to assume that the results of moving the children were simply due to mite free conditions.

On the other hand, the results of these experiments are the strongest evidence that changing the environment of children can lead to decreased symptoms and BHR. When the results were first reported in 1970 there was very little understanding that asthma was an inflammatory disease. Thus, the avoidance experiments in sanatoria have been a major part of the evidence (1) that conditions in houses are a *cause* of asthma, and (2) that avoidance measures can be an important form of treatment.

Detailed Studies on the Techniques Used for Controlling Allergens

If only our patients had the will and the means – avoidance is easy! Thus, an air-conditioned (i. e.,

Table 2. University of Virginia Allergy Clinic
Instructions for reducing exposure to house dust mites

Priority Objectives

1. Mattresses and pillows should be enclosed in a zippered, plastic cover or a vapor-permeable or a tightly woven air-permeable allergen-proof fabric. Damp wipe the mattress cover once a week.
2. Wash all bedding, including mattress pad, pillow cases, and blankets in hot cycle (~130°F) weekly. Comforters (or duvets) should be replaced with dacron or orlon, which can be washed with the bedding or covered with allergen-proof covers.
3. Small objects that accumulate dust, such as knickknacks, books, stuffed animals, and records, should be placed in drawers or closed cabinets. Clothing should be stored in drawers enclosed in plastic or in a closed closet. Unused clothing should be stored away from the bedroom.
4. Vacuum carpets each week using a vacuum cleaner with a double-thickness bag and effective filter (e. g., HEPA filter or electrostatic filter). The patient should either avoid vacuum cleaning or wear a mask during cleaning. In general, dust mite allergens will take about 20 minutes to fall after cleaning.

Medium Term Objectives

1. Removing carpets from bedrooms makes it much easier to control mites. This is because carpets are very difficult to clean and will tend not only to grow mites (in humid seasons) but also to act as a source to reinfest bedding, clothing, etc.
2. Replace curtains/drapes with washable cotton curtains or venetian/slat blinds.
3. Control humidity in the house: this can be achieved by increasing ventilation if the outdoor conditions are cold and/or dry; alternatively, reducing humidity can be achieved with central air conditioning. Dehumidifiers are helpful in basements. The objective is to keep relative humidity below 50%.
4. Carpets can be treated with acaricides (e. g., Acarosan) or 3% tannic acid though the use of these substances is controversial owing to short-lasting effects.

Choice of Houses/Apartments

1. Basements are not recommended for any allergic patients (in some cases moving out of a basement may be urgent because it is so difficult to control mite and/or fungal growth in the basement). Bedrooms should be upstairs.
2. Carpets fitted to a concrete slab, either in a basement or on the ground floor tend to become damp and remain damp. We recommend that all floors should have a primary polished floor (vinyl or wood) and carpets should be movable.
3. Upholstered sofas and chairs should be avoided.
4. Air filters on central air conditioning should be cleaned regularly. Good quality (e. g., electrostatic) filters may be helpful, but are no substitute for reducing available mite nests in the house.

---

low humidity) apartment with polished wooden floors, leather or wooden furniture, no animals, and a simple bedroom with covered mattress and pillows is easy to maintain (Table 2). Indeed, it is not difficult to maintain an "allergen-free" hospital provided helpful friends do not bring in stuffed toys and animals such as guinea pigs, rabbits, etc. The major problem is overcoming lifestyles that the family seems unwilling or unable to change. The biggest practical problems can be divided into two groups: (1) carpets, sofas, and bedding; (2) and animals.

Carpets, Sofas, and Bedding

Carpets and sofas represent an extraordinarily large reservoir of allergens, humidity and food for dust mites. Traditionally, carpets have been removed regularly and cleaned by beating (England and the United States), laying out in the sun (Finland), or putting out in the snow (Scandinavia). In France, rush matting in Versailles was composted or burned. Inherent in all these procedures is the ability to remove the carpet. Indeed, fitted or wall-to-wall carpets are a modern invention only conceived after the introduction of vacuum cleaners. Beating carpets and/or putting them out in the sun are effective methods of cleaning and killing mites [19]. The question then becomes; is it possible to clean and/or kill mites in a carpet that stays on the floor? Studies on vacuum cleaners have focused on the filtering capacity of the cleaner [20]. These studies showed that some vacuum cleaners leak more than others and show that double layer bags or additional filters, such as High Efficiency Particulate Air (HEPA) filters, may be highly effective. Recent studies evaluating vacuum cleaners recommended for allergic subjects have confirmed the importance

122

of filtration for minimizing allergen leakage [21]. Thus, the major negative effects of a vacuum cleaner can be minimized by good design. On the other hand, it is an illusion to imagine that cleaners can remove human debris from a carpet. All fitted carpets steadily *increase* in weight with time and this is due to accumulated material in the carpet. This debris provides nesting material and food for dust mites, but also makes it exceedingly difficult for acaricides to contact mites in a carpet. Steam cleaning has been recommended; indeed, the companies often claim that this treatment is effective against mites. However, steam cleaning is designed not to reach the bottom layers of a carpet, because these layers are often not colorfast, and water tends to bring up colors as well as old stains.

There are many different chemicals that will kill mites. These include benzyl benzoate, pirimiphos methyl, abamectin, and also some of the complex mixtures marketed as cockroach sprays [22–25]. In laboratory experiments benzyl benzoate or pirimiphos methyl will kill mites within a day. Thus, the problem is not *how* to kill mites but how to kill mites where they reside, i. e., within a carpet or sofa. With some effective acaricides the problem is compounded because the company is reluctant to market the chemical for domestic use; this has been true for pirimiphos methyl and abamectin. Thus, most acaricides for houses use benzyl benzoate, which has a long record of safe use with humans because it is a preservative for food and a traditional treatment for scabies mites. Benzyl benzoate has been marketed in three forms: as a moist powder ("fucht pulver"); as a foam; and in a liquid together with tannic acid. The foam appears to be ineffective on both mattresses and sofas [25, 26]. The powder form presents problems related to techniques for application; simply applying the powder and leaving it for a few hours is not effective. If the powder is brushed in, left overnight and brushed in again before vacuuming, it has a significant effect that may last up to 3 months. The liquid forms of benzyl benzoate or benzyl alcohol with tannic acid are not as effective as was originally hoped. This was attributed both to problems applying the fluid and to the chemicals being too dilute [25].

Tannic acid (TA) has been recognized for centuries as an important agent for crosslinking and denaturing proteins. Tannic acid works nonspecifically on proteins and it probably requires multiple "hits" with TA to denature a protein molecule. Tannic acid was first studied in detail by Dr. Green in Sydney who demonstrated its efficacy for mite al-

lergens [27]. Our group carried out detailed laboratory experiments to test the effects of TA on mite and cat allergens; the results illustrated several problems [28]. First, TA was ineffective when applied to high concentrations of cat allergen, and second, the presence of Fel d 1 inhibited the activity of TA against mite allergen in the same mixture. Problems with evaluating TA became apparent in handling dust samples from carpets that had been treated. Dried TA in the dust redissolves resulting in interference with assay measurements and further denaturion of protein in the dust; either of these effects can produce spuriously low allergen measurements. Adding bovine serum albumin (BSA) to house dust extracts caused precipitation of free TA and protected the assay. This is simply a technical problem, but the results illustrate well both the complex nature of interactions between TA and allergens, and potential problems in assessing the effects of chemicals on allergens in carpets. However, results of our studies suggested that TA is more likely to work if the carpet is cleaned first to reduce the total protein content and if it is applied as a 3% rather than 1% solution. Although TA has a reputation for staining, it can be produced in a form that does not stain. On the other hand, applying TA to basement carpets which are damp can bring out old stains creating further problems. In general, TA is an effective denaturing agent that has major effects on mite or cat allergens [29]. However, TA has no effect on live mites and the effects are short-lived. Combination with benzyl benzoate is appropriate but the correct mixture has not been established.

Sofas are a special problem both as a reservoir for allergen and as a mite nest. Approaches to mite allergen reduction include controlling humidity (sofas moved to Denver lose their mite population over about a year); freezing with liquid nitrogen (very effective but not practical); and designing a sofa with an impermeable barrier just below the fabric cover; this latter approach may be the best solution in the future. We recently tested the effectiveness of different fabrics in blocking both cat and dust mite allergens. Results showed that fine woven polyester fabrics (pore size 6 fm) efficiently blocked allergens tested while still allowing up to 40% of the airflow of control fabrics [30]. These results suggest that such fabrics could be effective alternatives to semipermeable or impermeable materials as allergen barriers.

Bedding is a primary target for allergen control owing to the high level of mite allergen exposure which may occur while sleeping [31]. Studies suggest that encasing bedding (i. e., mattresses and pillows) is an effective method for reducing allergen levels [30, 32–35]. Initially, materials used for encasings were made of vinyl or vapor-permeable fabrics which were uncomfortable. The recent availability of more comfortable, air permeable fabrics which are highly efficient at retaining allergens has made encasing bedding a reasonable approach for all patients in controlling exposure to allergens. It is now feasible to encase pillows with "breathable" fabrics which would prevent dust mite entry into bedding. However, it remains to be tested whether this approach is an efficient method for maintaining "allergen-free" bedding. Encasings should be wiped down each week with a damp cloth to remove any allergen, or washed. Clearly, it is necessary to control allergen levels in blankets and duvets which are not encased. A variety of laundry methods have been shown to be effective at reducing mite and cat allergens in bedding [36–38]. As a result of these studies, we recommend that patients wash their bedding in hot water on a weekly basis. It should be stressed that chemical treatments, e. g., acaricides, have not proved effective in treating mattresses [39].

Animals

Cats

Domestic animals have been recognized as an important source of allergens in house dust since the early 1920's. Indeed, patients usually give reliable histories of allergic reactions to cats and/or dogs. Despite this, even severely ill patients are often resistant to advice to replace live animals with porcelain ones. If the cat is removed from the house, it will still take weeks for allergen levels to decrease, reflecting the large reservoirs of cat allergen that accumulate in carpets, sofas, etc. [40, 41]. The major cat allergen, Fel d 1, is primarily produced in the skin and is probably carried on flakes of dander. These "flakes" appear to have two very important properties: first, they are sticky and become adherent not only to walls and other surfaces but also to clothing. This facilitates the transfer of cat allergen to other houses which may result in levels of Fel d 1 in houses without a cat comparable to those in houses with a cat, i. e., $\geq 20\,\mu g$ Fel d 1/g dust [42, 43]. Furthermore, it has recently been demonstrated that cat allergen can be airborne in houses without a cat [44]. This has very important consequences for avoidance, because most clinics do not consider the possibility that cat allergen is playing a role in symptoms if the patient states that they do not have a cat in the house. Second, particles carrying cat allergen behave aerodynamically as small particles [their actual size is not established but may be larger than their apparent $2\,\mu m$ diameter]. These particles or flakes remain airborne for hours and are almost always measurable in the air of undisturbed houses with a cat. Detailed studies on the falling rate of cat allergen after disturbance established that the aerodynamically "large" particles fall rapidly. However, increasing ventilation will remove small particles and tend to keep large particles airborne [45, 46]. Until recently it was considered pointless to try to control cat allergen exposure in a house with a cat. However, detailed study of Fel d 1 has indicated a range of useful steps and suggested that a radical change in the house could control cat allergen. The obvious measures are:

– Remove reservoirs such as carpets and sofas because very little allergen accumulates on polished floors, leather sofas, or wooden furniture.
– Keep the cat outside as much as possible.
– Use room air cleaners; these can reduce airborne cat allergen if the reservoirs are removed first. HEPA room air cleaners will remove almost all allergen particles from the air that passes through the filter.
– Wash the cat; at present the efficacy of washing cats is disputed. It has been observed repeatedly that sequential washing of cats yields progressively smaller quantities of Fel d 1 [47, 48]. The first experiments to study airborne allergen coming off a cat after washing also showed very clear results [45]. However, subsequent experiments by Klucka and his colleagues showed only a modest effect one week after washing [49]. We have carried out detailed experiments to assess the effects of different washing techniques on cats. The results showed that cats carry a large quantity of allergen (i. e., ~60 mg) and that even aggressive washing can only remove ~40–70% of this allergen. The allergen becoming airborne off cats is dramatically reduced 6 hours after washing but decreases do not persist for more than one week [50]. These results do not show that cats should not be washed, but suggest that the procedure will not control allergen release for more than a few days. Simple calculation of the allergen coming off a cat suggests that the amount coming off, i. e., ~1 µg/hour is ~0.02% of the allergen on the cat. Thus, the factors (e. g.,

electrostatic charge) controlling whether particles become airborne may be as important as the total quantity of Fel d 1 on the cat. However, use of a commercially available treatment to wipe on cats was not effective [49, 51].

Dogs

Obvious allergic reactions to dogs are less common than those to cats; however in areas where dogs are kept in houses, they can become an important source of allergens [52]. From preliminary results it appears that dog allergen becomes and remains airborne like cat allergen. Thus, it is likely that the same rules apply to dog allergen as to cat. Of course, many dogs are kept outside, which probably reduces the problem. Interestingly, in hotter climates (e. g., Virginia) it is normal practice to wash dogs regularly. A recent study has shown that washing the dog reduces recoverable allergen from dog hair and dander. However, as with cat allergen, reductions in Can f 1 are not maintained for more than a few days [53].

Rodents

The major source of allergen from rodents is urinary; in particular, the kidneys of male animals *leak* large quantities of protein into the urine. These urinary proteins have been studied, both in terms of the immune response and the form in which they become airborne. Although these experiments were carried out with laboratory animals, they are almost certainly relevant to caged animals at home. The main source of airborne rat allergen appears to be the bedding material. Further, the amount of allergen coming off the bedding is dramatically increased by *drying*. Particles in wet bedding probably stick together and fall rapidly [54]. The first line of treatment for all rodents in the house is eradication. However, controlling exposure to dried bedding is highly relevant to animal allergic laboratory workers, and may be relevant in some houses. Keeping cages out of bedrooms is essential and regular removal of the cage material may also help. Whether saliva is an important source of rodent allergen in the house is not clear, however biting by rats is a remarkably effective method of causing anaphylaxis in rat allergic individuals.

Insects – Cockroaches

The rapid development of immunochemistry of cockroach allergens between 1985 and today has made it possible to measure exposure and begin to study methods of controlling exposure [7, 55, 56]. Talking to patients who are allergic to cockroaches (as judged by skin tests), it is clear that they do not relate their symptoms to exposure to roaches. Furthermore, most of these patients, just like mite allergic patients, do not report rapid onset of symptoms on entering a house which is infested with roaches. In keeping with this, cockroach allergen is not found airborne in undisturbed houses. Thus, the airborne characteristics of cockroach allergens are similar to those of dust mites but not of cats. This suggests that environmental control should focus on reducing the allergen source rather than on air filtration. The highest levels of cockroach allergen have generally been found in kitchens. Although at present we don't have clear data on the effects of eradication measures on cockroach allergen, it is possible to extrapolate from eradication studies. The main approaches include:

– Fastidious cleaning to reduce food supplies, including enclosing all food and disposing of garbage rapidly.
– Closing all entry points with sealants.
– Killing roaches. The best approach is to use bait; traps only catch a small number and the sprays are irritating particularly to allergic individuals. With the best effort controlling cockroaches in some multi-dwelling buildings may be very difficult, but determined effort is usually successful and there is no reason for allowing infestation of a single dwelling unit.

Allergens That Are Primarily Outdoors: Fungi and Pollen

We are still in a difficult situation with indoor fungi because the methods proposed for measuring exposure are still very time consuming, i. e., microscopic examination of sticky rods. Furthermore, some of the key species cannot be distinguished by their spores, e. g., *Penicillium* and *Aspergillus*. Cultures are more time consuming and difficult to quantitate. It is clear that mold growth is an important problem in houses and can create a major problem for allergic patients. Surprisingly, the clearest association with asthma is for sensitization to Alternaria which is generally regarded as an outdoor mold [57–59]. The reason this seems surprising is because many of the *Alternaria* sensitive patients appear to have perennial rather than seasonal asthma implying that exposure is occurring indoors as has been suggested for pollen allergens [60]. Taken together, these observations suggest that *Alternaria* may be the most important outdoor allergen today. Recently, an assay has been developed for measuring the *Alternaria* allergen Alt a 1 allowing monitoring of environmental exposure to this allergen [61]. Measures for controlling fungal growth are well established and until detailed methods for studying the effects of exposure are developed, these measures should be advised.

Conclusions

Given that allergen avoidance is the primary anti-inflammatory treatment for asthma, it is clear that the treatment should be taken seriously. Furthermore, the ability to measure specific marker allergens in house dust has made it possible to test many of the measures advised to patients. During this process the advice given has become increasingly antigen specific. In general, avoidance can be classified as: (1) source reduction by elimination; (2) source reduction by physical barriers; (3) removing reservoirs; and (4) air filtration. The relative importance of these measures depends on the nature of airborne particles. However, the main reservoirs are very important (i. e., mattresses, pillows, carpets and upholstered furniture) because they act both as a nest for mites (and roaches) as well as a major site in which allergens accumulate. The second major issue is the "air handling"; this is a euphemism since domestic houses don't have controlled air entry, however the issues of humidity, temperature and ventilation rates are almost certainly central to the causes of increased asthma. If we could persuade families to run their houses colder and drier, then mite, cockroach and fungal problems would all decrease. It seems that houses should never be allowed to be hot, humid *and* have large reservoirs for growth of mold and mites. The choice is either to keep the house cool and dry or to remove carpets and sofas, and to cover mattresses and pillows. It is clear that the old model in the South of taking up all carpets in the spring and storing them for the summer was correct.

Address for correspondence:

Thomas AE Platts-Mills, MD PhD
Asthma & Allergic Diseases Center
Box 225 HSC
University of Virginia
Charlottesville, VA 22908
USA
Tel. +1 804 924-5917
Fax +1 804 924-5779
E-mail NKM8T@virginia.edu

References

1. Storm Van Leuven W, Einthoven W, Kremer W. The allergen proof chamber in the treatment of bronchial asthma and other respiratory diseases. Lancet 1927; i:1287–1289.

2. Rackemann FM. A working classification of asthma. Am J Med 1947; 3:601–609.

3. Voorhorst R, Spieksma FThM, Varekamp H, Leupen MJ, Lyklema AW. The house dust mite *(Dermatophagoides pteronyssinus)* and the allergens it produces: Identity with the house dust allergen. J Allergy 1967; 39:325–339.

4. Tovey ER. Methods and effectiveness of environmental control. J Allergy Clin Immunol 1999; 103:179–191.

5. Platts-Mills TAE, Thomas WR, Aalberse RC, Vervloet D, Chapman MD. Dust mite allergens and asthma: Report of a 2nd international workshop. J Allergy Clin Immunol 1992; 89:1046–1060.

6. Chapman MD, Aalberse RC, Brown MJ, Platts-Mills TAE. Monoclonal antibodies to the major feline allergen Fel d 1. II. Single step affinity purification of Fel d 1, N-terminal sequence analysis, and development of a sensitive two-site immunoassay to assess Fel d 1 exposure. J Immunol 1988; 140:812–818.

7. Arruda LK, Vailes LD, Mann BJ, Shannon J, Fox JW, Vedvick TS, Hayden ML, Chapman MD. Molecular cloning of a major cockroach *(Blattella germanica)* allergen, Bla g 2: Sequence homology to the aspartic proteases. J Biol Chem 1995; 270:19563–19568.

8. Pomes A, Melen E, Vailes LD, Retief JD, Arruda LK, Chapman MD. Novel allergen structures with tandem amino acid repeats derived from German and American cockroach. J Biol Chem 1998; 273:30801–30807.

9. De Blay F, Heymann PW, Chapman MD, Platts-Mills TAE. Airborne dust mite allergens: Comparison of Group II allergens with Group I mite allergen and cat allergen Fel d 1. J Allergy Clin Immunol 1991; 88: 919–926.

10. De Blay F, Kassel O, Chapman MD, Ott M, Verot A, Pauli G. Mise en evidence des allergenes majeurs des blattes par test ELISA dans la poussiere domestique. La Presse Med 1992; 21:1685.

11. Mollett JA, Vailes LD, Avner DB, Perzanowski MS, Arruda LK, Chapman MD, Platts-Mills TAE. Evaluation of German cockroach (Orthopetera: Blattellidae) allergen and its seasonal variation in low-income housing. J Med Entomol 1997; 34:307–311.

12. Kerrebijn KF. Endogenous factors in childhood CNSLD: Methodological aspects in population studies. In NGM Orie, R van der Lende (Eds), Bronchitis III (p. 38–48). The Netherlands: Royal Vangorcum Assen 1970.

13. Charpin D, Birnbaum J, Haddi E, Genard G, Lanteaume A, Toumi M, Faraj F, van der Brempt X, Vervloet D. Altitude and allergy to house dust mites: A paradigm of the influence of environmental exposure on allergic sensitization. Am Rev Resp Dis 1991; 143:983–986.

14. Boner AL, Niero E, Antolini I, Valletta EA, Gaburro D. Pulmonary function and bronchial hyperreactivity in asthmatic children with house dust mite allergy during prolonged stay in the Italian Alps (Misurina 1756m). Ann Allergy 1985; 54:42–45.

15. Platts-Mills TAE, Tovey ER, Mitchell EB, Moszoro H, Nock P, Wilkins SR. Reduction of bronchial hyperreactivity during prolonged allergen avoidance. Lancet 1982; 2:675–678.

16. Piacentini GL, Martinati L, Mingoni S, Boner AL. Influence of allergen avoidance on the eosinophil phase of airway inflammation in children with allergic asthma. J Allergy Clin Immunol 1996; 97:1079–1084.

17. Piacentini GL, Vicentini L, Mazzi P, Chilosi M, Martinati L, Boner AL. Mite-antigen avoidance can reduce bronchial epithelial shedding in allergic asthmatic children. Clin Exp Allergy 1998; 28:561–567.

18. Peroni DG, Boner AL, Vallone G, Antolini I, Warner JO. Effective allergen avoidance at high altitude reduces allergen-induced bronchial hyperresponsiveness. Am J Respir Care Med 1994; 6:1442–1446.

19. Tovey ER, Woolcock AJ. Direct exposure of carpets to sunlight can kill all mites. J Allergy Clin Immunol 1994; 93:1072.

20. Woodfolk JA, Luczynska CM, De Blay F, Chapman MD, Platts-Mills TAE. The effect of vacuum cleaners on the concentration and particle size distribution of airborne cat allergen. J Allergy Clin Immunol 1993; 91:829–837.

21. Vaughan JW, Woodfolk JA, Platts-Mills TAE. Evaluating vacuum cleaners recommended for allergic subjects. J Allergy Clin Immunol 1999; in press.

22. Arlian LG. Biology and ecology of house dust mites, Dermatophagoides spp. and Euroglyphus spp. Imm & All Clinics of N Am 1989; 9:339–356.

23. Mollet JA. Bioassay techniques for evaluating pesticides against Dermatophagoides spp. (Acari: Pyroglyphidae). J Med Entomol 1995; 32:515–518.

24. Mitchell EB, Wilkins S, Deighton JM, Platts-Mills TAE. Reduction of house dust mite allergen levels in the home: Use of the acaricide, pirimiphos methyl. Clin Allergy 1985; 15:235–240.

25. Hayden ML, Rose G, Diduch KB, Domson P, Chapman MD, Heymann PW, Platts-Mills TAE. Benzyl benzoate moist powder: Investigation of acaricidal activity in cultures and reduction of dust mite allergens in carpets. J Allergy Clin Immunol 1992; 89: 536–545.

26. Ehnert B, Lau S, Weber A, Wahn U. Reduction of mite allergen exposure and bronchial hyperreactivity. J Allergy Clin Immunol 1991; 87:320.

27. Green WF, Nicholas NR, Salome CM, Woolcock AJ. Reduction of house dust mites and mite allergens: Effects of spraying carpets and blankets with Allersearch DMS, an acaricide combined with an allergen reducing agent. Clin Exp Allergy 1989; 19:203–207.

28. Woodfolk JA, Hayden ML, Miller JD, Rose G, Chapman MD and Platts-Mills TAE. Chemical treatment of carpets to reduce allergen: A detailed study of the effects of tannic acid on indoor allergens. J Allergy Clin Immunol 1994; 94:19–26.

29. Woodfolk JA, Hayden ML, Couture N, Platts-Mills TAE. Chemical treatment of carpets to reduce allergen: A comparison of the effects of tannic acid and other treatment on proteins derived from dust mites and cats. J Allergy Clin Immunol 1995; 96:325–333.

30. Vaughan JW, McLaughlin TE, Perzanowski MS, Platts-Mills TAE. Evaluation of materials used for bedding encasement: Effect of pore size in blocking cat and dust mite allergen. J Allergy Clin Immunol 1999; 103:227–231.

31. Sakaguchi M, Inouye S, Yasueda H, Shida T. Concentrations of airborne mite allergen (Der I and Der II) during sleep. Allergy 1992; 47:55–57.

32. Nishioka K, Yasuea H, Saito H. Preventive effect of bedding encasement with microfine fibers on mite sensitization. J Allergy Clin Immunol 1998; 101:28–32.

33. Frederick JM, Warner JO, Jessop WJ, Enander I, Warner JA. Effect of a bed covering system in children with asthma and house dust mite hypersensitivity. Eur Respir J 1997; 10:361–366.

34. Owen S, Morganstem M, Hepworth J, Woodcock A. Control of house dust mite antigen in bedding. Lancet 1990; 335:396–397.

35. Chew G, Burge HA, Dockery D, Muilenburg M, Weiss S. Limitations of a home characteristics questionnaire as a predictor of indoor allergen levels. Am J Respir Crit Care Med 1998; 157:1536–1541.

36. McDonald LG, Tovey ER. The role of water temperature and laundry procedures in reducing house dust

mite populations and allergen content of bedding. J Allergy Clin Immunol 1992; 90:599–608.

37. Bischoff ER, Kniest FM. Mite-control and dust-removal by low temperature washing (86–104°F; 30–40°C)with a benzyl benzoate containing additive. Allergy Clin Immunol 1995; 95:263.

38. Tovey ER, McDonald LG. A simple washing procedure with eucalyptus oil for controlling house dust mites and their allergens in clothing and bedding. J Allergy Clin Immunol 1997; 100:464–466.

39. Carswell F, Birminham K, Oliver J, Crewes A, Weeks J. The respiratory effects of reduction of mite allergen in the bedrooms of asthmatic children – A double-blind controlled trial. Clin Exp Allergy 1996; 26:386–396.

40. Wood RA, Chapman MD, Adkinson NF,Jr., Eggleston PA. The effect of cat removal on allergen content in household-dust samples. J Allergy Clin Immunol 1989; 83:730–734.

41. Wood RA, Mudd KE, Eggleston PA. The distribution of cat and dust mite allergens on wall surfaces. J Allergy Clin Immunol 1992; 89:126–130.

42. Gelber LE, Seltzer LH, Bouzoukis JK, Pollart SM, Chapman MD, Platts-Mills TAE. Sensitization and exposure to indoor allergens as risk factors for asthma among patients presenting to hospital. Am Rev Resp Dis 1993; 147:573–578.

43. Sporik R, Ingram JM, Price W, Sussman JH, Honsinger RW, Platts-Mills TAE. Association of asthma with serum IgE and skin-test reactivity to allergens among children living at high altitude: Tickling the dragon's breath. Am J Res Crit Care Med 1995; 151:1388–1392.

44. Bollinger ME, Eggleston PA, Flanagan E, Wood RA. Cat antigen in homes with or without cats may induce allergic symptoms. J Allergy Clin Immunol 1996; 97(4):907–14.

45. De Blay F, Chapman MD, Platts-Mills TAE. Airborne cat allergen (Fel d 1): Environmental control with the cat in situ. Am Rev Respir Dis 1991; 143:1334–1339.

46. Luczynska CM, Li Y, Chapman MD, Platts-Mills TAE. Airborne concentrations and particle size distribution of allergen derived from domestic cats (Felis domesticus): Measurements using cascade impactor, liquid impinger and a two site monoclonal antibody assay for Fel d 1. Am Rev Resp Dis 1990; 141:361–367.

47. Ohman JL, Lowell FC, Bloch KJ. Allergens of mammalian origin: Characterization of allergen extract from cat pelts. J Allergy Clin Immunol 1973; 52:231.

48. Glinert R, Wilson P, Wedner HJ. Fel d 1 is markedly reduced following sequential washing of cats. J Allergy Clin Immunol 1990; 85:327.

49. Klucka GV, Ownby DR, Green J, Zoratti E. Cat shedding of Fel d 1 is not reduced by washings, Allerpet-C spray, or acepromazine. J Allergy Clin Immunol 1995; 95:1164–71.

50. Avner DB, Perzanowski MS, Platts-Mills TAE, Woodfolk JA. Evaluation of different techniques for washing cats: Quantitation of allergen removed from the cat and the effect on airborne Fel d 1. J Allergy Clin Immunol 1997; 100:307–312.

51. Perzanowski MS, Wheatley LM, Avner DB, Woodfolk JA, Platts-Mills TAE. The effectiveness of Allerpet-C at reducing the cat allergen Fel d 1 on a cat. J Allergy Clin Immunol 1997; 100:428–430.

52. Ingram JM, Sporik R, Rose G, Honsinger R, Chapman MD, Platts-Mills TAE. Quantitative assessment of exposure to dog (Can f 1) and cat (Fel d 1) allergens: Relationship to sensitization and asthma among children living in Los Alamos, NM. J Allergy Clin Immunol 1995; 96:449–56.

53. Hodson T, Custovic A, Simpson A, Chapman MD, Woodcock A, Green R. Washing the dog reduces dog allergen levels, but the dog needs to be washed twice a week. J Allergy Clin Immunol 1999; 103:581–585.

54. Platts-Mills TAE, Heymann PW, Longbottom JL, Wilkins SR. Airborne allergens associated with asthma: Particle sizes carrying dust mite and rat allergens measured with a cascade impactor. J Allergy Clin Immunol 1986; 77:850–857.

55. Pollart SM, Mullins DE, Vailes LD, Hayden ML, Platts-Mills TAE, Sutherland WM, Chapman MD. Identification, quantitation and purification of cockroach allergens using monoclonal antibodies. J Allergy Clin Immunol 1991; 87:511–521.

56. Chapman MD. Dissecting cockroach allergens. Clin Exp Allergy 1993; 23:459–461.

57. O'Hallaren MT, Yungigner JW, Offord KP, Somer MJ, O'Connell EJ, Ballerd DJ, Sachs MI. Exposure to an aeroallergen as a possible precipitating factor in respiratory arrest in young patients with asthma. New Eng J Med 1991; 324:359–363.

58. Halonen M, Stern DA, Wright AL, Taussig LM, Martinez FD. Alternaria as a major allergen in children raised in a desert environment. Am J Resp Crit Care Med 1997; 155:1356–1361.

59. Perzanowski MS, Sporik RB, Squillace SM, Gelber LE, Call R, Carter M, Platts-Mills TAE. Sensitization to Alternaria as a risk factor for asthma in school age children. J Allergy Clin Immunol 1998; 101:626–632.

60. Platts-Mills TAE, Hayden ML, Chapman MD, Wilkins SR. Seasonal variation in dust mite and grass pollen allergens in dust from the houses of patients with asthma. J Allergy Clin Immunol 1987; 79:791–791.

61. Sridhara S, Vailes LD, Weber B, Cromwell O, Chapman MD. A two-site ELISA for Alternaria allergen Alt a 1: Use for comparison of the major allergen content of fungal extracts. J Allergy Clin Immunol 1999; 103:S235.

Management of Severe Asthma in Children

Stanley J Szefler*, Joseph D Spahn*,**

Keywords: Severe asthma, corticosteroid insensitive asthma, corticosteroids, childhood asthma

Severe asthma in children is poorly understood in relation to its natural history, pathogenesis and treatment. Although limited information is available, principles of management for severe asthma can be extended based on experience in adult patients. Similar to severe asthma in adults, it is important to verify the diagnosis in children and evaluate for concomitant disorders, such as sinusitis and gastroesophageal reflux. Following this evaluation, the management of these patients requires the use of inhaled corticosteroids, administered in medium to high doses, as the cornerstone of management in combination with nonsteroid long-term controllers. This review will summarize the principles of evaluation and management of severe asthma in children and what areas need further study. Ongoing clinical research is needed to refine these management principles for these children who are at high risk for morbidity and mortality associated with asthma.

What Do We Know?

In understanding the management of severe asthma in children, it is important to improve our understanding of the natural history. We know that asthma can occur early in life. Current therapy, even in children, is based on the concept that chronic inflammation is a key feature of asthma, but there is very little information on the time of onset of inflammation and the mechanism for its initiation, progression, and persistence. There is a general feeling among asthma care specialists that early childhood asthma is underdiagnosed and undertreated. Current knowledge allows us to identify patients at high risk for asthma mortality. Information is now developing regarding patients at risk for chronic asthma, such as parental asthma, maternal smoking, atopic features and the presence of relevant allergens in the environment, and small lungs [1, 2].

One of the consequences of undertreatment may be a loss of pulmonary function (FEV_1) over time that is greater than that observed in patients without asthma, similar to that observed in chronic obstructive pulmonary disease and cystic fibrosis [3–5]. It is apparent that inhaled corticosteroids are effective in controlling asthma symptoms and reducing the intensity of the inflammatory response in studies conducted in adults with asthma. Since inhaled corticosteroids reduce asthma symptoms and lung function, it is likely that reduction in the inflammatory response also occurs in children with asthma. Unfortunately, inhaled corticosteroids appear to have limited long lasting and disease modifying effects. In other words, they are only effective as long as they are administered and for a short time (weeks to months) thereafter.

Two studies from the Dutch CNSLD Study Group sought to address this issue in children with moderate asthma. In the first study [6], the investigators sought to determine whether long-term budesonide therapy would result in clinical asthma remission during therapy. Of the 53 children originally randomized to receive budesonide, 60% achieved an 8-month clinical remission at some point during the three-year study. However, only one third were in remission upon completion of the study, and only 15% of the patients had a normal FEV_1 ($\geq 90\%$) and a normal PC_{20} value (> 150 μg). The authors concluded that although long-term budesonide therapy improved asthma symptoms and objective measures of asthma, it did not cure the disease.

This point was strengthened in their second follow-up study [7]. In this case, 28 children from the original cohort who had been on budesonide for 2–3 years were randomized to continue budesonide (8 patients; 600 μg/d) or to be completely tapered off budesonide (20 patients). All patients were

* Divisions of Clinical Pharmacology and Allergy and Immunology, Department of Pediatrics, University of Colorado Health Sciences Center, Denver, Colorado, USA; Helen Wohlberg & Herman Lambert Chair in Pharmacokinetics
** Department of Pediatrics, National Jewish Medical and Research Center, Denver, Colorado, USA

followed over a 6-month period. Eight of the 20 patients tapered off budesonide had to be withdrawn during the 6-month follow-up and 5 required prednisone secondary to poor asthma control compared to none in the budesonide group. In addition, much of the gain in lung function and bronchial hyperresponsiveness (BHR) that these children displayed while on 2–3 years of budesonide were lost by the end of the 6-month placebo period. Thus it appears as if inhaled corticosteroids can induce a short-lived clinical remission while on therapy. There is no known treatment that can consistently induce a lasting remission in the disease however, inhaled corticosteroids have a relatively slow offset of effect, compared to other long term controller medications [8]. Understanding the onset and progression of the inflammation, as well as its persistence, could provide insight into defining appropriate strategies for treatment depending on the stage of the disease [3].

Theories have developed that early intervention with inhaled corticosteroid therapy can be effective in preventing the progression of the disease and the risk for irreversible changes in the airways that could result in the persistence of symptoms [8–11]. Thus, there appears to be a "window of opportunity" that is critical for intervention. Patients with "difficult to control asthma" have evidence of persistent inflammation [12–14]. Their disease often has its onset in early childhood. Does this information suggest that children who manifest persistent inflammation in the presence of anti-inflammatory therapy could be at increased risk for disease progression? If so, it will be important to recognize these patients and provide more effective interventions at critical stages of their disease progression.

Given the paucity of published information on severe asthma in children, we recently performed a retrospective review of 164 consecutive adolescents admitted to our institution with the diagnosis of severe asthma [15]. The median age of the study population was 14.0 years with a median duration of asthma of 11.9 years. All were on high dose inhaled corticosteroid therapy (1500 µg/d) and roughly 50% also required maintenance oral corticosteroid therapy. Despite high dose inhaled and oral corticosteroid therapy, these children had evidence for ongoing airway inflammation as evidenced by elevated eosinophil cationic protein (ECP) levels (median 14.0 ng/ml, normal range 0–10) and airflow obstruction with an admission FEV_1 of 77% of predicted. In addition, nearly 3/4 of the children were atopic. Of some surprise, nearly 25% of the children were found to be corticosteroid insensitive as defined by a less than 15% improvement in their AM pre-bronchodilator FEV_1 following a course of high dose prednisone therapy. Corticosteroid insensitive asthmatics required a larger maintenance oral corticosteroid dose, required oral corticosteroid therapy at an earlier age, and were more likely to be African American than those adolescents with steroid sensitive asthma. In summary, our data would suggest that children with severe asthma had asthma for much of their lives and had evidence for ongoing disease activity despite aggressive inhaled and oftentimes oral corticosteroid therapy. In addition, a higher than expected number of these adolescents had a less than expected response to oral corticosteroid therapy and were termed corticosteroid insensitive. For a more complete discussion on our present understanding of corticosteroid insensitive asthma, see our review on this topic in this series of presentations [16].

The management of severe asthma in children poses some unique challenges. As is the case for the natural history of severe asthma in childhood, the available literature is a fraction of that published from research in adult patients. While some of the principles can be extrapolated from experience in managing adult patients, additional research is needed to determine if the pathogenesis of severe asthma is similar in children with severe asthma. Similar to adults with severe asthma, the cornerstone of management for severe asthma in children includes high dose inhaled corticosteroids. Dosage guidelines are available in the National Asthma Education and Prevention Program Expert Panel Report for the various inhaled corticosteroids and available delivery devices [2]. This treatment is combined with a long-acting nonsteroid controller medication either long acting inhaled β_2-agonist, sustained release theophylline, or long acting β_2-agonist tablets, and if necessary corticosteroid tablets or syrup long term. It is recommended to make repeated attempts to reduce systemic corticosteroid and maintain control with high-dose inhaled corticosteroid [1, 2]. It is extremely important that adherence to the treatment program be monitored.

A careful evaluation must be conducted for diseases that can masquerade as asthma, for example, vocal cord dysfunction, cystic fibrosis, congenital heart disease, etc. In addition, it is important that concomitant disorders, such as sinusitis and gastroesophageal reflux, be evaluated as these disorders can contribute to poor asthma control [17]. The clinician should be sure that an action plan is developed and that the patient is carefully following this plan. This along with frequent visits to review asthma control are key elements to reducing the oral and inhaled corticosteroid requirement, a necessity in minimizing the risk for significant adverse corticosteroid effects.

Although a preferred inhaled corticosteroid has not been defined to date, it seems reasonable that patients with severe asthma should be treated with a high potency inhaled corticosteroid, such as fluticasone propionate, to minimize the number of actuations administered. An inhaled corticosteroid administered with a delivery device that improves delivery to the lung, such as budesonide with the Turbuhaler device, is a reasonable alternative [2].

To minimize the dose of inhaled corticosteroid, long-term noncorticosteroid controllers can be added, as mentioned previously. It should be noted that the studies demonstrating an additive effect between inhaled corticosteroids and a long-term controller medication have been performed on adults with moderate to severe asthma [18, 19]. There has only been one study that evaluated this issue in childhood asthma. Verberne et al. [20], studied the effect of beclomethasone dipropionate (BDP) 400 µg/d vs. BDP 800 µg/d vs. BDP 400 µg/d plus salmeterol 100 µg/d in a group of 177 asthmatic children already on inhaled corticosteroid therapy. After 1 year, no significant differences in FEV_1, methacholine PD_{20} values, or symptom scores were noted. Each treatment resulted in improved baseline lung function (~5%) and reduced airway responsiveness (0.60 to 1.3 doubling doses). Of note, those on BDP 800 µg/d grew at a slower rate than the other 2 groups (mean height 3.6 cm for BDP 800 vs. 5.1 cm for BDP 400 + salmeterol, vs. 4.5 cm in the BDP 400 group). Of significance, BDP at a dose of 400 µg/d was as effective as either doubling the dose of BDP, or adding of salmeterol to the regimen. The results of this study differ from those performed in adults with asthma. The authors suggest that the adult studies recruited asthmatics with more severe and unstable disease as evidenced by their lower baseline lung function and greater symptoms upon entry into the study. Also of note, the improvement in airway responsiveness in the BPD 800 µg/d group was much greater than that seen in the adult studies where the dose of BDP was doubled. This would suggest that BHR can be altered to a greater extent in children than in adults.

Beyond high dose, high potency or increased pulmonary delivery of inhaled corticosteroids combined with a long-acting bronchodilator, it is not clear what the preferred additional long-term controller medication should be. There are no studies that evaluate the combination of high-dose inhaled corticosteroids with a long acting inhaled β_2-agonist, such as salmeterol, along with another long-term controller medication, for example a leukotriene modifier, theophylline, or nedocromil. Therefore, it is not known what combination is most effective in enhancing asthma control, resolving inflammation, and perhaps contributing to normalization of the airway. Studies are needed in this area to assist the clinician. In the absence of this information, the clinician should follow clinical parameters carefully in assessing the best combination of medications.

While environmental control can be helpful in the sensitized patient, immunotherapy should not be considered in severe asthma since it may incur a significant risk for adverse effects [21] and the beneficial effect, if any, is small. If a patient fails to respond or is unable to tolerate oral corticosteroid doses lower than 20 mg every other day with either prednisone or methylprednisolone, evaluation of corticosteroid pharmacokinetics, if available, can identify patients with incomplete corticosteroid absorption, failure to convert an inactive form (prednisone) to an active form (prednisolone), or rapid elimination [22, 23]. However, this is not a reason for poor response in all severe asthmatics since less than 25% of severe asthmatics show significantly increased clearance of either prednisolone or methylprednisolone. Most of the patients, both adults and children, with increased clearance have a specific reason for rapid elimination, such as a drug interaction with a medication that induces corticosteroid metabolism, for example the anticonvulsants, phenytoin, carbamazepine or phenobarbital, or rifampin.

Chronopharmacologic principles can be applied to optimize response to theophylline and corticosteroids [24–26]. For example, patients with nocturnal exacerbations may do much better with a single dose of a once daily sustained release theophylline preparation administered in the evening as compared to a standard twice daily preparation [24]. Children and rapid theophylline metabolizers appear to be prone to a reduction in serum theophylline concentrations during the night when the rate of elimination may exceed the rate of absorption [25]. An oral corticosteroid may also be more effective when administered in the late afternoon as compared to a morning dose [26].

Markers of inflammation, for example serum

ECP levels and circulating eosinophil counts, may be helpful in examining medication response in children with severe asthma when they are detectable [27]. In children with severe asthma, the marker can be measured before and after a one to two week course of oral corticosteroid therapy. A significant reduction in the marker should be noted following a course of prednisone therapy. Failure to respond to high dose corticosteroid therapy provides a strong base for incorporating trials of alternative anti-inflammatory or immunomodulator therapies, such as intravenous gammaglobulin, oral gold, or cyclosporine. Measurements of exhaled nitric oxide may also be useful as a measure of inflammation and response to therapeutic intervention, but even this measure has not been regularly incorporated in studies of severe asthma in children. Finally, in occasional circumstances a tissue biopsy approach may be considered in highly refractory patients. These studies should only be done in centers with experience in performing and interpreting biopsies from asthma patients. By the identification of tissue pathology, these studies could provide insight into the design of treatment options specifically suited to the pathology identified [28]. This could also lead to a differentiation of the disease among this patient population to guide the selection of individual patient treatment courses.

Several recent observations help to explain the limitations in response to conventional therapy in patients with severe asthma. Certain patients have been termed "corticosteroid resistant" or "insensitive" asthmatics. These patients are characterized by having a pre-bronchodilator FEV_1 less than 70% predicted while maintaining a bronchodilator response. Corticosteroid insensitivity is defined clinically by administering a course of oral prednisone, e. g., 40 mg per day (divided doses) for a minimum of 7 days, preferably two weeks, and observing the effect on morning pre-bronchodilator FEV_1 [14]. If the FEV_1 fails to increase by 15% or more then the patient is considered corticosteroid insensitive. See our accompanying review for more information on this topic [16].

It is not clear what corticosteroid dose should be administered in patients who are already receiving high dose oral and inhaled corticosteroid therapy. A trial of prednisone 40 mg per day for two weeks is usually given to assess the possibility of poor adherence to the maintenance regimen. If the patient fails to respond, the dose is generally doubled and the patient is monitored for an additional two weeks. If the patient responds to this high cortico-steroid dose, then the dose is gradually decreased while monitoring daily peak expiratory flow (PEF) to determine a threshold dose.

Studies of the corticosteroid insensitive patient population show that they have reduced glucocorticoid receptor (GCR) binding affinity, increased GCRβ concentrations, and failure to reduce inflammatory cells in bronchoalveolar lavage (BAL) fluid following a two week course of high dose oral prednisone therapy [14, 16, 29]. These abnormalities appear to be related to persistent inflammation despite high dose oral and inhaled corticosteroid therapy. Their course of treatment is often complicated by adverse effects of corticosteroid therapy, such as growth impairment, corticosteroid-induced osteoporosis, hypertension and obesity. In addition, some of these patients with severe asthma appear to have a neutrophil predominance [28] and additional studies are needed to determine if the neutrophils play a role in refractoriness to corticosteroid therapy and if a specific approach to altering neutrophil chemotaxis or activity would be an effective form of therapy. To date, clinical trials with the alternative anti-inflammatory and immunomodulator therapies are based on the symptom complex of the severe asthma patients and not specific pathology.

While examining corticosteroid insensitive asthma patients, it was also noted that a small proportion have a low GCR number [30]. This may be related to a genetic abnormality in the constitution of the receptor number. Other genetic abnormalities have been observed in the asthma population such as β-adrenergic receptor polymorphism [31] and 5-lipoxygenase polymorphism [32]. The prevalence of these abnormalities and clinical significance in the pathogenesis of severe asthma and refractoriness to treatment remains to be defined.

In addition, the clinician managing severe asthma in children must keep in mind the complicating effects of corticosteroids, especially high dose systemic corticosteroid therapy, such as growth impairment, osteoporosis, hypertension, and reduced neuromuscular function. The latter complication may interfere with the pulmonary assessment of the beneficial effects of anti-inflammatory and immunomodulating medications.

In children with severe asthma, who remain symptomatic despite optimal application of conventional therapy and management of concomitant disorders, studies are available primarily in adults demonstrating modest and inconsistent efficacy of alternative anti-inflammatory and immunomodulating drugs, such as methotrexate, gold, cyclosporine, and intravenous gammaglobulin, and macrolide antibiotics [33, 34]. In general, these studies indicate an ability to reduce oral corticosteroid requirements by approximately 50%, but with limited effect on improving pulmonary function and BHR. Most of the studies were not conducted at a time when it was customary to utilize high dose, high potency or enhanced delivery inhaled corticosteroids. In the presence of this form of treatment and especially in combination with other long-term controllers, these immunomodulator and alternative anti-inflammatory treatments are not very impressive. Intravenous gamma globulin can be effective in certain patients but its high cost is prohibitive. Methotrexate has limited efficacy and carries a risk for liver toxicity and immunosuppression. Cyclosporine has only been utilized in a limited study population and carries a significant risk for renal disease and hypertension. Oral gold has limited efficacy and gastrointestinal adverse effects can limit its use. In the limited number of studies where a placebo control is incorporated, there are responders and nonresponders to each of these treatments, but no methodology to predict who will respond favorably. These protocols have almost uniformly failed to incorporate methods to measure resolution of inflammation specifically with bronchial biopsy and bronchoalveolar lavage techniques [33, 34].

In studies where an indirect measure of resolving inflammation was incorporated, i.e., BHR, no change was observed following treatment with methotrexate or intravenous gammaglobulin. Biopsy studies in adults with severe asthma have stimulated a resurgence of interest in the use of macrolide antibiotics in the treatment of asthma with the recognition of mycoplasma and chlamydia-like organisms as a complicating feature of severe asthma [35–37]. Studies are needed with all of these agents to carefully define their benefits and risks, as well as the patients most likely to respond to the selected treatment. Therefore, all patients who require this form of alternative treatment should be directed to sites of clinical research with organized protocols.

What Do We Need to Know?

In order to effectively design treatment strategies for severe asthma in both children and adults it is obviously important to understand the pathophysiology of the disease. Several questions must be addressed

to improve our approach to management, including but not limited to the following: If severe asthma in children is a manifestation of persistent inflammation or different types of inflammation, what is the key driving force for this inflammatory response? If there are different types of persistent inflammation, can we match effective treatments to specific types of inflammation? Are there patients in whom steroid therapy may conceivably be disadvantageous? What diagnostic tests can be used to select those patients who will respond to alternative anti-inflammatory or immunomodulator therapies?

It is extremely important to understand the natural history of this form of asthma to not only determine whether it can be identified by measuring pulmonary function serially over time but also to determine methods to identify patients at risk for severe asthma and subsequently signal the need for early intervention. It is also important to move toward a categorization of the various forms of severe asthma. This is not only necessary for defining appropriate inclusion/exclusion criteria for clinical research but also for communication of results and extrapolation of studies to patient care. Although this categorization could be based on the symptom complex, perhaps a better alternative is the defined pulmonary pathology, or specific measures of pulmonary function. While pulmonary function via spirometry can be reliably measured in children great than 5 years of age, techniques must be defined to measure pulmonary function in younger children to assist in early recognition of severe airway compromise or progressive deterioration in pulmonary function.

Besides the available immunomodulators, anti-inflammatory, and antibiotic therapies, there are some new medications on the horizon that could be useful in altering the course of inflammation associated with severe persistent and refractory asthma. These medications include: anti-IgE, cytokine antagonists, adhesion molecule antagonists, selective agonists and antagonists of the neurogenic pathways, metalloproteinases, low molecular weight heparin, respiratory ant-sense oligonucleotides, and DNA vaccines.

How Do We Get the Answers?

Based on the complexity of the disease and the urgent needs for organizing the knowledge base, it would be very helpful to develop a working group or network to efficiently design and conduct clinical studies. This group should be multidisciplinary in order to address the many facets of severe asthma in children and produce guidelines for management. The advantages of such a network would be an organized approach to clinical research, shared resources, and adequate patient numbers to perform comprehensive studies. A registry of severe asthmatics could also be developed to conduct epidemiologic evaluation and assist in recruitment for clinical studies.

Clinical studies in severe asthma in adults and children should incorporate a standardized approach with all attempts being made to obtain as much information as possible to address specific questions without compromising safety, especially in children. As many available tools as possible should be used to understand the disease and evaluate response to treatment including pulmonary physiology (spirometry; bronchial challenge to methacholine, histamine, or exercise; and body plethysmography); biopsy; bronchoalveolar lavage; induced sputum; exhaled nitric oxide; and peripheral blood cell and plasma markers. Some, but not all, could be used in pediatric clinical studies.

More information is needed on the pathology of severe asthma in adults as well as children, if at all possible, to define the nature of the ultrastructural abnormalities. It is possible that aggressive courses of anti-inflammatory or immunomodulator therapy can suppress active inflammation, but airway remodeling may predispose the patient to residual symptoms secondary to persistent BHR or possibly, a noninflammatory based BHR. Obviously, more effort must be placed on understanding the pathophysiology of severe asthma to refine the selection of pharmacotherapy for this challenging group of patients. It is important to assess the effect of age, gender, duration of disease and race on response to medications, as well as risks of adverse effects [38, 39].

The core structure of a medication trial in severe asthma should consist of a multicenter, placebo controlled, randomized, and parallel design. Objective measures of response, such as pulmonary function measures and measures of airway inflammation should be incorporated to carefully evaluate responders and nonresponders within the treatment groups.

Studies with selected interventions should consist of two phases. In the first phase, the medication or corresponding placebo should be added with no change in concomitant therapy. The purpose of this phase is to assess the direct benefit of study medication as compared to placebo. The minimum time period to assess efficacy is usually 6 weeks, however this can be modified based on preliminary open label trials directly designed to evaluate the time of onset of effect. The second phase is where medication reduction can be evaluated, specifically oral corticosteroid therapy. The purpose is to assess the oral corticosteroid sparing effect of the trial medication. This phase usually takes a minimum of 3 months. Comprehensive measurements of pulmonary function and airway inflammation could be obtained prior to randomization and upon completion of each of the two study phases.

This type of design would permit pharmacologic trials to assess the effect of treatment on active inflammation vs. arrested progression, to identify major inflammatory cells and thus focus selection of treatment to correlate clinical response to alteration of inflammation, to assess the role of infection, and to assess the role of individual and combination therapy. The combination of careful clinical studies in children with established severe asthma and the coordination of programs to identify patients at risk and the identification of an appropriate intervention would go a long way to reduce the risk of this life threatening disease.

Acknowledgments

The authors wish to thank Maureen Plourd-Sandoval for assistance in preparing this manuscript.

Supported in part by Public Health Services Research Grants HL36577 and General Clinical Research Center Grant 5 MO1 RR00051 from the Division of Research Resources, and an American Lung Association Asthma Research Center Grant.

Address for correspondence:

Stanley J Szefler, MD
National Jewish Medical
and Research Center
1400 Jackson St.
Rm. J209
Denver, Colorado 80206
USA
Tel. +1 303 398-1193
Fax +1 303 270-2189
E-mail szeflers@njc.org

References

1. Global Initiative for Asthma. Global strategy for asthma management and prevention, NHLBI/NIH workshop report. In National Institutes of Health, National Heart, Lung, and Blood Institute, 1995, Publ. No. 95.

2. National Asthma Education and Prevention Program Expert Panel Report 2: Guidelines for the Diagnosis and Management of Asthma. In National Institutes of Health, National Heart, Lung, and Blood Institute, 1997, Publ. No. 97.

3. Peat JK. Asthma: A longitudinal perspective. J Asthma 1998; 35:235.

4. Weiss ST. Early life predictors of adult chronic obstructive lung disease. Eur Respir Rev 1995; 5:303.

5. Lange P, Parner J, Vestbo J, Schnohr P, Jensen G. A 15-year follow-up study of ventilatory function in adults with asthma. N Engl J Med 1998; 339:1194.

6. van Essen-Zandvliet EE, Hughes MD, Waalkens HJ, Duiverman EJ, Kerrebijn KF. Remission of childhood asthma after long-term treatment with an inhaled corticosteroid (budesonide): Can it be achieved? Dutch CNSLD Study Group. Eur Respir J 1994; 7:63.

7. Waalkens HJ, Van Essen-Zandvliet EE, Hughes MD, Gerritsen J, Duiverman EJ, Knol K, Kerrebijn KF. Cessation of long-term treatment with inhaled corticosteroid (budesonide) in children with asthma results in deterioration. The Dutch CNSLD Study Group. Am Rev Respir Dis 1993; 148:1252.

8. Haahtela T, Jarvinen M, Kava T, Kiviranta K, Koskinen S, Lehtonen K, Nikander K, Persson T, Selroos O, Sovijarvi A, et al. Effects of reducing or discontinuing inhaled budesonide in patients with mild asthma. N Engl J Med 1994; 331:700.

9. Agertoft L, Pedersen S. Effects of long-term treatment with an inhaled corticosteroid on growth and pulmonary function in asthmatic children. Respir Med 1994; 88:373.

10. Selroos O, Pietinalho A, Lofroos AB, Riska H. Effect of early vs late intervention with inhaled corticosteroids in asthma. Chest 1995; 108:1228.

11. Overbeek SE, Kerstjens HA, Bogaard JM, Mulder PG, Postma DS. Is delayed introduction of inhaled corticosteroids harmful in patients with obstructive airways disease (asthma and COPD)? The Dutch Chronic Nonspecific Lung Disease Study Groups. Chest 1996; 110:35.

12. Leung DYM, Martin RJ, Szefler SJ, Sher ER, Ying S, Kay AB, Hamid Q. Dysregulation of interleukin 4, interleukin 5, and interferon γ gene expression in steroid-resistant asthma. J Exp Med 1995; 181:33.

13. Wenzel SE, Szefler SJ, Leung DYM, Sloan SI, Rex MD, Martin RJ. Bronchoscopic evaluation of severe asthma. Persistent inflammation associated with high dose glucocorticoids. Am J Respir Crit Care Med 1997; 156:737.

14. Lee TH, Brattsand R, Leung DYM. Corticosteroid action and resistance in asthma. Am J Respir Crit Care Med 1996; 154:S1.

15. Chan MT, Leung DYM, Szefler SJ, Spahn JD. Difficult-to-control asthma: Clinical characteristics of steroid-insensitive asthma. J Allergy Clin Immunol 1998; 101:594.

16. Szefler SJ, Leung DYM. Severe persistent and corticosteroid insensitive asthma. In this volume.

17. Irwin RS, Curley FJ, French CL. Difficult-to-control asthma. Contributing factors and outcome of a systematic management protocol. Chest 1993; 103:1662.

18. Greening AP, Ind PW, Northfield M, Shaw G. Added salmeterol versus higher-dose corticosteroid in asthma patients with symptoms on existing inhaled corticosteroid. Allen & Hanburys Limited UK Study Group. Lancet 1994; 344:219.

19. Woolcock A, Lundback B, Ringdal N, Jacques LA. Comparison of addition of salmeterol to inhaled steroids with doubling of the dose of inhaled steroids. Am J Respir Crit Care Med 1996; 153:1481.

20. Verberne AA, Frost C, Duiverman EJ, Grol MH, Kerrebijn KF. Addition of salmeterol versus doubling the dose of beclomethasone in children with asthma. The Dutch Asthma Study Group. Am J Respir Crit Care Med 1998; 158:213.

21. Bousquet J, Michel FB. Specific immunotherapy in asthma: Is it effective? J Allergy Clin Immunol 1994; 94:1.

22. Spahn JD, Leung DYM, Szefler SJ. Difficult to control asthma: New insights and implications for management. In DYM Leung, SJ Szefler (Eds), Severe asthma: Pathogenesis and clinical management. New York: Marcel Dekker 1996, p. 497.

23. Hill MR, Szefler SJ, Ball BD, Bartoszek M, Brenner AM. Monitoring glucocorticoid therapy: A pharmacokinetic approach. Clin Pharmacol Ther 1990; 48:390.

24. Martin RJ, Cicutto LC, Ballard RD, Goldenheim PD, Cherniack RM. Circadian variations in theophylline concentrations and the treatment of nocturnal asthma. Am Rev Respir Dis 1989; 139:475.

25. Kossoy AF, Hill M, Lin FL, Szefler SJ. Are theophylline "levels" a reliable indicator of compliance? J Allergy Clin Immunol 1989; 84:60.

26. Beam WR, Weiner DE, Martin RJ. Timing of prednisone and alterations of airways inflammation in nocturnal asthma. Am Rev Respir Dis 1992; 146:1524.

27. Spahn JD, Leung DYM, Surs W, Harbeck RJ, Nimmagadda S, Szefler SJ. Reduced glucocorticoid binding affinity in asthma is related to ongoing allergic inflammation. Am J Respir Crit Care Med 1995; 151:1709.

28. Wenzel SE, Szefler SJ, Leung DYM, Sloan SI, Rex

MD, Martin RJ. Bronchoscopic evaluation of severe asthma. Persistent inflammation associated with high dose glucocorticoids. Am J Respir Crit Care Med 1997; 156:737.

29. Szefler SJ, Spahn JD, Wenzel SE, Leung DYM. Glucocorticoid insensitive asthma: Lessons for future asthma management. In AL Sheffer (Ed), Fatal asthma. New York: Marcel Dekker 1998, p. 307.

30. Sher ER, Leung DY, Surs W, Kam JC, Zieg G, Kamada AK, Szefler SJ. Steroid-resistant asthma. Cellular mechanisms contributing to inadequate response to glucocorticoid therapy. J Clin Invest 1994; 93:33.

31. Turki J, Pak J, Green SA, Martin RJ, Liggett SB. Genetic polymorphisms of the β_2-adrenergic receptor in nocturnal and nonnocturnal asthma. Evidence that Gly16 correlates with the nocturnal phenotype. J Clin Invest 1995; 95:1635.

32. In KH, Asano K, Beier D, Grobholz J, Finn PW, Silverman EK, Silverman ES, Collins T, Fischer AR, Keith TP, Serino K, Kim SW, De Sanctis GT, Yandava C, Pillari A, Rubin P, Kemp J, Israel E, Busse W, Ledford D, Murray JJ, Segal A, Tinkleman D, Drazen JM. Naturally occurring mutations in the human 5-lipoxygenase gene promoter that modify transcription factor binding and reporter gene transcription. J Clin Invest 1997; 99:1130.

33. Jarjour N, McGill K, Busse WW, Gelfand EW. Alternative anti-inflammatory and immunomodulatory therapy. In SJ Szefler, DYM Leung (Eds), Severe asthma: Pathogenesis and clinical management. New York: Marcel Dekker 1996, p. 333.

34. Spector SL. Treatment of the unusually difficult asthmatic patient. Allergy Asthma Proc 1997; 18:153.

35. Hahn DL. Intracellular pathogens and their role in asthma: Chlamydia pneumonia in adult patients. Eur Respir Rev 1996; 6:224.

36. Black PN. The use of macrolides in the treatment of asthma. Eur Respir Rev 1996; 6:240.

37. Kraft M, Cassell GH, Henson JE, Watson H, Williamson J, Marmion BP, Gaydos CA, Martin RJ. Detection of Mycoplasma pneumoniae in the airways of adults with chronic asthma. Am J Respir Crit Care Med 1998; 158:998.

38. Covar R, Leung DYM, Chan MTS, Spahn JD. Risk factors associated with glucocorticoid (GC) side effects in adolescents with severe asthma-revisited. J Allergy Clin Immunol 1999; 103:S61.

39. Spahn JD, Brown EE, Covar R, Leung DYM. Do African Americans display a diminished response to glucocorticoids (GCs)? J Allergy Clin Immunol 1999; 103:S62.

Asthma Self-Management Plan System of Care

Wendyl D'Souza, Neil Pearce, Julian Crane, Richard Beasley*

Keywords: Asthma, management, education

The development of self-management plans arose as clinicians tried to design better methods by which they could deliver asthma care and reduce the significant mortality and morbidity associated with this disease. The basic principles that resulted have been widely endorsed, with self-management plans now being considered essential in the long term management of adult asthma.

Self-management plans essentially focus on the early recognition of unstable or deteriorating asthma, by monitoring peak flow or symptoms. Through the use of written guidelines, patients are then able to determine when it is necessary to adjust therapy or obtain medical assistance. The use of self-management plans by patients with asthma has been shown to lead to improvements in asthma morbidity and a reduced requirement for acute medical treatment and hospital admission. However, it is acknowledged that more research is needed to clarify many different issues concerning their structure and implementation.

Many different systems of asthma self-management have now been developed, reflecting different management and educational practices. It is apparent that the needs of all patients cannot be met through the use of one particular version. Whatever plan is employed, the written guidelines need to reflect the health care system and cultural needs of the respective community in which it is introduced and must be tailored to meet the specific needs of individual patients.

Asthma self-management plans are currently recommended as being essential in the long term treatment of asthma [1–3]. Their importance originates from the knowledge that delays in recognising worsening asthma and initiating appropriate therapy are important factors contributing to morbidity and mortality from asthma [4, 5]. This has led to the development of self-assessment and self-management systems for the patient to follow, in accordance with predetermined written guidelines. Support for this approach is enhanced by the knowledge that the majority of asthma attacks occur in

the community and are self-managed by patients without immediate consultation with their general practitioner. Thus, if an impact is to be made on morbidity and mortality from asthma, a pre-arranged system of assessment and management of both severe attacks of asthma as well as the long term management of asthma needs to be established.

Basic Principles

The basic principles of the self-management plan system of care are outlined in Table 1. Fundamental to the success of this strategy is the ability of the patient to recognise a deterioration in asthma control. This requires the assessment of asthma severity through the educated interpretation of key symptoms and measurements of lung function. The development of nocturnal wakening is recognised to be a good marker of unstable asthma [6], whereas the poor response to the increased use of inhaled β-agonist therapy is an important marker of a severe attack requiring medical review [7]. Such "resistance" to high doses of β-agonist treatment in

Table 1. The basic principles of self-management in adult asthma.

1. Requirement for the objective assessment of asthma severity with the educated interpretation of key symptoms and peak flow recordings.
2. The use of regular inhaled corticosteroids and intermittent beta agonists for the long term treatment of asthma; the use of systemic corticosteroids, high dose inhaled beta agonists, oxygen therapy and medical review for severe asthma.
3. The integration of self-assessment and self-management with written guidelines for both the long term treatment of asthma and the treatment of acute severe asthma.

---

*   Department of Medicine, Wellington School of Medicine, Wellington, New Zealand

severe asthma is likely to reflect the major contribution of mucus plugging and airway mucosal oedema to the airways obstruction in this clinical situation. Domiciliary measurements of peak expiratory flow, with values expressed as a percentage of normal predicted or previous best achieved recordings, are also recommended for the objective assessment of the degree of airflow obstruction. Peak flow monitoring is of particular importance in the severe asthmatic, as they have been shown to have the worst perception of asthma severity [8].

Most self-management plans are based on the regular long term use of inhaled corticosteroid therapy in association with the early use of oral corticosteroids for major exacerbations. Inhaled β-agonists are the bronchodilator drugs of choice, with patients advised that they should be used "as required" to reverse episodes of symptomatic asthma, and that the increased requirement for inhaled β-agonist therapy indicates worsening asthma.

Prototype Plan

There are a number of systems of asthma self-management that have been developed, based on the basic principles outlined above. The self-management plan system which has been developed and promoted within New Zealand is outlined in Table 2 [9, 10]. In many respects the first two stages can be considered to provide guidelines for the long-term management of asthma. In particular the instructions to vary the dose of inhaled corticosteroid treatment in a stepwise manner in accordance with changes in asthma severity represents one practical method whereby the recommendations for the long-term treatment of chronic persistent asthma in adults can be implemented. The third and fourth stages provide guidelines for the treatment of severe asthma, with intensive treatment started by the patient in an attempt to prevent the development of a life-threatening attack. Thus, self-management plans represent one way in which the recommendations for acute severe and chronic persistent asthma can be brought together in a single framework.

Efficacy

Despite the consensus on both the necessity and the principles underlying the development of asthma self-management plans, it is only recently that their efficacy has been clearly established. The best assessment of their efficacy can be obtained from the recent systematic review of the literature of the effects of education of the asthmatic in self-management [11]. This review involved 24 randomised controlled trials in which self-management asthma education was studied, of which there were 17 studies which involved the assessment of written action plans. The meta-analysis of these studies identified

Table 2. Adult asthma self-management plan: What to do and when.

Step	Peak Flow	Symptoms	Action
1	> 80–85% best	Intermittent/few	Continue regular inhaled corticosteroid; inhaled β-agonist for relief of symptoms
2	> 60–70% best	Waking at night with asthma; symptoms of a "cold"	Increase the dose of inhaled corticosteroid; inhaled β-agonist for relief of symptoms
3	> 40–50% best	Increasing breathlessness or poor response to bronchodilator	Start oral corticosteroids and contact a doctor; inhaled β-agonist for relief of symptoms
4	< 40–50% best	Worse; no response to bronchodilator	Self-administer high dose inhaled β-agonist, call emergency doctor or ambulance urgently

This plan may need to be modified with respect to the amount of detail it provides and the specific drug treatment recommended at each stage. Likewise, the severity of symptoms chosen and the specific peak flow values recommended for each stage may need to be altered in accordance with physician preference and the asthmatic patient's individual needs.

138

that self-management involving provision of a written action plan led to a significant reduction in hospitalisations for asthma (odds ratio 0.35) whereas less intensive interventions did not work. Similar findings were observed with respect to emergency hospital visits, in which there was a significant trend for self-management education to reduce the proportion of asthmatics needing such visits, with the additional provision of a written action plan leading to a greater reduction. In those studies in which nocturnal asthma was examined, the greatest reduction was observed in those groups receiving a written plan. In contrast there was no effect on FEV_1 in those studies in which this outcome variable was measured.

In the four studies which compared peak flow with symptom-based management plans, equivalent efficacy was observed in terms of the proportion of subjects requiring hospitalisation, emergency room treatment or an unscheduled visit to the doctor. There were no significant differences found in the five studies in which a comparison was made between those plans in which there was self-adjustment of medication by the patient according to written, predetermined criteria, or on the basis of regular review by a doctor.

Issues Requiring Clarification

Although the efficacy of the asthma self-management plan system of care has been demonstrated, there are a number of issues which have yet to be clarified, as outlined in Table 3. While clarification will be obtained for some of these issues when specific studies are undertaken, some features such as which components of the plan lead to the best clinical outcomes may prove difficult to unravel, as the different features of the plans are so closely interrelated. The evidence to date suggests that it is likely that the greatest benefit from self-management plans will be obtained with the close integration of the different features of self-assessment and management [12, 13].

Recommended Use

One important issue on which a better understanding is emerging is that certain asthmatics may ben-

Table 3. Issues relating to the structure and implementation of asthma self-management plans that require further clarification.

1. Number of stages/levels
   e. g., 2, 3 vs 4 stage plans
2. Specific peak flow percentages indicating each stage
   e. g., < 60% or 70% to start oral steroids
3. Specific symptoms indicating each stage
   e. g., Nocturnal asthma, increasing beta agonist use and/or symptoms of a cold for recognizing worsening asthma
4. Role of other medications
   e. g., Long acting β-agonists, leukotriene antagonists, theophylline, sodium cromoglycate/nedocromil
5. The relationship between specific therapeutic responses and outcome
   e. g., Does increasing inhaled steroid dose in worsening asthma prevent further deterioration?
6. Which forms for different patient groups
   e. g., Adults versus children
7. Methods of implementation
   e. g., Doctor versus other health professionals
8. Intensity of implementation
   e. g., How much peak flow and symptom monitoring is optimal?

efit more than others from this system of care [14]. In particular, it is recognised that the greatest benefit is likely to be obtained in patients with chronic severe asthma, and that compliance is likely to be a major problem in patients with mild asthma. As a result, it is possible to make the following recommendations as a guide to the need for self-management according to asthma severity.

In mild asthma, an initial period of assessment with recording of asthma symptoms and peak flow rates is recommended, to educate the patient to recognise changes in asthma severity, to identify those with a poor perception of asthma severity, to determine the best recorded peak flow values, and to monitor the response to the introduction of prophylactic therapy. Following this initial period, it would be possible to develop an asthma self-management plan which simply provides patients with written instructions as to when to seek medical help in the situation of a severe asthma attack. Unless the patient has a poor symptomatic perception of asthma severity, the regular use of a more detailed self-management plan is not recommended at this stage, as it is unlikely to lead to a major improvement in asthma control and is unlikely to be undertaken by the patient (even if recommended).

In patients with moderate to severe asthma, a similar period of assessment is recommended for the same reasons as in mild asthma, and to allow for the development of a more detailed three or four stage asthma self-management plan. It is recommended that the amount of detail included will depend on the requirements of the patient and the degree of medical supervision that is deemed to be necessary. Patients should be advised to use the plan preferentially during periods of unstable asthma rather than during periods of good control. Patients who are identified as being poor perceivers of asthma severity on the basis of symptoms alone are particularly encouraged to use such a self-management plan system of care.

For patients with high risk asthma, for example, those with recent hospital admissions, a large diurnal variation of peak flow despite maximal therapy, or known brittle asthma, the regular use of peak flow monitoring and recording of symptoms in association with an asthma self-management plan is recommended, together with intensive medical and nursing supervision.

Summary

In summary, asthma self-management plans can now be recommended with confidence, due to the accepted principles on which they are based, and the evidence that their use by asthmatic patients leads to improvements in asthma morbidity and a reduced requirement for acute medical treatment and hospital admission. However, in recommending the use of asthma self-management plans it is also important to recognise that the requirements of individual asthmatic patients may vary considerably and that no single plan is likely to be suitable for every patient. As a result, the amount of detail plans provide, the specific drug treatment recommended at each stage and the percentage reduction in peak flow, or severity of symptoms chosen for the different therapeutic responses recommended, may need to vary, depending on the specific characteristics and needs of the asthmatic patient. Whatever plan is employed it needs to reflect the health care system, management practices and cultural needs of the community in which it is implemented.

Acknowledgments

The Wellington Asthma Research Group is supported by programme grants from the Health Research Council of New Zealand and the Guardian Trust. We thank Ms Denise Fabian for her expert secretarial assistance.

Address for correspondence:

Prof. Richard Beasley
Department of Medicine
Wellington School of Medicine
PO Box 7343, Wellington
New Zealand
Tel. +64 4 385-5589
Fax +64 4 389-5429
E-mail Beasley@wnmeds.ac.nz

References

1. British Thoracic Society, Research Unit of Royal College of Physicians, Kings Fund Centre, National Asthma Campaign. Guidelines for management of asthma in adults: I-Chronic persistent asthma. Br Med J 1990; 301:651–653.

2. Lenfant C. International Consensus Report on Diagnosis and Management of Asthma. National Heart, Lung and Blood Institute, National Institute of Health. US Department of Health and Human Services, Bethesda, MD, USA 1992.

3. Global Initiative for Asthma. Global strategy for asthma management and prevention NHLBI/WHO Workshop Report. National Institutes of Health, National Heart, Lung and Blood Institute 1996.

4. British Thoracic Association. Death from asthma in two regions of England. Br Med J 1982; 285:1251–5.

5. Rea HH, Sears MR, Beaglehole R, Fenwick J, Jackson RT, Gillies AJ, O'Donnell TV, Holst PE, Rothwell RP. Lessons from the national asthma mortality study: Circumstances surrounding death. NZ Med J 1987; 100:10–13.

6. Turner-Warwick M. On observing patterns of airflow obstruction in chronic asthma. Br J Dis Chest 1977; 71:73–86.

7. Windom HH, Burgess CD, Crane J, Pearce N, Kwong T, Beasley R. The self-administration of inhaled β-agonist drugs during severe asthma. NZ Med J 1990; 103:205–207.

8. Rubinfeld AR, Pain MC. Perception of asthma. Lancet 1976; 1:822–824.

9. D'Souza W, Crane J, Burgess C, Te Karu H, Fox C, Harper M, Robson B, Howden-Chapman P, Crossland L, Woodman K, Pearce N, Pomare E, Beasley R. Community-based asthma care: Trial of a "credit

card" asthma self-management plan. Eur Respir J 1994; 7:1260–265.

10. D'Souza W, Burgess C, Ayson M, Crane J, Pearce N, Beasley R. Trial of a "credit card" asthma self-management plan in a "high risk" group of patients with asthma. J Allergy Clin Immunol 1996; 97(5):1085–1092.

11. Gibson PG, Coughlan J, Wilson AJ, Abramson M, Bauman A, Hensley MJ, Walters EH. The effects of self-management education and regular practitioner review in adults with asthma. The Cochrane Database of Systematic Reviews. The Cochrane Library, Vol. 4, 1998.

12. Lahdensuo A, Haahtela T, Herrala J, Kava T, Kiviranta K, Kuusisto P, Peramaki E, Poussa T, Saarelainen S, Svahn T. Randomised comparison of guided self-management and traditional treatment of asthma over one year. Br Med J 1996; 312:748–752.

13. Ignacio-Garcia JM, Gonzalez-Santos P. Asthma self-management education program by home monitoring of peak expiratory flow. Am J Respir Crit Care Med 1995; 151:353–359.

14. Fishwick D, Beasley R. Use of peak flow-based self-management plans by adult asthmatic patients (editorial). Eur Respir J 1996; 9:861–865.

Indoor Air Pollution and Health Risks: An Overview

Wim A Zwart Voorspuij*

Keywords: Indoor air quality, respiratory ventilation, indoor pollution, air pollution, risk communication

The indoor environment is influenced by qualities of buildings and dwellings (e. g., ventilation and heating devices), emissions of materials indoors, behavior of occupants, and general quality of outdoor air. Health risks and effects can result from exposure to physical, chemical, and biological agents or combinations thereof. Health effects range from minor complaints such as short-term annoyance, vague discomfort, or irritation, to diseases such as asthma, COPD, infectious diseases (legionellosis), cancer, and even death. Psychosocial factors may contribute to some of these health effects. Moisture, lack of ventilation, combustion products from open fires, allergens, some housing and occupants characteristics, as well as a number of other conditions can contribute to respiratory disorders, especially in children.

It is important to offer risk information to the general public concerning the health risks of exposure to indoor air pollutants. The goal is to change their behavior, resulting in a more healthy indoor air quality. Other primary target groups are architects, constructors, building owners, and health care workers.

Recommendations are based on an abatement of exposure, an increase of indoor comfort, better ventilation and heating devices, good maintenance, public campaigns, legal regulation and implementation of guidelines.

Introduction

In industrialized countries people spend almost 80% of their time indoors, either at home or at work [1]. The indoor environment, including indoor air, thermal, and acoustic conditions, is influenced by the following conditions:

- Buildings: materials used, ventilation, and heating equipment;
- Emissions of materials and products within the building;
- Behavior of residents: smoking, ventilation, pets, noise;
- Outdoor air quality and outdoor noise.

Indoor air quality in buildings is generally worse than outdoor air quality because of energy-saving measures and the locking out of harmful things like noise, burglary, and outdoor pollution. The consequences of these factors are increased problems due to moisture and indoor air pollution, leading to health risks and other effects, not only in dwellings, but also in offices, schools, health-care institutions, and elsewhere.

In this article we look at the sources of exposure and the consequences for the health of exposed people.

Risk communication is a tool employed to make people aware of the health risks and to help them to understand the impact of these risks compared with other risks – and to be open to the available information to minimize the risks and to prevent health effects.

Healthy Indoor Air Quality

There are no hard and fast criteria for indoor air quality. The Air Quality Guidelines of the WHO refer to outdoor air quality [2]. But generally, good indoor air quality refers to thermal comfort (20–26°C with 40–50% relative humidity), odor comfort, and acceptable levels of biological, physical, and chemical agents in indoor air without creating risks to health of the occupants [3]. Inadequate control of these factors may cause health problems. In practice, control of the indoor environment is not easy. For instance, ventilation, a very important parameter, is a continual trade-off between climate control, air quality, and energy efficiency.

Carbon dioxide is considered an overall indicator of indoor air quality. Its concentration in indoor air represents the result of the production from metabolic activities of the occupants and other combustion sources in the building as well as the spread and removal from the ventilation system. A low

*   Dutch Association for Environmental Medicine, The Hague, The Netherlands

level of carbon dioxide usually corresponds to acceptably low level concentrations of other indoor contaminants. The concentration should not exceed 0.15%. Under normal conditions, in dwellings this requires a supply of fresh air of more than 12–15 m^3 per person per hour [4].

Occupants in the indoor environment are usually exposed to complex mixtures rather than a single pollutant. Assessment of exposure and health risk is therefore difficult. Standards should be determined for substances that may typically be released or concentrated in the indoor environment.

Agents Influencing the Indoor Environment

A classification of agents that can influence the indoor environment was made in accordance with a directive of the Commission of the European Union concerning exposure risks in the occupational environment.

Physical Agents and Health

The physical agents that influence the indoor environment are thermal factors (temperature of air and walls, airspeed, and humidity), daylight, noise, radiation, moisture, and ventilation.

Central heating and insulation measures can improve the comfort of houses, but can also influence other factors like the emission of formaldehyde from chipboard, the growth of biological agents, and limitations on natural ventilation. In specific situations adverse conditions can appear, such as draught or the greenhouse effect in rooms with large glass surfaces. Noises produced by neighbors, traffic, and industry are a problem in many houses.

Radioactivity is mainly caused by radon, which is a product of decay of radioactive isotopes of uranium, thorium, and potassium. These materials are present in different concentrations depending on the type of soil and geographical origin. Indoor concentration of radon is mainly determined by the infiltration of radon from outdoor air and from the underground via the crawl space or the basement, less from building materials.

Radiation caused by electromagnetic fields is a matter of increasing concern with the public. Sources are high-voltage cables, masts (radio, television, telephone), microwave ovens, etc.

Moisture in houses is a complex problem and is connected with mold growth. Related to this specific indoor problem are several other factors: architectural aspects like cold-bridges, crawl space, high level of groundwater, ventilation, heating behavior, and production of moisture indoors. High relative humidity can cause strong mold growth and the presence of house dust mites.

Insufficient ventilation is caused either by insufficient facilities or by insufficient use of these facilities. The consequence is an increase in indoor air pollution, moisture, and foul odors. The Dutch Health Council advises a ventilation minimum of 5 m^3/h per person per room.

Most of the physical factors are related to comfort and nuisance. When the indoor air quality is bad, people report unspecific symptoms like headache, fatigue, irritated mucous membranes, lack of concentration, sleep disorders, general malaise, etc. It is difficult to relate these symptoms to a specific cause. Improving the physical conditions sometimes can solve the problems, but the combination of low-quality housing with other factors like lifestyle, unemployment, and lack of education can play an important role in the health problems. Therefore, it is usually difficult to prove a causal relationship between any one environmental factor and disease on an individual level.

Exposure to radioactivity can cause a higher cancer risk, especially lung cancer after exposure to radon [5]. The health risk of exposure to electromagnetic fields of high-voltage cables and masts seems to be low, but the public concern is high and not enough research has been done, especially related to low exposure.

Chemical Agents and Health

Exposure to chemical air pollutants in homes can be ordered as follows:
- *Environmental tobacco smoke (ETS).* ETS is a complex mixture of compounds. Many of these are classified as carcinogenic or suspected carcinogenic, and many can effect health in other ways, for instance, by irritating mucous membranes and causing chronic obstructive pulmonary diseases (COPD) [6].
- *Indoor combustion.* Gas ranges and some water heaters have no means of diverting exhaust gases. The gaseous products enter the indoor air directly, causing peak concentrations during use. Nitrogen oxides (NO$_x$) and carbon monoxide

(CO) are of significance for health [7]. Organic products of combustion, like particulate matter, polycyclic aromatic hydrocarbons (PAH), and others are produced depending on the type of fuel and the conditions of the combustion process. Poorly maintained chimneys or leaking exhaust systems can be a source of indoor air pollution.

- *Building materials.* Chipboard can be a source of formaldehyde. Guidelines and improved production have prevented the risk of high indoor concentrations. Asbestos was used in the past in many buildings. Exposure to fibers should be avoided during renovation or demolition. Plasterboard can be a source of radon.
- *Household chemicals.* Cleaning products and hobbies can be the sources of different kinds of indoor air pollution like that from chlorine, solvents, chlorinated or aliphatic hydrocarbons, benzene, pesticides, etc.

Apart from general negative effects on health and well-being, changes in lung functions, allergic and hyperreactive symptoms, ETS is associated with throat cancer and lung cancer. Epidemiologic studies also prove a relationship of passive smoking and lung cancer [8]. Among children of smoking parents there is an increase in airway disorders like asthma and bronchitis [9].

Acute health effects can be expected by exposure to high concentrations of CO. In these cases poorly maintained gas installations or the lack of ventilation are the main causes.

Relatively high concentrations of nitrogen dioxide (NO_2) are related to a reduction of the lung function in children and a higher incidence of airway symptoms [7, 10, 11].

Some agents like benzene, PAH, asbestos, and nitrosamines are carcinogenic. Indoor concentrations of benzene and PAH may be above the acceptable risk level. Concentrations of volatile organic compounds (VOC) lie generally under the no-effect level.

Deposition change of particles and aerosols and their concentration in indoor air are decisive for real exposure. The nose, throat, and lungs are efficient filters for particles, although the deposition of toxic components in the higher airways can damage the mucous membranes [12]. Allergic reactions and local infections can occur. Not much is known about interactions between different components.

A number of agents can cause the nuisance of foul odors, which are related to unspecific symptoms as mentioned before.

Biological Agents and Health

House dust and aerosols can act as carriers for microorganisms and allergens of various origin. The presence of biological agents in indoor air is related to their possible growth, depending on the behavior of the occupants, for example, the presence of domestic animals, plants, vermin, use of a heating/ventilation/air conditioning (HVAC) system, production of water vapor, etc.

The biological agents in indoor air related to health problems are bacteria, viruses, fungus spores, and allergens.

Infections are caused by a wide range of microorganisms. A specific example is legionellosis. This bacteria multiplies in water between 25–50°C and is spread through aerosols, splashwaters, and droplets from hot-water installations, showers, humidifiers, and other places where water is present over a longer period. Inhalation can lead to a type of pneumonia that is not easy recognizable. The mortality rate is about 20% [13].

Allergies are most frequently observed in response to airborne allergens such as those from house dust mites and cockroaches, hair, feathers, and skin scales from domestic animals, molds and fungal spores, and microorganisms. In susceptible persons, exposure by inhalation, oral intake, or dermal contact can affect the airways, alimentary canal, nose, eyes, and skin. In recent years there has been a global increase in the prevalence of asthma, perhaps in connection with an increase in indoor air pollution [9, 14].

Sick Building Syndrome and Building-Related Illnesses

Currently, there is no generally accepted clinical definition of the sick building syndrome (SBS). Generally SBS refers to a broad range of symptoms and health complaints as clinical entities related to indoor environmental factors. These symptoms include irritation of mucous membranes (eyes, nose, upper airways, throat), neurotoxic effects (nausea, dizziness, headache, loss of coordination, fatigue, and irritability), respiratory disorders (wheezing, cough, chest tightness, and shortness of breath), skin dryness and irritation, and many other less specific complaints [15]. Psychosocial factors such as

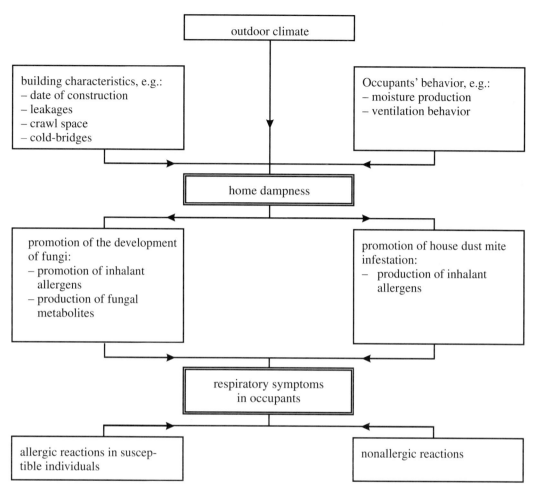

Figure 1. Outline of the theoretical causal relationships between home dampness and occupants' respiratory symptoms.

emotional concerns, work stress, and financial problems can also play a role. Some cases of SBS are thought to be primarily the result of psychological factors, including the response to odors [16]. One research program [17] found that there was an association of SBS with inadequate provision of fresh air without identifiable contaminants (50%) and with identifiable indoor or outdoor contaminants (40%); in the remaining cases the cause was not clear.

A building-related illness (BRI) is defined as a disorder related to indoor environmental factors, with appropriate clinical and laboratory findings [3]. BRIs, unlike SBS, are well-defined clinical entities with known causes, and they can be encountered also in other settings. BRIs include asthma (exposure to irritants and allergens), allergic rhinitis (exposure to allergens), hypersensitivity pneumonitis (exposure to biological agents or chemicals), humidifier fever (cough, dyspnea, and fever after exposure to aerosols containing biological agents like *Legionella pneumophila* or the amoeba *Naegleria gruberi*, or after exposure to chemicals), legionellosis (pneumonia after exposure to aerosols containing *Legionella pneumophila*), Pontiac fever (a nonpneumonic occurring illness after exposure to aerosols containing *Legionella* species), Q fever (an atypical pneumonia caused by *Coxiella burnetti*), and viral respiratory infections.

The mechanism of BRI may involve immunologic reactions, infectious processes, toxicity, and irritation.

The conclusion may be that the sources of indoor air environment are as diverse as the potential adverse health effects. Health concerns range from short-term annoyance, vague discomfort, or irritation to chronic diseases such as respiratory diseases, cancer, and even death. A combination of poor ventilation, moisture, and the presence of allergens can lead to an increased prevalence of respiratory symptoms among occupants of damp houses, especially among children [18]. Figure 1 shows the theoretical causal relationships between home dampness and respiratory symptoms and outlines the factors involved in this relationship [19].

Risk Communication

There are large inconsistencies in the acceptability of environmental risks [20]. To understand this phenomenon, it seems useful to describe the various hazards in a list of risk characteristics:
- voluntary – involuntary
- immediate effect – delayed effect
- alternatives available – no alternatives available
- risks known with certainty – risks unknown
- exposure essential – exposure a luxury
- occupational – nonoccupational
- common hazard – dread hazard
- affects average people – affects sensitive people
- is normally used as intended – likely to be misused
- consequences reversible – consequences irreversible

Risk communication is an instrument that can be used to offer information and make people aware of the such inconsistencies and make them deal with it.

There is a lack of effective strategies and processes for educating the public about indoor air quality. In many countries printed and video documents are available, but there is a need for communication with the public systematically and comprehensively at key times such as during the design or purchase of a home. The development of strategies for assuring consumer understanding of options and consequences, as key decisions are made with regard to residences, should be encouraged [21].

In the Netherlands several information programs have taken place. Brochures were printed, a video-tape was produced, presentations were given, and oral explanations were held during exhibitions. The main goals of these programs were to make the people aware of the health risks in the indoor environment and to influence their behavior, resulting in a more healthy indoor air quality. The main results of the evaluation of these programs showed that, although the programs were pointed at prevention, especially people with health problems or with problems from the HVAC system in their homes, were really interested. Public attention was present only during a short period of time after the information was given to the public. A change of behavior hardly occurred.

Legal regulation is only part of the solution. Regular national public information campaigns should be held especially to reduce children's exposure to ETS and indoor asthma triggers. In particular, it is necessary to convince smoking parents that they are not only endangering the health of their children acutely, but that they may also be causing chronic diseases in their children. Furthermore, occupants of dwellings with open sources of indoor fire, for example, open fire places or gas ranges, should be made aware that combustion always leads to the production of pollutants like carbon monoxide, nitrogen dioxide, and PAH. The resulting contamination can be reduced through an adequate supply of fresh air, a well-functioning chimney – in short effective ventilation.

People only are motivated to change their behavior if they understand that there is indeed a problem they can personally do something about, and when they can see the results, especially in a better health for themselves and their children. If these factors form the starting point of risk communication, maybe the results will be better than in earlier experiences.

Conclusions

- One general conclusion is that the indoor environment can be influenced by the quality of building materials, HVAC systems, indoor emissions, human behavior and outdoor environment.
- Indoor air pollution is related to many adverse health effects, ranging from short-term annoyance and vague discomfort to chronic diseases

such as respiratory diseases, cancer, and even death.
- Physical, chemical, and biological agents are sometimes linked.
- Many respiratory effects, especially among children, are thought to be the result of living in damp houses.
- Legal regulation and a good strategy for public information should lead to public awareness of health risks present in indoor air pollution and changing of behavior.

Recommendations

Considering the factors that influence the indoor environment, most of the recommendations are pointed at these sources:
- Architects should pay attention to the consequences of their designs, the construction and the operation of the building, and the HVAC systems. They should communicate with the constructors and the people who will live and work in those buildings [22].
- Plans should be available to occupants and building owners for appropriate HVAC and building maintenance.
- Information about the health risks of indoor air pollution should be available and provided both actively and passively to the population. Practical advice should to be given to eliminate or reduce exposure to physical, chemical, and biological agents. *Education is the best control technology for prevention.* Also the education of health-care workers is important, as they can appear as intermediates.
- Specific information about ventilation is needed, not only in situations with open sources of fire or special hobby activities, but in all cases. Attention should be paid to the consequences of sealing windows, doors, chinks, and ventilation openings in order to save energy, and to the need of short-term ventilation in dwellings and other buildings by opening windows from time to time (if possible).
- Regular campaigns should be held to emphasize the health risks of active and passive smoking.
- Examination of the effectiveness of risk communication activities should be done.
- Accepted guidelines for the ventilation of buildings and for agents harmful to indoor air quality

(such as formaldehyde, carbon dioxide, carbon monoxide, nitrogen dioxide, ozone, particulate matter, water vapor, and radon) should be implemented in workplaces, schools, hospitals and other indoor environments.
- Risk analysis based on health studies in combination with cost-benefit considerations should lead to standards that protect public health in the most effective and efficient way, using the best available technology.

Address for correspondence:

Wim A Zwart Voorspuij
City of The Hague
Dienst OCW/AGZ
P.O.B. 12652
NL-2500 DP The Hague
The Netherlands
Tel. +31 70 353-7159
Fax +31 70 353-7295
E-mail wzwart@knmg.nl

References

1. Lebowitz MD. Health effects of indoor pollutants. Annu Rev Public Health 1983; 4:203–221.

2. World Health Organization. Air quality guidelines for Europe. Copenhagen: WHO Regional Office for Europe 1987.

3. Canadian Association of Physicians for the Environment. Implications for human health: Indoor air quality. Briefing Paper 1995.

4. The Council of Environmental Advisors. Report on indoor air pollution. Federal Government of Germany, Ministry for the Environment 1987.

5. Biberman R, Lusky A, Schlesinger T, Margaloit M, Neeman E, Modan B. Increased risk for small cell lung cancer following residential exposure to low-dose radon: A pilot study. Arch Environ Health 1993; 48:209–212.

6. Smith CJ, Sears SB, Walker JC, DeLuca PO. Environmental tobacco smoke: Current assessment and future directions. Toxicol Pathol 1992; 20:289–303.

7. Alberts WM. Indoor air pollution: NO, NO_2, CO and CO_2. J Allergy Clin Immunol 1994; 94:289–294.

8. Tweedie RL, Mengersen KL. Lung cancer and passive smoking: Reconciling the biochemical and epidemiological approaches. Br J Cancer 1992; 66:700–705.

9. Infante-Revard C. Childhood asthma and environ-

mental risk factors. Am J Epidemiol 1993; 137:834–844.

10. Samet JM, Lambert WE, Skipper BJ, Cushing AH, Hunt WC, Young SA, McLaren LC, Schwab M, Spengler LD. Nitrogen dioxide and respiratory illness in infants. Am Rev Respir Dis 1993; 148:1258–1265.

11. Cuijpers CEJ, Swaen GMH, Wesseling GJ, Sturmans F, Wouters EFM. Adverse effects of the indoor environment on respiratory health in primary school children. Environ Res 1995; 68:11–23.

12. Bascom R. The upper respiratory tract: Mucous membrane irritation. Environ Health Persp 1991; 95:39–44.

13. Dennis PJ, Wright AE, Rotter DA, Death JE, Jones BPC. *Legionella pneumophila* in aerosols from shower baths. J Hygiene 1984; 93:349–355.

14. Jones AP. Asthma and domestic air quality. Social Sci Med 1998; 47:755–764.

15. Apter A, Bracker A, Hodgson M, Sidman J, Leung WY. Epidemiology of the sick building syndrome. J Allergy Clin Immunol 1994; 94:277–288.

16. Salvaggio JE. Psychological aspects of environmental illness, multiple chemical sensitivity and building-related illness. J Allergy Clin Immunol 1994; 94:366–370.

17. Samet JM, Spengler JD. Health effects and sources of indoor air pollution. Part II. Am Rev Respir Dis 1988; 137:221–242.

18. Verhoeff AP, van Strien RT, van Wijnen JH, Brunekreef B. Damp housing and childhood respiratory symptoms: The role of sensitization to dust mites and moulds. Am J Epidemiol 1995; 141:103–110.

19. Verhoeff AP. Home dampness, fungi and house dust mites, and respiratory symptoms in children. Erasmus University of Rotterdam. Thesis 1994.

20. Lindvall T. Assessing the relative risk of indoor exposures and hazards, and future needs. Indoor Air '87. Proceedings of the 4th International Conference on Indoor Air Quality and Climate, Berlin, August 17–21, 1987; 4:117–133.

21. American Thoracic Society Workshop: Achieving healthy indoor air. Am J Respir Crit Care Med 1997; 156:534–564.

22. Levin H. What architects can do to improve indoor air quality. Indoor Air '87. Proceedings of the 4th International Conference on Indoor Air Quality and Climate, Berlin, August 17–21, 1987; 4:17–26.

Asthma and Global Climate Change

John M Balbus*

Keywords: Asthma, climate, ecological change, environment, ecosystem

Global climate change is expected to result in direct and indirect changes in factors that are associated with asthma exacerbation. These factors include the weather (e. g., thunderstorms, sudden temperature or pressure changes), outdoor air pollutants (e. g., ozone, sulfur oxides, nitrogen oxides), and outdoor aeroallergens. Global climate change will manifest as highly variable climate change between regions, prohibiting generalizations about future changes in weather variables. A more active hydrologic cycle may produce more frequent and severe thunderstorms and cooling episodes. Warmer temperatures are associated with higher ozone concentrations. Lastly, pervasive climate changes are likely to alter dominant vegetation in specific regions, with secondary changes in aeroallergen timing and intensity. Whether some or all of these changes will have an impact on overall asthma incidence is highly uncertain. Indoor allergens and infection-related shifts in T-helper responses, which appear to play significant roles in the pathogenesis of asthma, are less likely to be affected by global climate change.

With the steady increase in asthma prevalence of the past two decades, a great deal of etiological research has been done to analyze the causes of asthma. Several theories have been proposed to explain this generalized increase of asthma prevalence in developed countries. Some have suggested a role for outdoor air pollution, especially ozone and particulates [1, 2]. Other authors have implicated increases in indoor air contaminants, including bioallergens such as cockroach feces and dust mites [1, 3]. A third theory attributes the increase to more frequent development of an atopic immune state, characterized by an increased Th2 ratio [4]. This immune shift is theorized to be due in part to decreased incidence of respiratory infections, such as measles virus and tuberculosis, in early life. Clearly, as asthma is a heterogeneous clinical entity with multiple causes, these three theories are not mutually exclusive, but in fact may all contribute to changes in asthma prevalence. The complexity of

the interactions potentially contributing to asthma has been described in an integrated model [5].

Just as multiple factors are likely to contribute to the initial development of asthma, the exacerbation of pre-existing asthma has been linked in epidemiologic studies to a wide variety of factors. These include respiratory infections (especially rhinovirus), indoor and outdoor air pollutants, indoor and outdoor allergens, and meterologic elements (temperature changes, barometric pressure changes, and thunderstorms). The public health burden due to asthma at any given point in time is related to both the prevalence of asthma and the existence and intensity of environmental triggers.

Because of the associations between a variety of atmospheric factors and asthma, the question arises as to how increasing levels of greenhouse gases and concomitant climate changes will affect the prevalence and severity of asthma. As the role of environmental factors in the initiation of asthma is still poorly understood, this paper will not emphasize possible impacts of climate change on asthma prevalence. Instead, the variety of mechanisms by which climate change may impact asthma exacerbation and severity will be explored.

Direct Influences of Meteorologic Factors on Asthma

A large body of observational evidence suggests that meteorologic factors are associated with exacerbations of asthma. These include rapid decrease in temperature, high barometric pressure, cold, dry air, and thunderstorms. Inhalation of cold air has been demonstrated to decrease lung function in asthmatics [6, 7, 8]. On a larger scale, the passage of cold fronts, particularly in the early fall, has been

*   The George Washington University, Washington, DC, USA

associated with increases in emergency room visits for asthma [9, 10]. In fact, the seasonal patterns of asthma almost universally show a strong annual peak in incidence occurring in the early fall. It should be noted that the increase in asthma exacerbations associated with an early fall cold front is most likely due to several intermediary factors. Associated winds may transport mold spores and pollens, certain respiratory viruses have their peak in the late summer and early fall, and the first use of indoor heating is likely to cause a peak in indoor allergens due to the disruption of settled dusts in heating ducts.

The relationship between asthma and barometric pressure is not clear, as some studies have shown associations with low pressure [11], some with high pressure [12], and some with rapid changes in pressure. The study by Jamason et al. [10], using synoptic classifications, found the highest risk air mass to be among those with highest barometric pressure. Further studies, using a variety of metrics of air pressure that reflect both absolute values and rapidity of changes, are needed to clarify this issue.

A substantial body of literature has documented an association between thunderstorms and "epidemics" or a sharp peak in asthma exacerbations requiring emergency room admission [11, 13, 14]. Specific factors have been implicated in these epidemics, including a high prevalence of sensitivity to grass pollens among patients presenting to emergency rooms. There are indications of sudden release of starch granules from grass pollens in sudden severe rains, lending further credence to the role of grasses in these epidemics. This raises the possibility that specific subpopulations may be particularly sensitive to climate-asthma interactions.

How might a changing climate regime affect these interactions? It is necessary to first describe the strengths and limitations of current climate modeling. Meteorologic factors of greatest importance to asthma exacerbation, such as sudden rain events, wind speed and direction, and passage of cold fronts, are not well modeled on a local scale with current methods. Thus, it must be admitted that the basis of predictions of such factors under climate change is expert judgment, with inherent limitations.

Current predictions of climate in general call for a more active hydrological cycle, which implies a greater frequency of severe rain events, including thunderstorms. Many forecasts have also predicted more frequent dry spells between rain events, which may further augment the role winds and rain

play in dispersing pollens and starch granules. Changes will vary widely between regions, with some areas receiving increases in rainfall frequency, others decreases. For the direct meterologic impacts, it is not possible at present to predict local changes in barometric pressure or thunderstorm frequency; it is unlikely that seasonal occurrences such as the first fall cold front will change substantially, although timing may change. To the extent that thunderstorms appear more frequently, thunderstorm associated outbreaks may be expected.

Indirect Influences of Meteorological Factors on Asthma

Aside from the direct role of temperature changes, winds and rains, the local climate and weather exert a strong influence on asthma triggers indirectly. These influences may be categorized as behavioral, impacts on pollutants, and impacts on bioallergens.

Behavioral Impacts

The role of behavioral impacts has been raised above in the context of human responses to the first fall cold snap. In general, human responses to weather dictate the constellation of environmental factors to which asthmatics are exposed. Thus, temperate summer weather increases time spent outdoors, elevating the importance of summertime air quality. Conversely, colder winter temperatures may lead to greater exposure to respiratory viruses due to several factors, including more time spent indoors, as well as greater survival of many viruses in colder temperatures. These changing exposure patterns may account for the wide variety and seasonal nature of associations between environmental factors (e. g., air pollutants, pollens, viral infections) and asthma.

Climate and Air Pollution Interactions

There are clear associations between concentrations of air pollutants and weather. Among the four pollutants most commonly associated with exacerbation of asthma (nitrogen oxides, sulfur oxides, ozone and particulates), specific weather situations may have varying effects. For example, temperature inversions are associated with the highest levels of particulates, NO_x, and SO_x. Ozone, on the other hand, is most impacted by elevated daytime temperatures, low wind speeds, and clear skies. This combination enhances the levels of volatile ozone precursors as well as photolysis rates [15]. The balance of these factors will be critical in determining how climate change affects ozone levels; the presence of positive (enhanced volatilization) and negative (increased fractional cloud cover) feedback loops complicates predictions. Estimates of the increases in ozone due to increased ambient temperatures range from 1 to 2% per 1°C [16]. Increases in tropospheric ozone would be expected to increase the risk of asthma exacerbation in at least a susceptible subpopulation of asthmatics.

Climate and Pollen Interactions

While many studies have investigated simple associations between air pollutants or aeroallergens and asthma, only recently have investigators systematically tried to determine relative contributions of pollutants and aeroallergens at the same time. Their results have been inconsistent. Delfino et al. [17] demonstrated independent associations between personal ozone exposure and inhaler use and between outdoor fungal spore counts and inhaler use. Pollens and fine particulates were not associated with asthma severity. Rosas et al. [18] found significant associations between grass pollens and fungal spores and asthma emergency admissions among different age groups. This study did not find similar associations between admissions and air pollutants (O_3, NO_2, SO_2, particulates). Other groups [19, 20] failed to show a strong association between pollen or fungal counts and asthma, but some of these studies were performed during the summer, when pollen counts are generally lower and air pollutant concentrations higher than the rest of the year.

The important question for this paper is whether climate factors affect the levels of aeroallergens that trigger or exacerbate asthma. There is a variety of direct and indirect evidence to suggest that climate, and by extension, long-term changes in climate, may affect pollen release and consequently pollen-related asthma. One such mechanism, thunderstorm-associated release of starch granules from grass pollens, has been discussed above.

Emberlin [21] addressed this question directly for Europe. Starting with current distributions of major allergenic plant species, he speculated on impacts for each species of predicted regional climate changes. His conclusions included northward extension of the ranges of olive, parietaria, and ragweed species, as well as more intense birch pollen seasons. Predictions for increased pollen release from grasses were tempered by an anticipated decrease in total land cover by these species due to land use changes. Emberlin did not address changes in asthma morbidity in this study. While local changes in pollen intensity, both increases and decreases, can be inferred, overall impacts for broader areas would be most uncertain. Gonzalez et al. [22] studied relations between climate factors and seasonal levels of grass pollens in Seville, Spain over a 10-year period. They found that intensity of the pollen season correlated with the amount of preseason rainfall, with spring peaks associated with low rainfall and high temperatures. Other studies have failed to show a consistent association between climate and pollen from year to year [23]. Precipitation is also likely to play an important role in the formation and release of fungal spores.

Longer-term changes in climate may have additional impacts on regional aeroallergens. Extensive changes in the global distribution of biomes have been predicted [24]. Depending on the rate with which changes occur, native plant species may have difficulty migrating over large distances, leading to greater proliferation of weed species. The impacts of such changes on regional asthma incidence are not possible to predict. It is conceivable that for certain populations in certain areas, a change in predominant grass or tree species, or the decline of a less common but potently allergenic species may lead to an improvement in asthma during the pollen season. Conversely, the confluence of climate changes (long dry spells punctuated by heavy rains) and proliferation of weed species may lead to more intense pollen seasons.

Summary

Asthma is a disease of complex etiology and pathophysiology, with a similarly complex web of triggers or modulators. Weather is clearly associated with short-term exacerbations of asthma, through sudden cooling, high winds, and conditions favorable for high air pollutant levels. Weather and climate are also primary drivers of exposure to a variety of aeroallergens, including pollens.

Unfortunately, those factors with the greatest impact on asthma, such as wind speed and direction, frequency of precipitation, and temperature inversions, are among the most difficult factors to predict with current climate models. This makes forecasting impacts of climate change on asthma extremely difficult. Moreover, the heterogeneity of asthmatics, combined with the regional variability of climate change, make simple conclusions of increases or decreases in asthma morbidity impossible. For example, changes in intensity of a specific pollen are likely to be local in nature, and only impact that subpopulation that is sensitized to that pollen. Asthma morbidity related to that particular allergen may increase or decrease, according to changes in pollen intensity. The rates of development of new asthma may not be greatly affected, even in the face of a decline of that specific pollen, if other allergens are present at the critical period of exposure. Increases in the levels of a nonspecific irritant, however, such as ozone, may be expected to have a more significant impact. As ozone is the air pollutant most likely to be affected by warmer temperatures, one would expect increases in ozone-related asthma morbidity in a generally warmer climate.

Our understanding of the two processes discussed in this paper, the etiology of asthma and the impacts of increased greenhouse gases, is rapidly growing. It is conceivable that as we understand the two processes better, we may be able to make specific recommendations to protect individuals in specific regions. These recommendations may involve avoidance of exposure at particular critical stages of development (i. e., avoidance of potent outdoor allergens, as well as other potent sensitizers, during infancy) or at particular parts of the year (i. e., enhanced prediction of extremely intense pollen seasons). At present, we may categorize the ways in which climate change may interact with asthma triggers, and only speculate how future changes in climate will affect the morbidity and mortality of this important disease.

Address for correspondence:

John M Balbus, MD, MPH
Dept. of Environmental and Occupational Health
2300 K St., N.W. #201
Washington, DC 20037
USA
Tel. +1 202 994-1734
Fax +1 202 994-0011
E-mail eohjmb@gwumc.edu

References

1. Utell MJ, Looney RJ. Environmentally induced asthma. Toxicol Lett 1995; 82–83:47–53.

2. Balmes JR. Asthma and air pollution. West J Med 1995; 163:372–373.

3. Becklake MR, Ernst P. Environmental factors. Lancet 1997; 350 Suppl 2:SII10–SII13.

4. Holt PG, Yabuhara A, Prescott S, Venaille T, Macaubas C, Holt BJ, Bjorksten B, Sly PD. Allergen recognition in the origin of asthma. Ciba Found Symp 1997; 206:35–49; discussion 49–55, 106–10:35–49.

5. Beggs PJ, Curson PH. An integrated environmental asthma model. Arch Environ Health 1995; 50:87–94.

6. Ramsey JM. Time course of bronchoconstrictive response in asthmatic subjects to reduced temperature. Thorax 1977; 32:26–28.

7. Deal ECJ, McFadden ERJ, Ingram RHJ, Breslin FJ, Jaeger JJ. Airway responsiveness to cold air and hyperpnea in normal subjects and in those with hay fever and asthma. Am Rev Respir Dis 1980; 121:621–628.

8. O'Byrne PM, Ryan G, Morris M, McCormack D, Jones NL, Morse JL, Hargreave FE. Asthma induced by cold air and its relation to nonspecific bronchial responsiveness to methacholine. Am Rev Respir Dis 1982; 125:281–285.

9. Erhardt C, Field F, Greenburg, L, Reed JIL. Asthma and temperature change: An epidemiological study of emergency clinic visits for asthma in three large New York hospitals. Arch Environ Health 1964; 8:642–647.

10. Jamason PF, Kalkstein LS, Gergen PJ. A synoptic evaluation of asthma hospital admissions in New York City. Am J Respir Crit Care Med 1997; 156:1781–1788.

11. Celenza A, Fothergill J, Kupek E, Shaw RJ. Thunderstorm associated asthma: A detailed analysis of environmental factors [see comments]. BMJ 1996; 312:604–607.

12. Garty BZ, Kosman E, Ganor E, Berger V, Garty L, Wietzen T, Waisman Y, Mimouni M, Waisel Y. Emergency room visits of asthmatic children, relation to air pollution, weather, and airborne allergens. Ann Allergy Asthma Immunol 1998; 81:563–570.

13. Bellomo R, Gigliotti P, Treloar A, Holmes P, Suphioglu C, Singh MB, Knox B. Two consecutive thunderstorm associated epidemics of asthma in the city of Melbourne. The possible role of rye grass pollen [see comments]. Med J Aust 1992; 156:834–837.

14. Venables KM, Allitt U, Collier CG, Emberlin J, Greig JB, Hardaker PJ, Highham JH, Laing-Morton T, Maynard RL, Murray V, Strachan D, Tee RD. Thunderstorm-related asthma – The epidemic of 24/25 June 1994. Clin Exp Allergy 1997; 27:725–736.

15. Walcek CJ. Temperature-related factors affecting

ozone formation in polluted areas. In Air & Waste Management Association 90th Annual Meeting. 1522, 1997, June 8–13; Toronto, Ontario (Canada). Pittsburgh, PA: Air & Waste Management Ass., 1997.

16. RT Watson, MC Zinyowera, RH Moss (Eds), Climate change 1995: Impacts, adaptations and mitigation of climate change: Scientific technical analyses. Cambridge: Cambridge University Press, 1996, p. 27.

17. Delfino RJ, Coate BD, Zeiger RS, Seltzer JM, Street DH, Koutrakis P. Daily asthma severity in relation to personal ozone exposure and outdoor fungal spores. Am J Respir Crit Care Med 1996; 154:633–641.

18. Rosas I, McCartney HA, Payne RW, Calderon C, Lacey J, Chapela R, Ruiz-Velazco S. Analysis of the relationships between environmental factors (aeroallergens, air pollution, and weather) and asthma emergency admissions to a hospital in Mexico City. Allergy 1998; 53:394–401.

19. Thurston GD, Lippmann M, Scott MB, Fine JM. Summertime haze air pollution and children with asthma [see comments]. Am J Respir Crit Care Med 1997; 155:654–660.

20. Epton MJ, Martin IR, Graham P, Healy PE, Smith H, Balasubramaniam R, Harvey IC, Fountain DW, Hedley J, Town GI. Climate and aeroallergen levels in asthma: A 12 month prospective study. Thorax 1997; 52:528–534.

21. Emberlin J. The effects of patterns in climate and pollen abundance on allergy. Allergy 1994; 49:15–20.

22. Gonzalez MF, Candau P, Tomas C, Morales J. Airborne grass (Poaceae) pollen in southern Spain. Results of a 10-year study (1987–96). Allergy 1998; 53:266–274.

23. Glassheim JW, Ledoux RA, Vaughan TR, Damiano MA, Goodman DL, Nelson HS, Weber RW. Analysis of meteorologic variables and seasonal aeroallergen pollen counts in Denver, Colorado. Ann Allergy Asthma Immunol 1995; 75:149–156.

24. Moreno RA, Skea J, et al. Industry, energy, and transportation: Impacts and adaptation. In Watson RT, Zinyowera MC, Moss RH (Eds), Climate Change 1995 Impacts, Adaptations and Mitigation of Climate Change: Scientific Technical Analyses. Cambridge: Cambridge University Press, 1996, p. 384.

Ecological Disaster Effect on the Respiratory Tract

Alexander G Chuchalin, Nickolai S Antonov, Olga Yu Stulova, Olga Yu Zaitseva*

Keywords: Epidemiology, ecology, space monitoring, pulmonary disease, environmental hazards

This investigation summarizes data of long-term surveys and results of international examinations of the state of the environment and lung disease morbidity. It provides the pertinent data and ecological monitoring results, the official medical statistics of lung diseases, and the results of natural examinations on the detection of the most widespread types of diseases of the respiratory system. The role of long-term risk factors, in particular industrial pollutants, cold, radionuclides, and smoking, are shown for both acute and chronic lung diseases.

The main idea of this report is the restoration of the health of persons living under unfavorable ecological conditions – in the critical zones of anthropogenic pollution.

Air pollution has both direct and indirect influences, causing acute pulmonary diseases in both children and adults with further development of chronic diseases. High pollutant content in the atmosphere is obviously one of the major risk factors for chronic nonspecific and acute respiratory disease. More than 30 million tons of harmful substances from industrial plants and almost 20 million tons from automobiles are annually released into the atmosphere in the Russian Federation, making the load per inhabitant at an intolerable level of 400 kg. According to regular monitoring information, the average annual concentration of dust, ammonia, fluorine hydride, nitrogen dioxide, soot, and other toxic ingredients, including permissible concentration of carbon disulfide, formic aldehyde, and benzpiren in 282 cities, exceeds the permitted concentrations by two or three times. Maximum concentration of contaminants in 94 cities of Russia exceeds permitted levels by a factor of ten. Special studies indicate that only 15% of urban population live in areas below the permissible atmosphere pollution level [1].

One of the most acute problems faced by Russian pulmonology research lies in conducting scientifically grounded epidemiological research and developing preventive programs for vast regions of this country in the light of the critical ecological situation in the majority of the country's regions. Utilization of satellites for environmental monitoring and anthropogenic influence on the environment is the most expedient way to estimate actual biospheric conditions. The outer-space facilities in this country for monitoring the earth's surface such as manned orbital stations, satellites of the "Resource" and "Space" type and others provide significant material for the solution of many environmental protection problems [2]. The major problem of designing charts of anthropogenic pollution of the environment was solved through the use of satellite information and digital interactive data processing methods worked out by the Space Ecology Research Center (Figure 1).

During 1993–1998, the Pulmonology Research Institute of the Russian Federation conducted joint studies with the cooperation of doctors, ecologists, and space engineers to solve the problem of medico-ecological project implementation with the purpose of restoring health quality and environment.

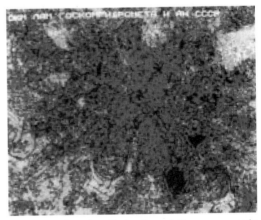

Figure 1. Urban air pollution from stationary sources in 1998 (kg/km^2).

---

* Pulmonology Research Institute, Moscow, Russia

154

Industrial giants of the Tula, Moscow, Lipetsk regions, and the Cherepovetsk complex (Vologda region) contribute greatly to the background pollution, including formation of a stream of pollutants, at the center of the European part of Russia. The air pollution center on the Middle Volga was formed in the Samara region. Volga-Kama and the Urals regions make up an excessive industrial pollution zone with the center in the Chelyabinsk region. Thus, particularly industrial influence determines the excessive background level of sulfur sulfate and the smaller amount of nitric nitrogen in this region. The Kemerovo region and the Norilsk Industrial Center are the largest industrial contributors to background atmospheric pollution in Siberia. The main sources of atmospheric pollution in the gas- and oil-producing districts of the Komi Republic and North Tyumen region (from pipeline compressor stations and the burning off of associated gas) lies far away from places of high residential population.

The number of respiratory cases and malignant tumors as well as number of newborns with a weight less than 2.5 kg were selected as the indices of a population's health condition in the industrial cities under review.

Space monitoring results suggested that the proportion of underweight newborns (less than 2500 g), the increase in the share of neoplasms in general morbidity, and death-rate increases in certain cities and regions are directly connected with environmental conditions. Presently, the rate of underweight newborns in certain cities of the Urals, Siberia, and Far East with high rate of environmental pollution is 6.8–11.3%, i. e., 3–5 times higher than, for example, that of the central part of the country. The increase in concentration of one, two, three, or four separate pollutants compared with the baseline (background) level is accompanied by an increase in respiratory diseases of 18–20% on average and by malignant tumor risk increase of 6–22%. The relative risk rate increases when a combination of pollutants is considered [3].

An analysis of the immune status of more than 10,000 healthy people, representing 56 cities of 19 regions of Russia, was conducted using a regimen of standard and unified tests. These regions differ by climate, geographical conditions, national and ethnic structure, level of industrial development and anthropogenic pollution, ecological situation, extraordinary living conditions, and other features. Average regional indices reflecting specific immunity features in each region, as well as generalized

data treated as normal were determined based on the average immunological status parameters. Some peculiarities were detected in the immunological status of the surveyed groups, depending on the type of industrial activity and on their contact with various anthropogenic factors. Regardless of the character of the industry and other extraordinary factors, the prevailing type of the immunological status is suppressive or mixed with suppression of the majority of indices [4].

These examinations conducted in different regions of the Russian Federation proved that the level of allergic diseases is directly connected with the environmental conditions.

A retrospective analysis of allergic morbidity in cities in which biochemical plants are located showed that increases in bronchial asthma are closely connected with the opening of new plants. Asthma epidemics have been registered within last 15 years in the cities of Kirishy, Angarsk, and Volgograd, where the biotechnological industry has been developed.

Thus, the opening of the Protein and Vitamin Complex (PVC) in Kirishy resulted in a major increase of bronchial asthma cases among adults (44.2 per 10 000 people) and other respiratory tract problems accompanied by asthma. These diseases developed in the initial four months following the opening of the PVC plant. Clinical patterns include asthmatic bronchitis or bronchial asthma with the development of dyspnea attacks, preceded by dry excruciating cough, dryness, itching, or burning of nasopharynx, sweating or acute respiratory disease. Dyspnea attacks were less often. The increase in morbidity did not differ from that found in epidemics of infectious diseases. The latent period was 4–5 months on level surfaces with absolute altitudes of 20–25 m, moderately cold climate, varying from marine to continental, with PVC production under prevailing winds with a protective zone of 3 km, an aggregate emission to the atmosphere of 2 tons of PVC dust and 40 kg of fungus producer clean culture together with air pollution by oxide of carboneum, phenolum, hydrogen sulfide 2–14 times in excess of permissible concentration.

It was important to discover the relationship between bronchial asthma morbidity and the population's need for medical assistance due to dyspnea attacks, and the production and rhythm of PVC operation. Indicators were increased dyspnea attacks of those patients who had previously had chronic or acute diseases with an asthmatic component, and pathological process in persons directly engaged in

PVC production, having the highest morbidity compared with other groups of people within the first year of allergenic component activity. Research showed that 23% of the residents and PVC workers in Kirishy had the diseases compared with 3% of the control group.

The analysis of allergic morbidity in Kirishy prior to and after the beginning of PVC production proved that there was an increase in bronchial asthma cases during the years of the gross violations of the plant's operation and parallel to the absence or poor operation of refining facilities. All this resulted in the release of protein paprine, which possesses high sensitizing activity. The bronchial asthma morbidity decreased upon improvement of PVC know-how in the refining facilities, and from 1981 onwards reached a level of 1.0–0.4 per 10,000 people, equal to the level before production of PVC.

Other increases in bronchopulmonary diseases among the population took place in Angarsk in October 1988 under unfavorable ecological conditions. Adult bronchial asthma morbidity in Angarsk increased by 4.5 times (33.0 per 10,000 people, the morbidity in children increased by 1.6 times (17.0 per 10,000) within this period. The number of cases of chronic pharyngitis, tonsillitis, and laryngotrachitis among children increased by 7.3 times, and bronchitis by 8 times within the same period of time.

The highest morbidity of lung disease accompanied by temporary work disability was, again, registered at PVC plants and exceeded indices by 1.5 times. The morbidity of people with work experience in this industry for over 10 years increased by 10 times.

These research results demonstrate the clear sensitizing activity of microbiological synthesis products, which, particularly when environmental protection laws are violated, may result in epidemic allergic disease outbreak with serious course, in the development of complications with extended work disability, and even in lethal outcome, without creating an immunosuppressive effect.

Geographic location must also be taken into account when evaluating lung disease morbidity. The further north the territory lies, the greater the prevalence of lung diseases. The immediate influence of low temperatures on the upper respiratory airways and the bronchopulmonary system is clearly seen after 3–5 years in newly arriving residents to the Northern regions, who develop so-called polar dyspnea together with hypertension of the pulmonary circulation.

Examinations revealed that the duration of lung diseases among residents of the far north and polar regions up to death is only half that of the residents of the European part of the country.

The closer the region is located to the East, with its continental climate, the higher lung disease morbidity is: From 2068 to 3030 per 10,000 people. However, this rule is partially broken in the Northwest region and, even more obviously, in the Central region. Thus, the registered morbidity in St. Petersburg is 220.6, and in the Leningrad region 2011 per 10,000 people. At the same time, the Moscow region, which is located to the South of the Leningrad region, has a higher incidence of lung disease (2443). Moscow also has the higher rate of these diseases (2564) than does St. Petersburg (2206). The above implies that other risk factors, the major one being air pollution, may be active besides natural climatic risk factors in certain territories.

Studies previously conducted in the regions with critical ecological conditions, namely, Moscow and Leningrad, revealed that the maximum zones of anthropogenic pollution are located in the industrial districts and along the highways of these cities.

A Moscow space ecological map shows the basic objects of anthropogenic pollution: ZIL, "Sickle and Hammer," "Dorohovsky Chemical Center" as well as other plants and highways. In fact, all of Moscow is covered with an aerosol anthropogenic mist. Three categories of respiratory disease prevalence were singled out based on the results of this research:

1. not exceeding the average level in Moscow;
2. exceeding the long-term level by no more than 10% (moderately excessive);
3. exceeding the average long-term level by more than 10%.

A comparison of the zones of extreme ecological problems and regions with maximum prevalence of lung diseases showed that they are almost identical (Figure 2). The following conclusions were thus made:

1. The ecogenesis of the respiratory system afflictions of Moscow residents is clearly connected with the city's anthropogenic air pollution.
2. The development of chronic respiratory diseases depends on the immediate influence of aerosol, pollutants, and small gas components of the atmosphere. In addition, indirect influence through the development of acute taints of respiratory trajectories is possible.

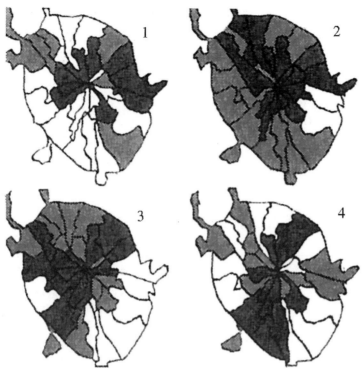

Figure 2. Map of anthropogenic air pollution over the Moscow region and respiratory diseases in 0–14-year-old children in Moscow. 1: Influenza and AVRD; 2: Pneumonia; 3: Bronchial asthma; 4: Chronic bronchitis and other COPD.

■ = category 1: average annual long-term level;

▦ = category 2: increase over average level by no more than 10%;

□ = category 3: increase over average level by more than 10%

3. Control examinations conducted in the critical zones revealed extremely high indices of respiratory disease prevalence, some of which were significantly higher than the average data of the Ministry of Health of Russia.

The "Pulmobile" program was created with the purpose of examining the population to detect the true prevalence of obstructive pulmonary problems as well as the formation of risk groups among the residents of the regions under unfavorable ecological conditions.

"Pulmobile" constitutes a mobile laboratory that assists in conducting and operating active diagnostic and preventive public health care work. The epidemiological and economic importance of similar programs has been proved in other countries (Germany, The Netherlands, Austria, Brazil, the Philippines). The "Pulmobile" mobile laboratory has the proper equipment, thus making it possible to conduct high-quality, prompt, and complete lung-function screening in accordance with European standards.

One of the Moscow regions with critical ecological conditions is "ZIL," the largest metal works in Russia, where the "Pulmobile" program was first tested by us. The employees of the Pulmonology Research Institute conducted epidemiological research of respiratory disease prevalence among the workers and employees, including testing the immunological status and the sanitary-hygienic characteristics of working places and the surrounding territory for a period of 3 years. The basic components characteristic of the air composition were siliceous dust, excessive temperature and humidity, heat radiance, the influence of which is directly connected with length of service.

An analysis of the relationship between incidence of obstructive syndrome and length of work under hazardous conditions among the workers and employees of these industrial plants showed a high rate of affliction and a decrease in number of healthy persons.

The statistical results of the examinations allow us to propose tentative terms of a working plan on the conversion of primary tags of pulmonary pathology into actual disease.

Epidemiological research conducted by the specialists of the Pulmonology Research Institute has made it possible to detect early symptoms of airway

Table 1. Harmful factors of metallurgical industry.

	Max. allowed concentration (mg/m^3)	Concentration in workplace
1. Siliceous dust	2	3–29
2. Formaldehyde	0.5	2.2–5.5
3. Lead	0.01	0.64–0.85
4. Abrasive dust	6	0.9–21.5
5. Pivotal mixt.	17–36	32–146
6. Mould mixt.	6	10.2–42.8
7. Bentonid	2	2.8–70.8
8. Fireproof mixt.	2	62

Table 2. Appearance of lung diseases symptoms in "dust profession" workers.

Concentration in workplace (mg/m^3)	Occupational time (years) Initial signs	Interim period	Disease
10–12.5	5.7 ± 2.2	8.3 ± 1.9	10.8 ± 2.4
3.7–7.5	7.3 ± 4.1	9.7 ± 3.0	13.4 ± 1.8
8.7–24.3	5.4 ± 1.8	7.8 ± 2.3	9.7 ± 1.6
2.7–10.5	12.7 ± 2.8	14.6 ± 3.5	18.7 ± 4.8

pathology in 30% of workers, which is twice the official statistics figures. And 12.3% of the examined people who considered themselves healthy turned out to be suffering from chronic obstructive bronchitis, 13% from bronchial asthma, and 14% from airway hyperresponsiveness.

During the immunological examination it was determined that the immunological status of metal-industry workers differs from that of the above group; specifically, there is a decrease in the absolute number of T-lymphocytes and their subpopulations. The humoral immunity factors were less subject to changes: IgM concentration was clearly decreased, whereas IgA and IgE concentration – which testify to extended allergen activity – increased.

Thus, a comprehensive analysis of immunological indices of the workers and employees in metal-industry factories, including clinical and functional signs of disease and allergic status, reveal both precursory symptoms of respiratory tract pathology and signs of a chronic infectious process (otolaryngological organs pathology, acute respiratory viral infections).

The next stage of "Pulmobile" program took place in the Povolzhsky region, one of the largest industrial regions of Russia, with extremely unsat-isfactory ecological and sanitary-hygienic conditions.

The sanitary and epidemiological monitoring service revealed that in 1997 the average annual formic aldehyde concentration amounted to 2.3–6 MAC (Maximum Allowable Concentration), nitrogen dioxide to 1.3–2.3 MAC, and dust to 1.3–2 MAC. Average annual concentration of ammonia was 1.5–2.5 MAC, hydrogen chloride and phenolum 1–1.5 MAC. The concentration of fluorine hydride gas in the atmosphere equaled 1.5–2.2 MAC, benzapyrene 1–3 MAC, carbon disulfide 2.6 MAC.

Industrial power plants as well as chemical and petroleum works are the most dangerous sources of atmospheric pollution. A considerable share of air pollution is caused by transportation: 30%. Annually, some 800,000 tons of harmful agents are emitted by stationary sources and about 200,000 tons by other sources. The composition of exhausts consists of solid agents (smoke, dust, etc.): 75,000 tons; gases and fluids (liquids): 739,000 tons, including sulfurous anhydride 170,400 tons; carbon monoxide: 143,200 tons; nitric oxides: 8,400 tons; hydrocarbons: 105,400 tons; organic compounds: 133,400 tons; other substances: 9,300 tons.

63,000 residents of 8 areas of the Povolzhsky region were examined with the help of "Pulmobile" mobile lab, and a databank was created. The following results were obtained:

– 12.5% of the people examined (7896) had different degrees of lung function disorder. While 6.9% of people knew that they suffered from airway diseases and had sought medical treatment, in 5.6% of the cases this diagnosis was made for the first time. It is noteworthy that many patients knew nothing about their respiratory disease before the examination; either they underestimated it or because of the lack of information did not pay attention to obvious signs of illness (chronic cough, sputum, labored respiration due to obstruction).

– Young women and mature men are in greater danger of getting these diseases. The success of broncholytic therapy among the smokers is less than among the nonsmokers, and there is no success at all with respect to the fluctuation of mostly responsive parameters of final expiration flow (MEF75). Drug therapy makes no sense in case of continued smoking.

One may conclude from the results of these examinations that the incidence of obstructive pulmonary diseases is much higher than the information received from people seeking medical care.

An examination of the epidemiology of different diseases in one district of the Povolzhsky region showed that, in addition to poor ecological conditions, there is an increase in most acute and chronic diseases. It suffices to quote the child mortality rates in some cities: from 17.0 up to 29.7 per 1000 (1996)! A comparison of the indices of bronchopulmonary disease prevalence among 660 children in the regions with the mostly ecologically unfavorable districts (close to transportation highways and railways) with medical statistics data resulted in the following:

- incorrect diagnosis of acute diseases in 27.6% of the cases,
- late diagnosis in 12.5%,
- incorrect diagnosis of formation of chronic obstructive diseases amounted to 63%, during the periods of developed clinical pattern to 29%,
- incorrect recognition of diseases of the congenital bronchus and lung pathology 89%.

The obtained results and official data available were analyzed in the attempt to apply correction factors to the statistical data on seeking out assistance, in order to get reliable indices of the prevalence of lung tract diseases.

The correction factor for bronchial asthma was 2.9; for chronic bronchitis it was 3.8, i. e., with reference to the statistical data in the region the approximate number of bronchial asthma patients was 92.4 per 10,000 persons, for chronic bronchitis 516.8 per 10,000 persons, as opposed to 30.8 and 136, respectively. The ecological correction factor for the most unfavorable districts turned out to be 3.1 (for the elderly and children) according to preliminary calculations compared to average indices.

An analysis of information content of the factors contributing to rise and development of chronic obstructive pulmonary diseases of healthy and sick persons was conducted with the help of statistical calculations to make their role more precise.

The following contributing factors were determined to have the highest information content: heredity (3.06), congenital lung pathology (2.95), decreased organism resistance to infection according to the anamnesis data, without giving concrete expression, of the immune system defect (2.05), polyvalent allergy (3.8), age (men 19 to 25 years old: 1.05; men 54 to 60 years old: 1.9; women 23 to 28 years old: 1.25; women 44 to 50 years old: 1.96);

unfavorable ecological environment (1.1), housing (1.96).

A clear increase of acute and chronic diseases in general, primarily of the respiratory tract, parallel to negative ecological conditions, was detected in the results of the examinations conducted, i. e., lung pathology may be considered an index of ecological health.

We initiated a new quality in ecological pulmonology on the basis of work in the regions with negative ecological conditions, by analyzing the increase and structure of respiratory diseases among the workers at the Chernobyl atomic power station's (following the failure) and the influence of the risk factors, in the main the duration and intensity of radiation.

The period of work to eliminate the consequences of the failure of this power plant started in the second half of May 1986. It was characterized by near-to-ground atmosphere contamination due to secondary dust formation as a result of natural wind forces and human activity in the contaminated territories. Thus, a considerable number of people, primarily those participating in the containment, were exposed to radionuclides through inhalation and through external radiation. The deposition of inhaled radionuclides was confirmed by detection of "hot" particles in the pulmonary tissue of the people who died within the first year after the Chernobyl failure. This deposition of aerosol particles was confirmed by Brookhaven National Laboratory and Lawrence Berkeley National Laboratory.

The program of epidemiological examination of these workers and the control group included the following:

- A questionnaire of the European community on coal and steel (1987 edition) to detect respiratory signs, with the additionally developed group of questions on the health conditions of persons who reside near or worked in Chernobyl, aimed at examining regularities and peculiarities of the lung pathology of the former workers;
- An examination of external breath function according to European standards;
- Consultation of a pulmonology specialist;
- Selection of a group for complete examination and monitoring with subsequent stationary treatment;
- Statistical processing of the material.

The analysis of the results of the examinations made in accordance with the special additional group of questions concerning each person's terms

Table 3. The beginning of cough and breathlessness after the completion of work in Chernobyl.

Time of onset	Cough	Breathlessness
1986 to 1988 (in 2 years)	39.5%	24.1%
1989 to 1991 (in 5 years)	40.7%	48.3%
1992 to 1994 (in 8 years)	19.8%	27.6%

of stay and place of operations in the power plant revealed signs of acute inhaled affection of respiratory organs during the period of work in the Chernobyl zone. We also tried to determine the emergence and prevalence of pulmonary diseases within a period of time after the failure.

The examined workers of the failure were exposed to radiation during operations on the plant, mainly due to the extended inhalation of "Chernobyl aerosol."

The above was confirmed by the fact that only 38.6% of the workers utilized individual protection appliances (respirators: 27.1%, overalls: 13.7). Moreover, 17.6% of these workers used the indicated aids only extremely irregularly.

Health complaints, in particular complaints about the condition of respiratory organs, were made by 66.7% of the surveyed workers during the time of employment in the Chernobyl zone. The most frequent complaints were dry cough (58.3%), itching and pharyngalgia (62.4%), voice wheezing (43.9%).

The signs of acute problems in respiratory organs of 53% of the workers who developed complaints during their stay at the plant, were cut off after evacuation from the Chernobyl zone. The signs persisted in 13.7% of the workers, and this particular group directly traced the emergence of lung disease to their stay in the Chernobyl zone. 39.3% of the people surveyed reported the emergence of a constant cough after participation in the cleanup operations, and 28.2% the appearance of dyspnea.

A study of the time patterns of the basic signs of lung diseases (cough and dyspnea) revealed that the basic peak of morbidity among the workers occurred in 1989–1990, i. e., 3–4 years after their participation in the cleanup operations. First, there emerged a cough with sputum, and later, usually after a year, dyspnea appeared during exercise stress, characteristic of this group of surveyed people.

On the basis of the functional criteria of airway obstruction in 16.6% of the workers and 9.8% of the surveyed group, we detected a decrease in forced expiratory volume in the first second below the 80% norm. One should note that for the majority of the persons surveyed the decrease of this index was within 75–65% FEV_1 from normal. Cough with sputum developed approximately 4 years after termination of the cleanup was the basic clinical sign, accompanying functional changes. It is interesting to note that, according to the survey, frequent relapses, lingering and flaccid respiratory viral infections were characteristic of the same group of people.

Early diagnosis of lung functional disorders with the help of a number of diagnostic measures (anamnesis data, clinical signs, and functional examinations) constitute the integral part of any examination. However, the analysis of functional indices does not necessarily reveal deviations from normal values. In particular, 109 workers (33.3%) complained about breathing difficulties, chest hissing and wheezing, dyspnea attacks after irritation, allergic diseases or responses in an anamnesis, without deviations of lung function; there were 35 similar cases (29.6%) in the control group. When a bronchoprovocation challenge test with metacholin was performed, 18.8% of the surveyed workers and none of the control group had a FEV_1 drop by 20% and more.

This medical and ecological project, including space ecological monitoring, ground-level estimate of the ecological situation, and screening epidemiological examinations to detect bronchopulmonary diseases will enable us to improve considerably the quality of diagnostic and early detection of diseases. It will make it possible to carry out preventive programs to improve environmental ecological conditions and actively implement treatment and prophylactic programs directed at improving patients' quality of life. The creation of medical ecological maps, revealing critical zones of anthropogenic pollution and regions of high prevalence of respiratory diseases, has started a qualitatively new trend of medical and ecological analysis on the basis of scientifically grounded connections between human health and the environment. The examinations conducted convincingly showed that respiratory system diseases may be considered indicators of ecological disaster.

Address for correspondence:

Alexander G Chuchalin
11th Parkovaya St., 32/61
Moscow 105077, Russia
Tel. +7 095 465-5264
Fax +7 095 465-5364
E-mail chuchalin@rhhf.ru

References

1. Belyakov VD. Methodical bases of medico-economic regionation. In Regional problems of Russian population health, 1993, p. 6–21.
2. Chuchalin AG, Novikov YK. Eco-epidemiological monitoring of towns with the use of space satellite technology. Allergy Clin Immunol News 1992; 4(1): 7–10.
3. Feshbakh M. Environmental and health atlas of Russia. Moscow: PAIMS 1995, p. 19–23.
4. Khaitov RM, Pinegin BV, Istamov HI. Immunological status of different Russian region population. In Ecological Immunology, Moscow, 1995, p. 53–59.
5. Avitsin AR, Zhavoroncov AA, Marachev AG, Milovanov AP. Pathology of man in North. Moscow, Medicine, 1985, p. 416.

Asthma and Rhinitis: A Systemic Disease

Judah A Denburg*

Keywords: Asthma, rhinitis, cytokines, hemopoiesis

The bone marrow actively participates in the production of IgER-positive inflammatory cells (eosinophils, basophils, mast cells), which are typically recruited to tissues in atopic individuals. Understanding the signalling between the tissue and the bone marrow at the molecular level may well open up new avenues of therapy for allergic inflammation. These studies also indicate the critical involvement of the bone marrow in the development of eosinophilic airways inflammation, pointing out the systemic nature of these conditions and their potential biological underpinnings. Hemopoietic events originating in the bone marrow are potential targets for long-term therapy of rhinitis and asthma, and corticosteroids may have to exhibit a "beneficial" systemic activity in the optimal treatment of upper and lower airway inflammation.

Asthma and Rhinitis: A Biological Link

While substantial epidemiological, neurophysiological, and clinical evidence exists for a relationship between allergic rhinitis and asthma, the precise mechanisms for cell recruitment through a common pathway to both upper and lower airways in allergic inflammation have not yet been fully delineated. One potentially important systemic, contributing mechanism to cell recruitment in both allergic rhinitis and asthma is the bone marrow, since it can provide an ongoing source of differentiating inflammatory cells (eosinophils, basophils, and mast cells in particular) to the upper and lower airways.

Peripheral Blood Progenitors

We have previously demonstrated the clinical relevance of eosinophil-basophil (Eo/B) progenitors in the blood of patients with a variety of allergic airways disorders, especially those with allergic rhinitis, nasal polyposis and asthma. In these patients, fluctuations in basophil/eosinophil progenitors (CFU-Eo/B) in the peripheral blood are observed: higher out of season, increased after allergen exposure [1–7].

In Situ Hemopoiesis

Inflamed tissues from patients with allergic rhinitis and nasal polyposis produce hemopoietic cytokines which promote the differentiation and maturation of CFU-Eo/B, as well as of mast cell progenitors; we have termed this tissue-driven response "*in situ* hemopoiesis" [8–14].

The nasal polyp model has served to emphasize that a specific tissue microenvironment, in which IgER-positive inflammatory cells such as eosinophils and mast cells are abundant, can be the repository of both hemopoietic growth factors and of inflammatory cell progenitors. Supporting this is our recent observation that mononuclear cells bearing the hemopoietic stem cell marker for CD34, are present within nasal polyp tissues, can be isolated therefrom and are an enriched source of CFU-Eo/B [7, 15].

Bone Marrow Progenitors

We have turned our attention recently to hemopoietic events taking place simultaneously in the bone marrow and airways in subjects with nasal polyposis and/or asthma, utilizing hemopoietic colony assays for Eo/B, as well as flow cytometric analyses of progenitors expressing surface α-receptor subunits for IL-3, IL-5, and GM-CSF [1, 2].

---

* Clinical Immunology & Allergy, McMaster University, Hamilton, Ontario, Canada

Lineage-Specific Markers for Eosinophils-Basophils

Steps in lineage commitment of Eo/B progenitors involve the expression of IgERs in a potentially orderly fashion. Observations we have made regarding the induction of differentiation of Eo/B in leukemic cell lines demonstrate both IgER and IL-5R expression at relatively early stages of differentiation of this lineage [16–18].

In studies of CD34+ progenitors induced to differentiate to Eo/B lineage from human cord blood samples, Rottem et al. demonstrated the appearance of IgERI by flow cytometry [19, 20]. We have recently demonstrated the upregulation of IL-5R on cord blood CD34+ cells, and its suppression by retinoic acid [21, 22]. Although the relationship and timing of the acquisition of IgER and other lineage markers such as IL-5R is not yet clear, the results of previous and current studies suggest an orderly sequence of appearance of the lineage-specific markers on developing Eo/B progenitors. More detailed knowledge of this sequence could form the basis for novel therapeutic approaches targeting hemopoietic mechanisms in allergic inflammation.

Communication Between the Bone Marrow and Airways

The specific communication between the airway and the bone marrow, which leads to upregulation of IL-5Rα on CD34+ progenitors *in vivo*, is not yet known. We have recently found that IL-5Rα and other markers of this lineage can be induced on clone 15 HL-60 cells *in vitro* [18, 22]; recent evidence points to IL-5 itself as a potential regulator of IL-5Rα expression (Tavernier J, personal communication). Indeed, several studies in murine models of allergen-induced airways inflammation suggest that hemopoietic factors such as IL-5 and/or granulocyte-macrophage colony stimulating factor (GM-CSF) may be critical in signalling the bone marrow to produce more cells committed to the Eo/B lineage [23, 24]. The finding that both in humans and mice, bone marrow transplantation can transfer the atopic diathesis, with its attendant eosinophil- and mast-cell-rich inflammatory response, to previously nonatopic recipients, supports the view that progenitor cells in the bone marrow, in addition to immunocompetent cells such as T-cells, may be the source of this transplantable atopy [25–27].

Effects of Inhaled Corticosteroids on Hemopoietic Events: Studies in a Canine Model

Intranasal and inhaled corticosteroids modulate both local (i. e., in nasal polyp tissue) and systemic numbers and activation of Eo/B progenitors. Indeed, studies in a canine model of allergen-induced bronchial hyperresponsiveness showed an upregulation of myeloid progenitors after airway allergen challenge; this was abrogated by pretreatment with inhaled corticosteroids [28]. In this model, a serum hemopoietic activity, which acts on the bone marrow to elicit further upregulation of myeloid progenitors, is released following allergen provocation; this also could be blocked by pretreatment with inhaled corticosteroids [29–31]. At the same time, actively dividing (presumably hemopoietic) cells appear in both the blood and bronchoalveolar lavage fluid within 24 hours of the airway allergen challenge [32]. These results indicate an active link between the airways and hemopoiesis during allergic inflammation, and suggest a "beneficial" systemic effect of inhaled corticosteroids on hemopoietic mechanisms and inflammatory cell recruitment to the airways.

Studies in Human Asthma and Rhinitis

Inhaled corticosteroids have also been used to study the contribution of the bone marrow to allergic inflammation in human subjects: An exacerbation of asthma, which can be provoked by controlled withdrawal of inhaled corticosteroids, is attended by an increase in circulating CFU-Eo/B, at the time of first development of symptoms [33, 34]. Thus, the bone marrow is sensitive to inhaled corticosteroids, actively releasing progenitors to be recruited to the upper and lower airways. Recently, we have shown increases in CD34+ mononuclear cell populations within nasal polyps after intranasal corticosteroids [15]. This tissue elevation of progenitors after topical corticosteroids, implies a block in differentiation, consistent with an ongoing contribution of hemopoiesis to the process of inflammatory cell maturation in the tissue.

Finally, in studies we have just completed, inhaled corticosteroids deposited in the lung of atopic asthmatics developing late-phase responses to inhaled allergen are capable of downregulating the airway inflammatory response comprising eosinophils and mast cells [35, 36], as well as reducing baseline numbers of more primitive progenitor cells. However, the specific upregulation of IL-$5R\alpha$ on CD34$^+$ cells in the bone marrow in these same individuals is not apparently affected by inhaled corticosteroids [32, 37–39]: a single allergen challenge still could induce upregulation of IL-$5R\alpha$ cells in the bone marrow, despite pretreatment (for one week) with inhaled corticosteroids. This suggests that an ongoing, *chronic* inflammatory response in the marrow requires more sustained treatment with inhaled corticosteroids. Further studies are in progress to examine this.

own growth factors such as IL-5 and GM-CSF, thus perpetuating the inflammatory process [35]. The chief goal of therapy in these conditions may well be to give sufficient anti-inflammatory and hemopoietic-modulating therapy so as to achieve blunting of the bone marrow contribution to the development of allergic inflammation.

Acknowledgment

This research was supported by a grant from the Medical Research Council of Canada

Address for correspondence:

Dr Judah A Denburg
Department of Medicine, HSC 3V46
McMaster University
1200 Main Street West
Hamilton, ON L8N 3Z5
Canada
Tel. +1 905 521-2100, ext. 76714
Fax +1 905 521-4971
E-mail denburg@fhs.csu.mcmaster.ca

The Bone Marrow in Allergic Inflammation: A Target for Anti-Inflammatory Therapy

We have proposed that the bone marrow is an ongoing source of chronic inflammation that seeds atopic tissues with cells capable of maturing into the effector cells of allergy [3]. Therapies directed at the bone marrow, whether via an effect of inhaled corticosteroids or, more specifically, through antagonism of hemopoietic cytokine receptors for factors such as IL-5, or anti-IgE therapy which could theoretically interfere with maturation of Eo/B progenitors, need to be considered in the treatment of chronic allergic inflammation. Recent findings on the specific Eo/B-lineage inhibitory effects of retinoic acid may provide new insights in this regard [22, 40]. A corollary of these observations is that allergic inflammation is a systemic process in which the bone marrow actively contributes to maintain and sustain disease and symptoms. Eo/B progenitors and mature cells can both acquire an altered, autostimulatory and chronic inflammatory phenotype, expressing IgERs and producing their

References

1. Denburg JA, Dolovich J, Harnish D. Basophil mast cell and eosinophil growth and differentiation factors in human allergic disease. Clin Exp Allergy 1989; 19:249–254.
2. Denburg JA, Woolley M, Leber B, Linden M, O'Byrne P. Basophil and eosinophil differentiation in allergic reactions. J Allergy Clin Immunol 1994; 94: 1135–1141.
3. Denburg JA, Inman MD, Leber B, Sehmi R, O'Byrne PM. The role of the bone marrow in allergy and asthma. Allergy 1996; 51:141–148.
4. Denburg JA, Telizyn S, Belda A, Dolovich J, Bienenstock J. Increased numbers of circulating basophil progenitors in atopic patients. J Allergy Clin Immunol 1985; 76:466–472.
5. Otsuka H, Dolovich J, Befus AD, Bienenstock J, Denburg JA. Peripheral blood basophils, basophil progenitors, and nasal metachromatic cells in allergic rhinitis. Am Rev Respir Dis 1986; 133:757–762.
6. Otsuka H, Dolovich J, Befus AD, Telizyn S, Bienenstock J, Denburg JA. Basophilic cell progenitors, nasal metachromatic cells, and peripheral blood basophils in ragweed-allergic patients. J Allergy Clin Immunol 1986; 78:365–371.

7. Otsuka H, Dolovich J, Richardson M, Bienenstock J, Denburg JA. Metachromatic cell progenitors and specific growth and differentiation factors in human nasal mucosa and polyps. Am Rev Respir Dis 1987; 136:710–717.

8. Ohnishi M, Ruhno J, Bienenstock J, Dolovich J, Denburg JA. Hematopoietic growth factor production by cultured cells of human nasal polyp epithelial scrapings: Kinetics, cell source, and relationship to clinical status. J Allergy Clin Immunol 1989; 83:1091–1100.

9. Ohnishi M, Ruhno J, Bienenstock J, Milner R, Dolovich J, Denburg JA. Human nasal polyp epithelial basophil/mast cell and eosinophil colony-stimulating activity: The effect is T-cell-dependent. Am Rev Respir Dis 1988; 138:560–564.

10. Ohnishi M, Ruhno J, Dolovich J, Denburg JA. Allergic rhinitis nasal mucosal conditioned medium stimulates growth and differentiation of basophil/mast cell and eosinophil progenitors from atopic blood. J Allergy Clin Immunol 1988; 81:1149–1154.

11. Denburg JA, Dolovich J, Ohtoshi T, Cox G, Gauldie J, Jordana M. The microenvironmental differentiation hypothesis of airway inflammation. Am J Rhinology 1990; 4:29–32.

12. Cox G, Ohtoshi T, Vancheri C, Denburg JA, Dolovich J, Gauldie J, Jordana M. Promotion of eosinophil survival by human bronchial epithelial cells and its modulation by steroids. Am J Respir Cell Mol Biol 1991; 4:525–531.

13. Vancheri C, Gauldie J, Bienenstock J, Cox G, Scicchitano R, Stanisz A, Jordana M. Human lung fibroblast-derived granulocyte-macrophage colony stimulating factor (GM-CSF) mediates eosinophil survival in vitro. Am J Respir Cell Mol Biol 1989; 1:289–295.

14. Vancheri C, Ohtoshi T, Cox G, Xaubet A, Abrams JS, Gauldie J, Dolovich J, Denburg J, Jordana M. Neutrophilic differentiation induced by human upper airway fibroblast-derived granulocyte/macrophage colony-stimulating factor (GM-CSF). Am J Respir Cell Mol Biol 1991; 4:11–17.

15. Kim YK, Uno M, Hamilos DL, Beck L, Bockner B, Schleimer R, Denburg JA. Immunolocalization of CD34 in nasal polyposis. Effect of topical corticosteroids. Am J Respir Cell Mol Biol 1999; 20:388–397.

16. Hutt-Taylor SR, Harnish D, Richardson M, Ishizaka T, Denburg JA. Sodium butyrate and a T lymphocyte cell line-derived differentiation factor induce basophilic differentiation of the human promyelocytic leukemia cell line HL-60. Blood 1988; 71:209–215.

17. Plaetinck G, Van der Heyden J, Tavernier J, Faché I, Tuypens T, Fischkoff S, Fiers W, Devos R. Characterization of interleukin 5 receptors on eosinophilic sublines from human promyelocytic leukemia (HL-60) cells. J Exp Med 1990; 172:683–691.

18. Lundahl J, Sehmi R, Hayes L, Upham J, Howie K, Denburg JA. Induction of eosinophilic differentiation involves a selective up-regulation of β-7 integrin (abstract). J Allergy Clin Immunol 1998; 101:S219.

19. Rottem M, Barbieri S, Kinet JP, Metcalfe DD. Kinetics of the appearance of FcεRI– bearing cells in interleukin-3-dependent mouse bone marrow cultures: Correlation with histamine content and mast cell maturation. Blood 1992; 79:972–980.

20. Rottem M, Hull G, Metcalfe DD. Demonstration of differential effects of cytokines on mast cells derived from murine bone marrow and peripheral blood mononuclear cells. Exp Hematol 1994; 22:1147–1155.

21. Upham J, Hayes L, Leber B, O'Byrne P, Denburg J. Retinoic acid inhibits eosinophil- basophil differentiation of hematopoietic progenitor cells (abstract). Am J Respir Crit Care Med 1997; 155:A624.

22. Upham JW, Hayes LM, Sehmi R, Denburg JA. Retinoic acid selectively inhibits IL-5 receptor expression during differentiation of hemopoietic progenitor cells (abstract). J Allergy Clin Immunol 1998; 101:S214.

23. Gaspar Elsas MI, Joseph D, Elsas PX, Vargaftig BB. Rapid increase in bone-marrow eosinophil production and responses to eosinopoietic interleukins triggered by intranasal allergen challenge. Am J Respir Cell Mol Biol 1997; 17:404–413.

24. Ohkawara Y, Lei XF, Stampfli MR, Marshall JS, Xing Z, Jordana M. Cytokine and eosinophil responses in the lung, peripheral blood, and bone marrow compartments in a murine model of allergen-induced airways inflammation. Am J Respir Cell Mol Biol 1997; 16: 510–520.

25. Agosti JM, Sprenger JD, Lum LG, Witherspoon RP, Fisher LD, Storb R, Henderson WR. Transfer of allergen-specific IgE-mediated hypersensitivity with allogeneic bone marrow transplantation. N Engl J Med 1988; 319:1623–1628.

26. Hamelmann E, Oshiba A, Paluh J, Bradley K, Loader J, Potter TA, Larsen GL, Gelfand EW. Requirement for CD8+ T cells in the development of airway hyperresponsiveness in a murine model of airway sensitization. J Exp Med 1996; 183:1719–1729.

27. Hamelmann E, Oshiba A, Schwarze J, Bradley K, Loader J, Larsen GL, Gelfand EW. Allergen-specific IgE and IL-5 are essential for the development of airway hyperresponsiveness. Am J Respir Cell Mol Biol 1997; 16:674–682.

28. Woolley MJ, Denburg JA, Ellis R, Dahlback M, O'Byrne PM. Allergen-induced changes in bone marrow progenitors and airway responsiveness in dogs and the effect of inhaled budesonide on these parameters. Am J Respir Cell Mol Biol 1994; 11:600–606.

29. Inman MD, Denburg JA, Ellis R, Dahlback M, O'Byrne PM. Allergen-induced increase in bone marrow progenitors in airway hyperresponsive dogs: Regulation by a serum hemopoietic factor. Am J Respir Cell Mol Biol 1996; 15:305–311.

30. Inman MD, Denburg JA, Ellis R, Dahlback M, O'Byrne PM. The effect of treatment with budesonide or PGE2 *in vitro* on allergen-induced increases in canine bone marrow progenitors. Am J Respir Cell Mol Biol 1997; 17:634–641.

31. Inman MD, Sehmi R, O'Byrne PM, Denburg JA. The role of the bone marrow in allergic disease. In Denburg JA (Ed), Allergy and allergic diseases: The new mechanisms and therapeutics. Totowa, NJ: Humana Press, 1998, pp. 85–102.

32. Wood LJ, Inman MD, Denburg JA, O'Byrne PM. Allergen challenge increases cell traffic between bone marrow and lung. Am J Respir Cell Mol Biol 1998; 18:759–767.

33. Gibson PG, Wong BJ, Hepperle MJ, Kline PA, Girgis-Gabardo A, Guyatt G, Dolovich J, Denburg JA, Ramsdale EH, Hargreave FE. A research method to induce and examine a mild exacerbation of asthma by withdrawal of inhaled corticosteroid. Clin Exp Allergy 1992; 22:525–532.

34. Gibson PG, Dolovich J, Girgis-Gabardo A, Morris MM, Anderson M, Hargreave FE, Denburg JA. The inflammatory response · in asthma exacerbation: Changes in circulating eosinophils, basophils and their progenitors. Clin Exp Allergy 1990; 20:661–668.

35. Gauvreau GM, O'Byrne PM, Moqbel R, Velazquez J, Watson RM, Howie KJ, Denburg JA. Enhanced expression of GM-CSF in differentiating eosinophils of atopic and atopic asthmatic subjects. Am J Respir Cell Mol Biol 1998; 19:55–62.

36. Gauvreau GM, Doctor J, Watson RM, Jordana M, O'Byrne PM. Effects of inhaled budesonide on allergen-induced airway responses and airway inflammation. Am J Respir Crit Care Med 1996; 154:1267–1271.

37. Wood LJ, Inman MD, Watson RM, Foley R, Denburg JA, O'Byrne PM. Changes in bone marrow inflammatory cell progenitors after inhaled allergen in asthmatic subjects. Am J Respir Crit Care Med 1998; 157: 99–105.

38. Sehmi R, Howie K, Sutherland DR, Schragge W, O'Byrne PM, Denburg JA. Increased levels of CD34[+] hemopoietic progenitor cells in atopic subjects. Am J Respir Cell Mol Biol 1996; 15:645–654.

39. Sehmi R, Wood LJ, Watson R, Foley R, Hamid Q, O'Byrne PM, Denburg JA. Allergen-induced increases in IL-5 receptor a-subunit expression on bone marrow-derived CD34[+] cells from asthmatic subjects. A novel marker of progenitor cell commitment toward eosinophilic differentiation. J Clin Invest 1997; 100: 2466–2475.

40. Leber BF, Denburg JA. Retinoic acid modulation of induced basophil differentiation. Allergy 1997; 52: 1201–1206.

Heterogeneity of Responses to Antiasthma Treatment

Ana R Sousa, Tak H Lee*

Keywords: Asthma, glucocorticoids, resistance, β_2-agonists, leukotriene antagonists

Asthma is a complex clinical syndrome with multiple genetic and environmental factors contributing to its phenotypic expression. This adds to the complexity when addressing heterogeneity in the response to anti-asthma treatment. Currently, there are three main lines of treatment available: (1) inhaled glucocorticoids which suppress asthmatic inflammation; (2) β_2-agonists, which are very effective bronchodilators and act predominantly on airway smooth muscle; (3) cysteinyl-leukotriene inhibitors. Among the sources of variability that can cause heterogeneity in the response to treatment are the degree of underlying inflammation, such as in glucocorticoid resistance, and polymorphisms in the genes encoding the drug target, such as β_2-adrenoceptor and 5-lipoxygenase gene promoter polymorphisms.

Introduction

Bronchial asthma is a disease characterized clinically by episodic symptoms of wheeze, dyspnoea and chest tightness. Physiological abnormalities include a variable reduction in airflow which is secondary to increased airway resistance and bronchial hyperresponsiveness (BHR) to specific and non-specific agents such as allergen and histamine, respectively. Pathologically, even in the mildest of cases, there is evidence for airway inflammation with a cellular infiltrate of mononuclear cells and eosinophils into the airway mucosa. These cells are present in increased numbers and are activated to secrete proinflammatory cytokines that may be pertinent to the pathophysiology of the asthmatic process.

Currently, there are three main lines of treatment available: (1) inhaled glucocorticoids; (2) β_2-agonists; and (3) leukotriene inhibitors. Bronchial asthma is a heterogeneous disorder but even in patients with an apparently identical clinical phenotype, response to drug treatment may be remarkably variable. It is common for some patients to respond in a salutary fashion to a given treatment while others fail to manifest such a response. Heterogeneity of response to drug therapy can be observed in all three main line of asthma treatment presently used. Elucidation of this heterogeneity of response will contribute to a greater understanding of the immunopathology of bronchial asthma and may lead to the development of new drugs.

Glucocorticoid Therapy

Glucocorticoids (GC) are the mainstay of treatment for bronchial asthma and inhaled GCs are now the appropriate first-line treatment for patients who require inhalation with β-agonists more than once daily as recommended in national and international guidelines [1–3]. Short-term treatment with high dose oral prednisolone dramatically improves the clinical, physiological and pathological changes of asthma in most cases. It has been shown that prednisolone 40 mg orally daily for 14 days will reverse the reduction in forced expired volume in 1 second (FEV_1) to baseline in asthmatic exacerbations in most subjects. In addition a similar course of prednisolone is associated with an improvement in methacholine-induced BHR and a reduction in bronchoalveolar lavage (BAL) eosinophilia.

Both low and high dose inhaled GCs improve symptoms and lung function in newly-diagnosed asthmatic children and adults to a greater degree than that provided by β_2-agonists alone in studies up to 2 years. In addition, inhaled GCs attenuate the accelerated decline in lung function seen in asthmatic subjects and recent evidence suggests that a delay in the initiation of GC therapy lessens the subsequent GC response and so may contribute

* Department of Respiratory Medicine and Allergy, Guy's, King's College and St Thomas' Medical School, Guy's Hospital, London, UK

to an eventual sub-optimal response to GC. Therefore, earlier introduction of GCs in asthma may have important disease-modifying effects and this is reflected in the current British and American Thoracic Society Guidelines [2].

Glucocorticoid Resistance in Asthma

In recent years there has been increasing recognition of a group of asthmatic patients who do not appear to benefit from glucocorticoid therapy, i. e., the GC-resistant (GR) asthmatic [4].

GC responsiveness is probably a continuous spectrum with individuals who demonstrate GC resistance falling at one end of a unimodal distribution. For clinical purposes, the failure of an asthmatic patient to improve FEV_1 by 15% from a baseline of $\leq 75\%$ predicted after an adequate dose (e. g., ≥ 40 mg prednisolone) for an adequate duration of time (e. g., 1–2 weeks) would satisfy the definition for GC resistance, despite demonstrating greater than 15% reversibility to an inhaled β_2-agonist and provided compliance was ensured.

This is a pragmatic definition, which nevertheless is useful because it defines a sufficiently high dose of glucocorticoid and a duration of usage after which physicians would feel uncomfortable in maintaining patients on continuous systemic GCs. Furthermore, irrespective of whether GC resistance is part of a continuum of GC responsiveness or whether it is a distinct population, the definition stated above allows research to be conducted on patients at polar extremes of the clinical spectrum of asthma.

GR asthma was first described by Schwartz and colleagues in 1967 [5]. In 1981 Carmichael described 58 subjects with chronic asthma who were clinically resistant to prednisolone therapy [6]. Compared with GS subjects, these patients had a longer duration of asthma, a more frequent family history of asthma, poorer morning lung function, and a greater degree of bronchial reactivity. These early clinical studies suggested that both genetic (family history of asthma) and environmental (longer duration of asthma) factors may play a role in the pathogenesis of this condition.

Primary Glucocorticoid Resistance

Target tissue resistance to steroid hormones implies inability or decreased sensitivity of the tissues to respond to these hormones. This resistance can be transient or permanent, incomplete (partial) or complete, and compensated or noncompensated. The best recognized syndromes of GC resistance are in patients with primary glucocorticoid resistance [7, 8]. In these rare syndromes end-organ resistance to cortisol results in increased cortisol and ACTH levels. Increased ACTH stimulates excess adrenal androgens and mineralocorticoids. The resultant clinical syndromes can range from subtle biochemical abnormalities to the full blown syndrome [9]. Abnormalities reflecting androgen excess include virilization, infertility, acne and precocious puberty while abnormalities reflecting mineralocorticoid excess include hypertension, hypocalaemia and metabolic alkalosis. Many of these end-organ resistant syndromes have been shown to be due to polymorphisms in the primary structure of the glucocorticoid receptor [10]. The prevalence of polymorphisms in the general population is thought to be very low as the glucocorticoid receptor is highly conserved. Patients who exhibit relative or absolute resistance to the anti-inflammatory effects of GCs do not typically demonstrate these clinical or biochemical abnormalities. Furthermore, their prevalence in the general population is much greater than that of expected polymorphisms in the glucocorticoid receptor. Therefore it is unlikely that significant abnormalities in the primary structure of the glucocorticoid receptor can account for "anti-inflammatory" resistance or that, if present, these subtle polymorphisms would not affect the metabolic functions of GCs.

Cellular Abnormalities in GR Asthma

In view of the lack of evidence for any gross biochemical abnormality in these patients subsequent studies focused on the role played by peripheral blood mononuclear cells in GR asthma. Many studies have now demonstrated that GR asthma is associated with impaired *in vitro* and *in vivo* responsiveness of monocytes and T lymphocytes to the suppressive effects of GCs [11].

In an *ex vivo* study, complement receptor expression on monocytes from GS subjects was reduced as compared with cells from untreated patients. The reduction in complement receptor expression induced by prednisolone was not observed in the monocytes of those patients exhibiting GR asthma. Also, methylprednisolone, which substantially inhibited growth of colonies from phytohaemagglutinin-stimulated mononuclear cells of GS asthmatics, had little effect on colony growth from the mixed mononuclear cells of GR asthmatic individuals. In subsequent crossover experiments the origin of this *in vitro* resistance was found to be monocyte-, rather than lymphocyte-derived. In contrast to nonasthmatic controls, we have shown that monocyte supernatants from asthmatic subjects generated a neutrophil priming activity (NPA) which was selectively suppressed *in vitro* in a dose-dependent and rank order fashion by glucocorticoid treatment in the GS, but not in the GR, group [12, 13]. The degree of *in vitro* suppression by GCs of NPA correlated significantly with *in vivo* airways responsiveness to oral prednisolone in the GS group. Physicochemical analysis has shown this activity to be a 3kD heat and pronase sensitive molecule which may be related to the low molecular weight chemokine family. In addition we have demonstrated that the enhanced monocyte expression of the activation antigens, complement receptors 1 and 3 and class 2 molecules, seen in bronchial asthma is suppressed by hydrocortisone in GS, but not in GR asthmatic subjects [14].

Glucocorticoid resistance is not cell specific and there is evidence for T lymphocyte dysfunction in GR asthma. Corrigan has shown enhanced interleukin-2 (IL-2) and HLA-DR receptor expression on peripheral T lymphocytes in GR as opposed to GS asthma [15]. In addition he has shown that PHA-induced T cell proliferation and the elaboration of IFN-γ and IL-2 from mitogen-stimulated T lymphocytes was inhibited by dexamethasone in GS, but not in GR subjects [16]. Interestingly cyclosporin-A was seen to partially reverse this *in vitro* resistance, suggesting a potentially therapeutic role for this treatment in GR asthma.

A recent study by Leung and colleagues has demonstrated a 2-fold increase in the glucocorticoid receptor b isoform in PBMCs derived from GR asthmatics as compared to GS subjects [17].

We have provided evidence for an *in vivo* defect in the responsiveness of the macrophage-T-cell interaction to the suppressive effects of GCs in GR asthma. We have used the classical tuberculin cutaneous delayed hypersensitivity immune response to investigate *in vivo* defects in mononuclear cell function in 9 GR and 6 GS asthmatic subjects who demonstrated sensitivity to intradermal purified protein derivative (PPD) of Mycobacterium tuberculosis [18]. In a double-blind, crossed-over, placebo-controlled study, patients were given oral prednisolone/placebo starting on day 0, a predetermined intradermal dose of PPD on day 7 and on day 9 the site of the induration was measured and biopsied for immunohistochemical analysis. There was no difference in skin induration between the GS and GR groups during the placebo limb of the study. Prednisolone significantly suppressed the cutaneous induration in the GS but not in the GR group. As compared to placebo, there was suppression by prednisolone of the number of macrophages, eosinophils and T memory cells in the GS, but not in the GR group. There was no significant suppression by prednisolone in the number of neutrophils or monocytes/immature macrophages in either group. There was no difference in ICAM-1, VCAM-1 and ELAM-1 expression in blood vessels or epidermis between the GS and GR groups with no suppression by prednisolone in either group. These findings suggest a generalized *in vivo* defect in the responsiveness of cellular immune mechanisms to the suppressive effects of GCs in steroid-resistant asthma. The differential suppressive effects of GCs on cellular recruitment in the PPD response between the GS and GR individuals are not due to modulation of expression of endothelial adhesion molecules.

Further evidence for *in vivo* abnormalities in GR asthma comes from a study by Brown et al. who demonstrated that the cutaneous vasoconstrictor response to beclomethasone dipropionate was significantly reduced in patients in GR asthma as opposed to patients with either mild or severe steroid-dependent GS asthma suggesting that cells other than mononuclear cells may demonstrate impaired steroid responsiveness in this condition [19].

In a recent study Leung has examined the effects of a 1 week course of prednisolone on BAL cells obtained from patients with GR asthma using *in situ* hybridization [20]. GR subjects had elevated cell numbers expressing IL-2 and IL-4 before prednisolone treatment as compared to the GS subjects. In contrast to GS subjects prednisolone failed to suppress IL-4 and IL-5 expression in the GR subjects. In addition, prednisolone treatment increased IFN-γ mRNA +ve cells in GS group, but suppressed it the GR group. Therefore, the airway cells from patients with GR compared with GS asthma have different patterns of cytokine gene expression and distinct responses to GC therapy.

Tissue Specificity of Glucocorticoid Resistance in Asthma

We have examined whether the lack of clinical response to GCs seen in GR bronchial asthma is reflected in abnormalities of endogenous cortisol secretion and in the sensitivity of the hypothalamic-pituitary-adrenal (HPA) in GR subjects by using a modification of the standard dexamethasone suppression test in response to 0.25 and 1 mg oral dexamethasone [21]. Five GS and 5 GR asthmatic subjects were studied on two occasions one month apart. On the first limb of the study subjects received 0.25 mg of oral dexamethasone and on the second limb 1 mg was administered. Urinary cortisol was measured by fluorimetry after extraction and plasma cortisol and ACTH levels were estimated by ELISA and immunoradiometric assays, respectively. On day 1, a 24-hour urine was collected for estimation of urinary free cortisol. On day 2, a fasting blood was taken at 09.00 for estimation of plasma cortisol and ACTH. At 23.00, 0.25 mg (1 mg) of dexamethasone was taken orally by each subject. On day 3, blood was taken at 09.00 and at 15.00 for similar estimations. Plasma ACTH and cortisol levels were not significantly suppressed in either group after 0.25 mg dexamethasone but were equally suppressed in both groups to undetectable levels by 1 mg dexamethasone. These data indicate that GR asthma is not reflected in an altered secretory rate of endogenous cortisol or in a different sensitivity of the HPA axis to dexamethasone suppression. In order to assess whether GR asthmatic patients are equally at risk from the side effects of GCs on bone metabolism, GS and GR asthmatic patients received prednisolone 40 mg orally for five days. Prednisolone suppressed osteocalcin equally in both the GS and GR groups [22]. These two studies indicate that "nonimmune" tissue responds normally to GCs in GR asthma and that these subjects are therefore equally at risk of Cushingoid side effects. We speculated that the presence of inflammation in these cells is a necessary prerequisite for the unmasking of the resistant profile.

Glucocorticoid Bioavailability in GR Asthma

Interest has also focused on whether impaired bioavailability of GCs can account for the differences in therapeutic responses in steroid-dependent and steroid resistant asthma. May et al. measured the pharmacokinetic profile of a single dose of 15 mg oral prednisolone in 12 steroid dependent asthmatic subjects by radioimmunoassay (RIA) and found no inter-individual differences in these subjects with respect to C_{max}, plasma half life and area under the concentration/time curve and concluded that differences in prednisolone bioavailability is not a factor

in determining the dose required to control asthma [23]. Rose and colleagues observed that the plasma protein binding, distribution and clearance of prednisolone are not responsible for the large prednisolone requirement of steroid-dependent asthmatics. He extended the above studies to GC dependent and resistant asthmatic children and again found no difference in bioavailability parameters. We have examined the pharmacokinetic profile of an oral dose of 40 mg prednisolone in GS and GR asthmatic subjects [24]. We found that there was no significant difference in AUC, C_{max} and estimated clearance values between the normal group studied and each of the asthmatic groups. This implies that clinical GC resistance in asthmatic subjects is not reflected in any gross abnormality of the absorption or elimination of prednisolone. These data are in agreement with pharmacokinetic studies carried out in GR asthma by other groups who observed no differences in estimated clearance values of a single dose of oral prednisolone between groups of well characterized GR and GS asthmatic subjects [16].

Glucocorticoid Receptor Characteristics in GR Asthma

Competitive binding studies on nuclear extracts derived from peripheral blood monocytes using [^{3}H]-dexamethasone have demonstrated no difference in the K_d, R_o or nuclear translocation of the activated receptor complex between GS and GR asthmatics [13]. We have shown that GC resistance in bronchial asthma cannot be explained by abnormalities in receptor nuclear translocation, density or binding affinity. It is possible that the phenomenon of GC resistance may be a heterogeneous. Indeed, a 4-fold reduction in receptor binding affinity has been described in T cells however, the authors concluded that such a small reduction in K_d was insufficient to explain the gross difference in GC responsiveness at the clinical level [16]. Similarly, Sher et al. have described two patterns of ligand binding abnormalities in their group of CR asthmatics termed type 1 and 2 [25]. The more common type 1 defect was associated with "Cushingoid side effects," reduced K_d, normal receptor numbers, localization to T cells, reversibility with serum deprivation and was IL-2- and IL-4-dependent. The less common type 2 defect was associated with reduced receptor density with a normal K_d, was irreversible and was seen in the total mononuclear cell population. Type 1 defect is acquired as a result of longstanding inflammation whereas the type 2 defect is more likely to be a genetic defect.

We have demonstrated a reduction in the binding of the activated glucocorticoid receptor complex to its GRE using gel retardation assay in mononuclear cells from GS, GR and nonasthmatic control subjects [26]. Dexamethasone was seen to induce a significant rapid and sustained 2-fold increase in GRE binding in the mononuclear cells from the GS subjects and nonasthmatic control subjects that was markedly reduced over all time points in the GR subjects. These data have recently been confirmed by other investigators who have suggested that this defect may occur as a result of an IL-2- and IL-4-dependent increase in the proinflammatory GRβ isoform [17]. These data suggested that there may be a mutation(s) in the primary structure of the glucocorticoid receptor, particularly in its DNA-binding domain.

We have tested whether the reduction in DNA binding of the glucocorticoid receptor is due to polymorphisms in its primary structure using the sensitive technique of chemical mutational analysis (CMA) [27]. Using this technique we did not detect any base pair mismatch between the 6 GS and 6 GR patients and the corresponding wild type glucocorticoid receptor, despite a 100% detection of control mutations indicating that the defect in GR asthma does not lie in the structure of the GR. This was further confirmed by dideoxy sequencing using linear PCR elongation and chain termination [28]. Therefore, a defect in the primary structure of the glucocorticoid receptor does not account for the reduction of *in vitro* DNA binding and prompted us to further examine the binding characteristics of receptor-DNA interaction. Subsequent Scatchard analysis indicated that the defect in the GR subjects was underpinned by a reduction in the numbers of nuclear translocated glucocorticoid receptors available for DNA interaction. This was despite there being an equal amount of nuclear translocated receptors available on the basis of previous ligand binding experiments. These data indicated to us that the DNA binding sites of the glucocorticoid receptors were being competed out, possibly by proinflammatory transcription factors. These factors are bound by glucocorticoid receptor DNA binding sites and so prevent their subsequently activating cytokine genes and thereby inflammation. Thus the reduction in the "read-out" of DNA binding of the GRE may reflect the presence of excess proinflammatory activity rather than a direct problem with positive gene transcription *per se*. It is therefore im-

portant to review the mechanisms of negative gene regulation by GCs.

Transcription Factor Interactions in GR Asthma

We have examined whether the functional abnormality of reduced DNA binding of the glucocorticoid receptor in GR asthma is caused by increased activity of proinflammatory transcription factors [29]. We examined the activities of AP-1, NF-κB and CREB using gel shift assays in unstimulated PBMCs from GR and GS subjects and found that AP-1-, but not NF-κB- and CREB-, DNA binding was significantly increased 2-fold in the GR subjects. In order to further understand these mechanism we sequenced the c-jun and c-fos major components of AP-1 and found not evidence of polymorphism in their primary structure. We have recently shown that T lymphocytes and monocytes from GR subjects generate a 2-fold excess of Fos protein which is secondary to an increase in the c-fos transcription rate [30]. We were able to suppress glucocorticoid receptor-DNA binding in GS subjects to levels seen in GR subjects by a PMA inducible factor which we have shown by co-immunoprecipitation studies to be c-Fos. Therefore GR subjects generate excess c-Fos which results excess AP-1 activity [31]. This would result in perpetuation of AP-1-mediated inflammation and would render the therapeutic effects of GCs less effective by sequestration of glucocorticoid receptors within the nucleus.

We then used the tuberculin-induced model of dermal inflammation to evaluate the effect of corticosteroids in regulating components of AP-1 *in vivo* on 9 GS and 6 GR asthmatic subjects for the regulatory components of AP-1 before and after 9 days of either of 40 mg prednisolone or placebo. Significantly greater expression of c-FOS, phosphorylated c-JUN and phosphorylated JUN amino terminal kinase (JNK) protein has been identified in GR than GS subjects. Corticosteroids suppressed phosphorylation of c-JUN and JNK in the GS Group, but enhanced phosphorylation of c-JUN and JNK in the GR Group [32].

Whatever the mechanism, there is excess AP-1 activity in GR asthma. This molecular observation is consistent with the clinical observation that prolonged untreated asthma renders the subsequent response to GCs less effective. We would suggest that this is as a result of chronic unopposed AP-1-mediated inflammation. Therefore, early suppression of inflammation by GCs would predict a more favourable outcome in asthma by early suppression of AP-1-mediated inflammation.

β_2-Agonist Therapy

β_2-Adrenoceptor agonists are recommended for first line use as bronchodilator therapy in asthma [33, 34]. Short and long acting β_2-agonists exhibit protective effects against a variety of direct and indirect bronchoconstrictor stimuli. However, regular treatment with β_2-agonists is associated with tachyphylaxis to the functional antagonism against bronchoconstrictor stimuli. There is evidence to show that inhaled corticosteroids and long-acting β_2-agonists given on a regular basis have addictive effects in improving long-term asthma control. The debate about the safety of regular β-agonist use in asthma has evolved substantially over the past decade. In spite of epidemiological data suggesting an association between β-agonist use and asthma deaths and an early study suggesting decreased asthma control on regular fenoterol, the overwhelming message from subsequent, large clinical studies, especially with the newer long-acting β-agonists, as been reassuring [35].

β_2-Adrenoceptor Polymorphism

One of the remaining issues in this debate is whether there might be a subgroup in the asthmatic population which does not benefit from regular β_2-agonist use, or which may be more vulnerable to rapid deterioration. One potential source of such an anomalous response could be genetic polymorphisms within the β_2-adrenoceptor (β_2AR) gene. This gene was cloned in 1987 and is situated on the long arm of chromosome 5 (5q 31–33) and has no introns. Nine polymorphisms have been described within the single coding region, although five are degenerate. The four remaining polymorphisms result in single aminoacid substitutions: Glycine for arginine at aminoacid 16, glutamate for glutamine at aminoacid 27, methionine for valine at 34 and isoleucine for threonine at position 164. Aminoacids 16 and 17 lie in the extracellular N-terminal domain, whereas aminoacids 34 and 164 are in the transmembrane spanning regions. These polymorphisms have been found with equal frequency in normal and asthmatic populations [36] and are

unlikely to be a cause of asthma *per se*, although they may influence the phenotype of the illness once it is expressed.

In vitro studies have shown that these polymorphisms have potential functional consequences. The Ile-164 polymorphism results in a major decrease in agonist binding affinity and coupling to adenylate cyclase. Polymorphisms Gly-16 and Glu-27 did not affect receptor binding or coupling but markedly altered agonist-promoted receptor down-regulation and functional desensitisation. Gly-16 enhanced this down-regulation, whereas Glu-27 protected against it.

The Ile-164 polymorphism is thought to be fairly uncommon, and there have been no studies on the corresponding phenotype. However, with a frequency of 3–6% of the population this may have major consequences at a population level.

There are a number of recent clinical studies relating to the Gly-16 and Glu-27 polymorphisms, because they are present in large numbers of the general population, perhaps over 50% for Gly-16 and over 25% for Glu-27, with quite strong linkage disequilibrium between them. A relatively early report suggested that homozygous Gly-16 was associated with a more severe asthma phenotype [36], but this has not been supported by more recent studies [37]. Gly-16 has also been associated with nocturnal asthma [38] and in children it has been reported to be associated with decreased bronchodilator response to an inhaled β_2-agonist [39].

The potential protective Glu-27 polymorphism has indeed been reported to be associated with decreased airway reactivity in asthma [40] but it did not seem to influence nocturnal asthma [38] or bronchodilator responsiveness [39]. The Gln-27 allele, on the other hand, has been associated with elevated IgE levels and with an increase in self reported asthma in children.

Lipworth et al. [41] have recently reported that Gly-16 increased the propensity for bronchodilator desensitization after regular formoterol, although whether such tachyphylaxis actually occurs has been quite controversial, with most groups failing to find any drop-off in the bronchodilator effectiveness of β-agonists when they are used long term. Tachyphylaxis to bronchoprotection, however is a very real phenomenon but may not have any great clinical relevance, at least for most patients. Lipworth et al. pursued this issue further and have investigated the relationship of the common β_2AR polymorphisms to the fall-off in protection afforded by β_2-agonists against induced bronchoconstriction when in regular use (bronchoprotective subsensitivity or tachyphylaxis). β_2-agonist subsensitivity occurred irrespective of variations in $\beta_2 AR$ phenotype. The Glu-27 polymorphism was not protective. although this may have been confounded by its linkage disequilibrium with Gly-16. Indeed, with lower doses of formoterol the Gln-27 polymorphism may be relatively protective, but this could just reflect lesser association with Gly-16. At lower doses of formoterol, whereas the Gly-16 homozygotes showed uniform marked loss of protection, there was a much greater spread when Arg-16 allele was present.

Further studies should be performed on these polymorphisms using lower dose of formoterol, preferably 12 mg as used in clinical practice and with salmeterol, which as a partial-agonist, is less likely than formoterol to induce tachyphylaxis as easily, and so may highlight any Gly-16 susceptibility and give further insight into heterogeneous response to β_2-agonist treatment [42].

Anti-Leukotriene Therapy

The newly released family of specifically targeted asthma treatments, namely agents that interfere with the synthesis or action of the leukotrienes, provide a previously unavailable method to identify a subset of patients in whom leukotrienes are key contributors to the expression of the asthma phenotype.

The 5-lipoxygenase (5-LO) pathway is the name given to the series of biochemical reactions which result in the transformation of arachidonic acid, which is esterified in membrane phospholipids, into leukotrienes [43].

There are a number of observations suggesting that leukotrienes contribute to the pathogenesis of asthma. Firstly they can induce many of the abnormalities seen in asthma, including airway obstruction, bronchovascular leakage, mucus gland secretion, and granulocyte chemotaxis [44, 45]. Secondly they are, on a molar basis, among the most potent effector molecules known to cause airway obstruction. Thirdly, Leukotriene E_4 (LTE$_4$), an end-product of leukotriene metabolism, can be recovered in increased amounts from the urine of individuals with allergic asthma after antigen challenge [46, 47]. In addition, elevated levels of urinary LTE$_4$ are present in over two-thirds of patients presenting for the emergency treatment of asthmatic airway obstruction [44].

Leukotriene action may be pharmacologically modulated by antagonism at the receptor site or by biosynthesis inhibition. Leukotriene B_4 receptor antagonists have not yet been evaluated in humans, but LTD$_4$ receptor antagonists have been developed for use in human trials. Inhibition of 5-lipoxygenase (5-LO) biosynthesis is effected either by direct interference with its enzymatic properties, or by secondary inhibition of its interaction with FLAP.

At present, several antileukotriene drugs have been approved for the treatment of asthma. Zileuton, an inhibitor of 5-lipoxygenase, zafirlukast, pranlukast and montelukast are inhibitors of the action of LTD$_4$ at its receptor. A large number of clinical trials have been completed with these agents, establishing their efficacy in the treatment of spontaneous or induced asthma. All drugs have been shown to provide a superior effect, when compared to placebo, in the treatment of patients with mild-to-moderate asthma.

The leukotriene inhibitors will not supplant β-agonists since their acute bronchodilator effects are not as marked as those of β-agonists. Their use in more severe asthma is currently under study. Agents active on the 5-LO pathway such as zileuton and zafirlukast are an alternative to inhaled steroids for patients who are using β-agonists as their primary asthma treatment. The efficacy of these drugs is clearly established in this setting. It also seems likely, but not as yet clearly established, that they will be effective adjunctive therapy in patients whose asthma is poorly controlled despite use of inhaled steroids at a low dose. There is reason to believe that this class of agents will be effective preventive therapy for patients with exercise-induced asthma; an additional important indication for the use of these agents is the treatment of aspirin-induced asthma. Furthermore, heterogeneity of the response to treatment could be related with heterogeneity of the clinical manifestation of asthma.

5-Lipoxygenase Gene Promoter Polymorphisms

The failure of a patient with asthma to respond to antileukotriene treatment provides evidence consistent with the hypothesis that leukotrienes are not critical to the expression of the asthmatic phenotype in that patient.

Among the pharmacogenetic causes of this clinical phenotype are genetic variants that downregulate gene expression of 5-LO. A family of polymorphisms exists in the core promoter of the 5-LO gene [48]. They consist of an alteration in the number of tandem Sp1 and Egr-1 (early growth response protein) consensus binding sites, from the deletion of one or two or addition of one zinc finger binding sites in the region 176 to 147 upstream from the ATG translation start site . The wild type contains five such tandem repeats. Five-lipoxygenase promoter reporter constructs containing these polymorphisms display less capacity for promoter binding and direct less gene transcription than constructs containing the wild-type 5-LO core promoter. Such polymorphisms may explain the heterogeneous therapeutic response to 5-LO inhibition in asthmatic patients.

Summary

Our understanding of asthma and its therapy has changed markedly over the last few years, particularly with the application of molecular and cell biology and the discovery of new and more specific pharmacologic tools. It is timely to use these novel technologies to elucidate the mechanism(s) of heterogeneity of responsiveness to drug therapy, as this may provide insight into optimal targeting of drug therapy to subgroups of asthmatic patients. This may, in turn, provide greater understanding of underlying pathogenetic mechanisms.

Address for correspondence:

Professor TH Lee
Dept Respiratory Medicine and Allergy
5th Floor Thomas Guy House
Guy's Hospital
London SE1 9RT UK
Tel. +44 171 955-4571
Fax +44 171 403-8640
E-mail tak.lee@kcl.ac.uk

References

1. Barnes PJ. Drug-therapy – inhaled glucocorticoids for asthma. N Engl J Med 1995; 332:868–875.

2. International consensus report on the diagnosis and management of asthma. International Asthma Management Project. Clin Exp Allergy 1992; 22:1–72.

3. The British Thoracic Society Guidelines on the management of asthma. Thorax 1993:S1–S24.

4. Lane SJ, Lee TH. Mechanism and detection of glucocorticoid insensitivity in asthma. Allergy Clin Immunol Int 1997; 9:165–173.

5. Schwartz HJ, Lowell FC, Melby JC. Steroid resistance in bronchial asthma. Ann Int Med 1968; 69: 4493–4498.

6. Carmichael J, Paterson IC, Diaz P, Crompton GK, Kay AB, Grant IWB. Corticosteroid resistance in chronic asthma. Br Med J 1981; 282:1419–1422.

7. Chrousos GP, Deterawadleigh SD, Karl M. Syndromes of glucocorticoid resistance. Ann Int Med 1993; 119:1113–1124.

8. Bronnegard M, Carlstedt-Duke J. The genetic basis of glucocorticoid resistance. Trends Endocrinol Metabolism 1995; 6:160–164.

9. Karl M, Chrousos GP. Familial glucocorticoid resistance – An overview. Exp Clin Endocrinol 1993; 101:30–35.

10. Hurley DM, Accili D, Stratakis CA, Karl M, Vamvakopoulos N, Rorer E, Constantine K, Taylor SI, Chrousos GP. Point mutation causing a single amino-acid substitution in the hormone binding domain of the glucocorticoid receptor in familial glucocorticoid resistance. J Clin Invest 1991; 87:680–686.

11. Lane SJ. Pathogenesis of steroid-resistant asthma. Br J Hosp Med 1997; 57:394–398.

12. Wilkinson JRW, Crea AEG, Clark TJH, Lee TH. Identification and characterization of a monocyte-derived neutrophil-activating factor in corticosteroid-resistant bronchial asthma. J Clin Invest 1989; 84:1930–1941.

13. Lane SJ, Lee TH. Glucocorticoid receptor characteristics in monocytes of patients with corticosteroid-resistant bronchial-asthma. Am Rev Respir Dis 1991; 143:1020–1024.

14. Wilkinson JR, Lane SJ, Lee TH. Effects of corticosteroids on cytokine generation and expression of activation antigens by monocytes in bronchial asthma. Int Arch Allergy Appl Immunol 1991; 94:220–221.

15. Corrigan CJ, Brown PH, Barnes NC, Tsai JJ, Frew AJ, Kay AB. Glucocorticoid resistance in chronic asthma – Peripheral-blood lymphocyte-T activation and comparison of the lymphocyte-T inhibitory effects of glucocorticoids and cyclosporin-A. Am Rev Respir Dis 1991; 144:1026–1032.

16. Corrigan CJ, Brown PH, Barnes NC, Szefler SJ, Tsai JJ, Frew AJ, Kay AB. Glucocorticoid resistance in chronic asthma – Glucocorticoid pharmacokinetics, glucocorticoid receptor characteristics, and inhibition of peripheral blood T cell proliferation by glucocorticoids *in vitro*. Am Rev Respir Dis 1991; 144:1016–1025.

17. Leung DYM, Hamid Q, Vottero A, Szefler S, Surs W, Minshall E, Chrousos G, Klemm DJ. Association of glucocorticoid insensitivity with increased expression of glucocorticoid receptor β. J Exp Med 1997; 186: 1567–1574.

18. Sousa AR, Lane SJ, Atkinson BA, Poston RN, Lee TH. The effects of prednisolone on the cutaneous tuberculin response in patients with corticosteroid-resistant bronchial asthma. J Allergy Clin Immunol 1996; 97:698–706.

19. Brown PJ, Teelucksingh S, Matusiewicz SP, Greening AP, Crompton GK, Edwards CRW. Cutaneous vasoconstrictor response to glucocorticoids in asthma. Lancet 1991; 337:576–580.

20. Leung DYM, Martin RJ, Szefler SJ, Sher ER, Ying S, Kay AB, Hamid Q. Dysregulation of interleukin-4, interleukin-5, and interferon-γ gene-expression in steroid-resistant asthma. J Exp Med 1995; 181:33–40.

21. Lane SJ, Atkinson BA, Swaminathan R, Lee TH. Hypothalamic-pituitary-adrenal axis in corticosteroid-resistant bronchial asthma. Am J Respir Crit Care Med 1996; 153:557–560.

22. Lane SJ, Vaja S, Swaminathan R, Lee TH. Effects of prednisolone on bone turnover in patients with corticosteroid resistant asthma. Clin Exp Allergy 1996; 26:1197–1201.

23. May CS, Caffin JA, Halliday JW, Bochner F. Prednisolone pharmacokinetics in asthmatic patients. Br J Dis Chest 1980; 74:91–92.

24. Rose JQ, Nickelson JA, Ellis EF, Middleton E, Jusko WJ. Prednisolone disposition in steroid-dependent asthmatic children. J Allergy Clin Immunol 1981; 67:188–195.

25. Sher ER, Leung DYM, Surs W, Kam JC, Zieg G, Kamada AK, Szefler SJ. Steroid-resistant asthma – Cellular mechanisms contributing to inadequate response to glucocorticoid therapy. J Clin Invest 1994; 93:33–39.

26. Adcock IM, Lane SJ, Brown CR, Peters MJ, Lee TH, Barnes PJ. Differences in binding of glucocorticoid receptor to DNA in steroid-resistant asthma. J Immunol 1995; 154:3500–3505.

27. Lane SJ, Arm JP, Staynov DZ, Lee TH. Chemical mutational analysis of the human glucocorticoid receptor cdna in glucocorticoid-resistant bronchial asthma. Am J Respir Cell Mol Biol 1994; 11:42–48.

28. Lane SJ. Mechanism of glucocorticoid resistance in chronic bronchial asthma [PhD]. University of London, 1994.

29. Adcock IM, Lane SJ, Brown CR, Lee TH, Barnes PJ. Abnormal glucocorticoid receptor activator protein-1 interaction in steroid-resistant asthma. J Exp Med 1995; 182:1951–1958.

30. Lane SJ, Adcock IM, Barnes PJ, Lee TH. Increased c-Fos synthesis in mononuclear-cells from patients with corticosteroid resistant asthma. J Allergy Clin Immunol 1996; S97:529 (abstract).

31. Lane SJ, Adcock IM, Richards D, Hawrylowicz C, Barnes PJ, Lee TH. Corticosteroid-resistant bronchial asthma is associated with increased c-Fos expression in monocytes and T lymphocytes. J Clin Invest 1998; 102:2156–2164.

32. Sousa AR, Lane SJ, Lee TH. In vivo resistance to corticosteroids in bronchial asthma is associated with enhanced phosphorylation of jun amino terminal kinase (Jnk) and failure of prednisolone to inhibit Jnk phosphorylation. Am J Respir Crit Care Med 1999; 159: A632.

33. National Asthma Education and prevention programme. Expert Panel Report II. Guidelines for the diagnosis and management of asthma, National Institutes of Health publication. 1997; 97:4051–4055.

34. The British Guidelines On Asthma Management. Thorax 1997; 52:S1–S21.

35. Taylor DR, Town GI, Herbison GP, Boothman-Burrell D, Flannery EM, Hancox B, Harre E, Laubscher K, Linscott V, Ramsay CM, Richards G, Cowan J, Holbrook N, McLachlan C, Rigby S. Asthma control during long-term treatment with regular inhaled salbutamol and salmeterol. Thorax 1998; 53:744–752.

36. Reihaus E, Innis M, MacIntyre N, Liggett SB. Mutations in the gene encoding for the β2-adrenergic receptor in normal and asthmatic subjects. Am Resp Cell Mol Biol 1993; 8:334–339.

37. Dewar JC, Wheatley AP, Venn A, Morrison JFJ, Britton J, Hall IP. β2-adrenoceptor polymorphisms are in linkage disequilibrium but are not associated with asthma in an adult population. Clin Exp Allergy 1998; 28:442–448.

38. Turki J, Pak J, Green SA, Martin RJ, Liggett SB. Genetic polymorphisms of the β2-adrenergic receptor in nocturnal and nonnocturnal asthma. J Clin Invest 1995; 95:1635–1641.

39. Martinez FD, Graves PE, Baldini M, Solomon S, Erickson R. Association between genetic polymorphisms of the β2-adrenoceptor and response to albuterol in children with and without a history of wheezing. J Clin Invest 1997; 100:3184–3188.

40. Hall IP, Wheatley A, Wilding P, Liggett SB. Association of the Glu-27 β2-adrenoceptor polymorphism with lower airway reactivity in asthmatic subjects. Lancet 1995; 345:1213–1214.

41. Lipworth BJ, Hall IP, Aziz I, Tan KS, Wheatley A. β2-adrenoceptor polymorphism and bronchoprotective sensitivity with regular short and long-acting β2-agonist therapy. Clin Sci 1999; 96:253–259.

42. Walters EH, Walters JAE. A genetic twist to the β2 agonist debate. Clin Science 1999; 96:219–220.

43. Samuelsson B. Leukotrienes: Mediators of immediate hypersensitivity reactions and inflammation. Science 1983; 220:568–575.

44. Drazen JM, O'Brien J, Sparrow D, Weiss ST, Martins MA, Israel E, Fanta CH. Recovery of leukotriene-E4 from the urine of patients with airway obstruction. Am Rev Respir Dis 1992; 146:104–108.

45. Piper PJ. Leukotrienes and the airways. Eur J Anaesthesiol 1989; 6:241–255.

46. Taylor GW, Taylor I, Black P, Maltby NH, Turner N, Fuller RW, Dollery CT. Urinary leukotriene E4 after antigen challenge and in acute asthma and allergic rhinitis. Lancet 1989; 1:584–588.

47. Sladek K, Dworski R, Fitzgerald GA, Buitkus KL, Block FJ, Marney SR Jr., Sheller JR. Allergen-stimulated release of thromboxane A2 and leukotriene E4 in humans. Effect of indomethacin. Am Rev Respir Dis 1990; 141:1441–1445.

48. In KH, Asano K, Beier D, Grobholz J, Finn PW, Silverman EK, Silverman ES, Collins T, Fischer AR, Keith TP, Serino K, Kim SW, De Sanctis GT, Yandava C, Pillari A, Rubin P, Kemp J, Israel E, Busse W, Ledford D, Murray JJ, Segal A, Tinkleman D, Drazen JM. Naturally-occurring mutations in the human 5-lipoxygenase gene promoter that modify transcription factor binding and reporter gene transcription. J Clin Invest 1997; 99:1130–1137.

Severe Persistent and Corticosteroid Insensitive Asthma

Stanley J Szefler*, Donald YM Leung*,**

Keywords: Severe asthma, steroid resistant asthma, corticosteroids, glucocorticoid receptor, glucocorticoid receptor β

Asthma is now characterized in several stages, specifically intermittent, mild persistent, moderate persistent, and severe persistent. The most concerning level, severe persistent asthma, is associated with continual symptoms, frequent exacerbations, frequent nocturnal symptoms and low and highly variable pulmonary function. Corticosteroids are anti-inflammatory drugs used in the treatment of asthma and very effective in almost all asthma patients. However, a subset of asthmatics referred to as "corticosteroid-insensitive" or "resistant" fail to experience clinical improvement when treated with even high dose corticosteroids. The purpose of this chapter will be to review our current understanding and management of severe persistent asthma, especially the form that is corticosteroid insensitive. Understanding the mechanisms which give rise to relative corticosteroid insensitivity have important clinical implications for the management of asthma and other allergic disorders characterized by tissue inflammation.

Introduction

The National Heart, Lung and Blood Institute Expert Panel has characterized asthma as chronic airway inflammation associated with several levels of severity including intermittent, mild persistent, moderate persistent and severe persistent [1]. Severity is based on the patient's frequency of symptoms, the presence and frequency of nocturnal exacerbations, along with their level and variability of pulmonary function. The most concerning category, severe persistent asthma, is characterized by continual symptoms, limited physical activity and frequent exacerbations. These patients also have frequent nocturnal symptoms. Their pulmonary function is less than or equal to 60% of predicted as measured by FEV_1 or peak expiratory flow (PEF) with greater than 30% variability in PEF [1]. Pharmacotherapy consists of high dose inhaled corticosteroids combined with one or more nonsteroid long term controllers, such as a long-acting beta agonist, theophylline or possibly a leukotriene modifier.

Corticosteroids (CS) are highly effective anti-inflammatory drugs used frequently in the treatment of asthma. The clinical efficacy of these drugs result from an array of effects on chronic and acute airways inflammation [2, 3]. These include immunosuppressive effects on inflammatory cell trafficking into the lung, reduction of inflammatory cell survival, diminished airway mucus production, an inhibitory effect on inflammatory mechanisms including the increased gene transcription of anti-inflammatory proteins and cytokines. Asthmatics, however, vary in their response to CS. Although almost all patients respond to continuous treatment with inhaled or systemic CS, a small proportion of asthmatics have poorly controlled asthma even following treatment with high doses of oral prednisone or its equivalent. These patients account for a large proportion of the hospitalizations and emergency room visits due to asthma.

The purpose of this review will be to briefly summarize our current understanding of the management and mechanisms associated with the most severe forms of persistent asthma, especially those contributing to CS insensitivity. Understanding the mechanisms which give rise to CS insensitivity have important clinical implications for the management of asthma and other allergic disorders

* Divisions of Clinical Pharmacology and Allergy-Immunology, Department of Pediatrics, National Jewish Medical and Research Center, Denver, Colorado, USA; Helen Wohlberg & Herman Lambert Chair in Pharmacokinetics
** Department of Pediatrics, National Jewish Medical and Research Center, Denver, Colorado, USA

characterized by tissue inflammation. It is important to evaluate patients with severe persistent asthma very carefully in order to confirm the diagnosis of asthma and identify and manage concomitant conditions which may confound their asthma. If the diagnosis of CS insensitive asthma is made, then alternative anti-inflammatory approaches must be considered.

Clinical Presentation of Corticosteroid-Insensitive Asthma

The diagnosis of "corticosteroid-insensitive" asthma is based on clinical and physiologic responses to CS. Such patients have several distinguishing features. By clinical definition, these patients frequently have difficult-to-control persistent asthma characterized by continual respiratory symptoms, nocturnal exacerbations, chronic airflow limitation (FEV_1 < 70% of predicted), and a poor clinical and spirometric response to oral CS therapy [4]. To understand what constitutes an adequate trial of systemic CS therapy, Kamada et al. [5] studied the response of asthmatic children whose baseline morning pre-bronchodilator FEV_1 was < 70% predicted prior to a course of prednisone therapy. Over 60% of patients demonstrated a > 15% improvement of their morning pre-bronchodilator FEV_1 within 3 days, and 93% showed a significant improvement within 10 days of starting CS therapy. In this study, extending the course of therapy over 10 days did not lead to a significantly greater improvement in FEV_1.

In a workshop centered on the understanding of CS insensitive asthma, it was proposed that CS-insensitive asthma should be defined by the failure to improve baseline morning pre-bronchodilator FEV_1 by greater than 15% predicted following at least 7–14 days of 20 mg twice daily oral prednisone or its equivalent [6]. Although some patients might respond to higher doses of prednisone given for longer periods of time, such doses are undesirable due to the significant risk for adverse systemic effects.

Patients with CS-insensitive asthma should have a bronchodilator response of greater than 15% improvement in FEV_1 consistent with the American Thoracic Society criteria for diagnosis of asthma. For asthmatic patients who fail to respond to systemic CS, it is important to rule out other respiratory conditions which mimic the symptoms of asthma or confounding factors which contribute to difficult management (Table 1). These conditions must be thoroughly studied and, if present, appropriate management instituted prior to making the diagnosis of CS-insensitive asthma.

The actual percentage of total patients with CS-insensitive asthma is unknown since investigations have been focused on patients with relatively severe asthma. Furthermore, many asthmatics are not regularly monitored for changes in pulmonary function before and after a defined prednisone course. Most patients with mild to moderate persistent asthma may have spontaneous recovery of their asthma irrespective of whether a course of systemic CS are given or not. It is generally thought that CS-insensitivity is rare affecting less than 5% of all asthmatics [7]. Of interest, our recent study in patients with severe or difficult-to-control asthma found nearly 25% of patients fulfilled the criteria of CS insensitivity [8]. Therefore, in poorly controlled asthma, CS insensitivity must be considered.

Table 1. Diagnostic considerations in severe persistent asthma.

Alternative diagnosis (e. g., vocal cord dysfunction, cystic fibrosis, anatomic abnormalities, interstitial lung disease, foreign body, bronchiolitis obliterans, etc.)
Concomitant conditions (e. g., sinusitis, gastroesophageal reflux)
Persistent allergen exposure
Poor adherence to prescribed management course, i. e., environmental control, medications
Inadequate dose of long-term controller medications
Corticosteroid pharmacokinetic abnormality
   Rapid elimination
   Poor delivery to the site of action
   Incomplete absorption of oral glucocorticoid
Immunologic mechanisms contributing to persistent airway inflammation
Abnormal GCR number or function
Increased glucocorticoid receptor-β expression

Mechanisms of Corticosteroid Response and Insensitivity

Considerable information is now available on the nature of the glucocorticoid receptor (GCR), molecular mechanisms involved in CS response, and

Table 2. Immunologic features of corticosteroid-insensitive asthma.

---

1. T cells:
    - Increased levels of T cell activation unresponsive to corticosteroids
    - Decreased capacity of corticosteroids to inhibit PHA-induced T cell proliferation *in vitro*
    - Increased IL-2 and IL-4 gene expression in the airways
    - Failure to decrease production of airway IL-2, IL-4, and IL-5 after corticosteroids
    - Increased expression of peripheral blood and airway GCRβ
2. Eosinophils
    - Persistent eosinophilia following treatment with corticosteroids
3. Monocytes
    - Failure of corticosteroids to suppress production of a monocyte derived factor which primes neutrophils for enhanced LTB_4 production
    - Persistent IL-8 production despite corticosteroid treatment
    - Increased expression of AP-1
4. Neutrophils
    - Increased airway neutrophilia
    - Increased LTB_4 production

From [9]. Reprinted with permission.

cellular responses in CS sensitive asthma, as well as GCR abnormalities in CS-insensitive asthma ([6, 9], Table 2).

Patients with CS-insensitive asthma have decreased cellular immune responses to courses of high dose systemic CS. These abnormalities involve their T cells, monocytes and eosinophils such that CS treatment is less effective in suppressing the activation of these cells from CS-insensitive asthmatics as compared to CS-sensitive asthmatics. The most frequently used laboratory assay for CS-insensitivity has been the demonstration that PHA-induced proliferation of peripheral blood T lymphocytes in CS-sensitive, but not in CS-insensitive, asthmatics is inhibited by dexamethasone [10, 11]. The failure of CS to inhibit T cell activation in CS-insensitive asthmatics is consistent with the observation that they have increased expression of the CD25 (IL-2 receptor) and HLA-DR activation antigens on peripheral blood T-cells [12]. It has also been found that dexamethasone fails to inhibit PHA induced IL-2 and IFN-γ production in cells from CS-insensitive asthmatics. In contrast, synthesis of these cytokines by T cells from CS-sensitive asthmatics are inhibited by dexamethasone. It should be noted, however, that the immunosuppressant, cyclosporin A, and the macrolide antibiotic, troleandomycin (TAO), inhibit proliferation and cytokine production by T cells from CS-insensitive asthmatics [11, 12]. This is of clinical importance because while CS-insensitive asthma is associated with poor responsiveness to CS, these patients can be sensitive to other anti-inflammatory and immunomodulator drugs, such as cyclosporine, used in the treatment of severe, difficult to control asthma.

We have also examined bronchoalveolar lavage (BAL) airway cells from both CS-sensitive and CS-insensitive asthmatics, prior to and after a one week course of daily high dose (20 mg twice a day) prednisone [13]. At baseline, there were no significant differences between BAL total eosinophil counts or numbers of activated T cells in CS-insensitive versus CS-sensitive asthmatics. However, after prednisone therapy, the anticipated decrease in numbers of BAL eosinophils activated T cells was observed in CS-sensitive, but not CS-insensitive, asthmatics.

Additional studies were carried out to determine the cytokine mRNA expression in BAL cells. At baseline, BAL cells from CS-insensitive, as compared to CS-sensitive, asthmatics had a significantly higher number of cells expressing mRNA for IL-2 and IL-4. However, no significant differences between these two patient populations were observed in the expression of IL-5 mRNA at baseline. After prednisone therapy, BAL cells from CS-sensitive, but not CS-insensitive, asthmatics demonstrated a significant decrease in cells expressing IL-4 mRNA and IL-5 mRNA. However, CS therapy did not affect IL-2 mRNA expression in either group of asthmatic patients.

Sousa et al. [14] also demonstrated decreased inhibition by prednisone of macrophage, T cell and eosinophil infiltration into the cutaneous tuberculin response in CS-insensitive, as compared to CS-sensitive, asthmatics. Thus, these patients have a global defect in the responsiveness of their immune effector cells to CS. This CS-insensitivity is generally localized to their immune cells because other tissues, e. g., the hypothalamic-pituitary and bone, are CS sensitive, indicating that these patients are at risk for severe adverse effects with prolonged courses of high dose CS therapy [15, 16].

Based on our investigations of peripheral blood mononuclear cells (PBMC) GCR binding studies we were able to identify at least two forms of CS-insensitive asthma: an acquired form (Type I) and a primary form (Type II) [17 and Table 3]. The majority of patients with CS-insensitive asthma have

Table 3. Clinical and laboratory features of corticosteroid-insensitive asthma.

Features	Type I (acquired)	Type II (primary)
AM cortisol*	Suppressed	No
Cushingoid side effects*	Yes	No
GCR ligand and DNA binding affinity	Reduced	Normal
GCR number	Normal/High	Low
Reversibility of GCR defect	Yes	No
IL-2, IL-4 effect on PBMC GCR receptor	Sustains abnormality	No effect

* Characteristic observed on high dose systemic steroids.
From [9]. Reprinted with permission.

the Type I or acquired defect. These patients develop significant side effects, including adrenal suppression, cushingoid changes and osteoporosis, when treated chronically with high dose systemic CS. They have a decreased ligand and DNA GR binding defect affecting their mononuclear cells, particularly T cells, that reverses when their cells are incubated in culture medium in the absence of cytokines [17–19]. In contrast to this Type I acquired form of CS-insensitive asthma, PBMC from another group of patients termed Type II or primary CS-insensitive asthma have normal GR binding affinity but extremely low numbers of GCRs [17] that do not demonstrate any changes in GR binding when incubated in culture medium alone. The low

GCR number in this form of CS-insensitive asthma patients appears to be an irreversible defect. Patients with the Type II defect are also more refractory to the adverse systemic effects of CS suggesting that the low number of GCRs are also present in other tissues (Table 3).

A potential mechanism for CS insensitivity (Type I form) is based on studies demonstrating that alternative splicing of the GR pre-mRNA generates a second GCR, termed GCRβ, which does not bind to CS and antagonizes the transactivating activity of the classic GCR [19]. The increased expression of GCRβ could therefore account for CS-insensitive asthma. Indeed, we have reported that CS-insensitive asthma is associated with a significant increase in the number of peripheral blood and BAL cells expressing GCRβ (Figure 1) [19, 20]. The expression of GCRβ is inducible by the combination of IL-2 and IL-4, and markedly increased in BAL cells as compared to PBMC of CS-insensitive asthmatics. Interestingly, GCRβ expression is markedly increased in the T cell subset as compared to other cell types found in BAL or PBMC of patients with CS-insensitive asthma.

Recently, Wenzel et al. [21] carried out bronchoscopic studies of the inflammatory cell infiltrate in patients with severe asthma who were dependent on high-dose oral CS (mean ± SEM FEV_1 = 58 ± 6% predicted despite daily prednisone treatment of ≥ 20 mg/d for more than one year), and compared them to patients with moderate asthma (mean

GCR β Expression in Bronchoalveolar Lavage Cells

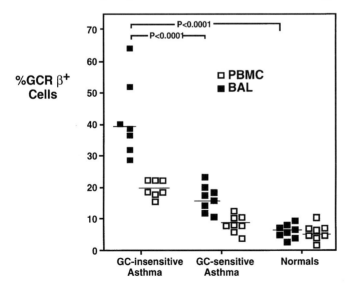

Figure 1. Percent GRβ+ cells in freshly isolated PBMC vs BAL from corticosteroid-insensitive asthmatics vs corticosteroid-sensitive asthmatics and control subjects. PBMC were processed and stained for GRβ immunoreactivity using an immunocytochemistry technique with a specific antibody to GRβ (modified with permission from [20]).

$\pm$ SEM FEV$_1$ = 65 $\pm$ 3% predicted but not requiring prednisone therapy) versus normal controls. The concentration of eosinophils in BAL fluid was highest in the moderate asthmatics not on prednisone, with little difference in eosinophils between normal controls and severe asthmatics. In contrast, the severe asthmatics demonstrated a significantly higher concentration of neutrophils in BAL than either the moderate asthmatics or the normal controls. Patients with severe asthma were also found to have significantly higher levels of leukotriene B4 and thromboxane, which respectively can induce neutrophil chemotaxis and airway hyperreactivity [22]. These studies indicate a novel form of inflammation in severe symptomatic asthmatics chronically treated with high dose oral CS.

It remains to be determined whether these findings are due to a different pathologic form of asthma, a direct response to high dose CS or a response to an infectious trigger. As noted above, so-called CS-insensitive asthma is associated with a relative CS-insensitivity of T lymphocytes. Thus, it might be expected that treatment of such patients with a prolonged course of high-dose systemic CS could reduce the eosinophil/T lymphocyte driven process but leave behind, or even augment, a neutrophil-mediated process. Indeed, it is well established that neutrophils are CS resistant and CS may even activate neutrophils.

Management of Severe Persistent Asthma

The management of severe persistent asthma patients, especially those with steroid insensitivity, poses a considerable challenge for the clinician. A systematic, stepwise approach is important for a successful outcome (see Table 4). The first step is to obtain a thorough history, physical examination and appropriate laboratory tests to confirm the diagnosis of asthma and rule out concomitant medical disorders which can complicate the management of patients with severe persistent asthma, such as vocal cord dysfunction [23].

The second step is to develop a written action plan for acute exacerbations. Emphasis should be placed on appropriate use of rescue medications such as bronchodilators and when to notify the physician. A written care plan should also be used to summarize routine prophylactic medications in-

Table 4. Stepwise approach to managing severe persistent asthma.

1. Examine for concomitant medical disorders, e. g., VCD, sinusitis, and GE reflux
2. Prepare written action plan
3. Evaluate for psychosocial factors including adherence to prescribed treatment
4. Review medication technique
5. Instruct on environmental control
6. Control nocturnal exacerbations
   – Salmeterol
   – Formoterol
   – Theophylline
7. Modify inhaled glucocorticoid therapy
   – increase dose
   – increase frequency of administration
   – introduce more potent inhaled glucocorticoids, i. e., fluticasone propionate
   – improve lung delivery of inhaled glucocorticoid, i. e., budesonide via Turbuhaler
8. Evaluate corticosteroid pharmacokinetics and cell response
   – Split-dosing regimen
   – 3 pm dosing
   – Monitor for adverse effects
9. Alternative therapy
   – Cyclosporine
   – Gold
   – Intravenous immune globulin

cluding recommendations for pre-treatment programs for exercise and anticipated exposure to irritants or allergens. If a patient has difficulty in following the recommendations or appears to be intentionally noncompliant, a psychological evaluation may be needed to identify psychosocial features that interfere with adherence to the treatment regimen, including learning disabilities, family dysfunction, depression, anxiety, etc.

The third step is to rule out psychosocial factors affecting the illness. A large proportion of patients with severe persistent asthma have an inadequate response to therapy simply due to poor adherence with recommended therapy. The basis for noncompliance is complex and can range from simple forgetfulness, in which case a medication diary or pill box is useful, to the inability to pay for the medications. Alternatively, poor adherence could be due to a severe psychologic problem such as depression which could impair the patient's ability to function and adhere to a suggested medical regimen. Correction of these underlying problems are important to ensure adherence to therapy. In addition, it is important to keep the medication regimen as simple as possible, prioritize recommendations, educate the patient regarding their asthma management and adjust the dosing schedule to the patient's lifestyle.

The fourth step is to review the patient's technique of medication administration. This should be incorporated as a routine part of the physical examination as patients often forget proper inhaler technique. Spacer devices should be used to optimize medication delivery and reduce adverse effects of medications. New breath actuated, dry powder or metered dose inhalers can be used to compensate for inadequate technique. For inhaled steroids, a mouth rinsing procedure and expectoration of the mouth rinse should be used to minimize systemic steroid absorption.

The fifth step is to assure appropriate environmental control at home, in school and at work. The focus should be on areas where the patient spends the highest proportion of time, for example, the bedroom, or areas of high indoor allergen exposure. A number of studies have demonstrated that atopic patients who live with animals at home require higher doses of steroids to maintain control of their asthma [24]. In support of these observations, we reported that exposure to allergens reduces GCR binding affinity in PBMCs from atopic asthmatics [25].

The sixth step is to maximize anti-inflammatory and bronchodilator therapy for control of nocturnal exacerbations. Inhaled salmeterol or formoterol administered at bedtime can be very useful in controlling nocturnal asthma. Oral theophylline can also be used as well in the treatment of nocturnal asthma. In this case, chronopharmacologic principles can be applied to optimize response to theophylline. Patients with nocturnal exacerbations may do better with a single dose of a once daily sustained release preparation administered in the evening as compared to a standard twice daily preparation [26, 27]. Children and rapid theophylline metabolizers appear to be prone to reduction in serum theophylline concentrations during the night [28].

The seventh step is to modify inhaled CS therapy in an effort to reduce requirements for systemic CS therapy. One approach would be to increase the dose and frequency of inhaled CS. This is based on the assumption that high dose inhaled CS are more effective and also that adverse CS effects are less than those commonly associated with high dose systemic CS therapy. The majority of patients with CS insensitive asthma have the acquired form which is associated with reduced GCR binding affinity. Studies of their T cells indicate a shift to the

right in their dose response to CS rather than an absolute resistance [29]. Thus, higher doses of CS or a change to CS with a higher GCR binding affinity, such as fluticasone propionate, or higher lung delivery, such as budesonide via the Turbuhaler device, is a reasonable approach to gain control of their asthma.

The eighth step is to evaluate systemic CS pharmacokinetics and other cellular mechanisms to determine the basis of CS insensitivity in these patients. The purpose of these studies is to determine whether there is incomplete CS absorption, failure to convert to an active form, rapid elimination, reduced glucocorticoid receptor number or binding affinity, or a combination of abnormalities [30, 31]. This evaluation is particularly important in a patient who fails to demonstrate the anticipated adverse effects of long-term, high-dose CS therapy. Measurements of plasma CS concentrations can also be used in an assessment of compliance. Patients with poor absorption of prednisone, frequently respond well to oral liquid steroid preparations or alternatively a change to a different systemic CS, such as methylprednisolone. In patients with rapid CS elimination, a split dosing regimen, with the second dose of the day administered in the afternoon, should be considered. In such patients, the morning dose should be titrated, then convert afternoon dose to morning dose, then attempt to reduce to alternate day therapy.

We are also beginning to incorporate markers of inflammation, for example, exhaled nitric oxide, plasma eosinophilic cationic protein and serum sIL-2 receptors, to examine medication response [32, 33]. This is most useful before and after a one to two week course of oral glucocorticoid therapy. Failure to respond with persistent elevated levels of inflammation despite treatment with high dose prednisone provides a strong basis for incorporating alternative therapies.

It is important to monitor patients carefully for adverse effects related to CS therapy and initiate measures to minimize their effect. For example, CS-induced osteoporosis can be monitored with bone densitometry. Attention should be placed on providing adequate dietary calcium and vitamin D, as well as other therapeutic interventions as indicated [34].

The final step is to consider alternative anti-inflammatory and immunomodulator approaches. This is of particular importance in patients with the Type II or primary form of CS insensitive asthma who have a generalized primary resistance to CS therapy. Unfortunately, there have been no well-controlled studies of alternative therapies in CS-insensitive asthma. Treatment with gold, cyclosporine, and intravenous immunoglobulin, have been reported to have steroid sparing effects, and may be potentially useful in patients who fail steroid therapy [35–37]. Limited information from *in vitro* studies suggest that T cells from CS insensitive asthma will respond to the immunosuppressive actions of cyclosporine thus providing a rationale for use of this agent in the management of these patients [12].

To date, studies of these medications have not systematically incorporated bronchial biopsies and BAL to verify resolution of inflammation although several case reports have now demonstrated decreased airway inflammation in CS-insensitive asthmatics treatment with intravenous immunoglobulin or cyclosporin [38, 39]. An organized program with carefully designed protocols and a larger numbers of patients is needed to understand the role of these alternative anti-inflammatory therapies in the treatment of CS-insensitive asthma and to identify a hierarchy of medication selection for patients with severe persistent asthma.

In the future, more information is also needed on the pathology of "difficult to control" asthma to determine whether there are ultrastructural abnormalities present that may be irreversible [40, 41]. In this regard, it is possible that aggressive courses of anti-inflammatory or immunomodulator therapy can suppress acute inflammation, but airway remodeling may predispose the patient to residual symptoms, and the development of irreversible airway disease. Of greater concern is the possibility that the persistent symptoms in certain patients could be related to noninflammatory airways hyperresponsiveness. Obviously, more effort must be placed on understanding the pathophysiology of severe persistent asthma to refine the selection of pharmacotherapy for this challenging group of patients.

There have been no systematic studies examining the long-term prognosis of severe persistent asthma, especially CS-insensitive asthma. The major concern with this group of patients is that they are at high risk for morbidity and mortality due to asthma. During acute exacerbations of their asthma, patients with Type I or acquired CS insensitive asthma require much higher doses of intravenous CS than CS sensitive asthmatics to gain control of their inflammation. This places them at higher risk for steroid-induced side effects. In patients with

Type II or primary CS-insensitive asthma, high doses of intravenous CS is also worth trying, but it is possible that they will require alternative anti-inflammatory therapy. It should be emphasized that CS insensitive asthmatics do respond to bronchodilator therapy and that such medications should be instituted early as rescue therapy. Finally, the presence of high level persistent airway inflammation in this group of asthmatics predisposes them to the development of airway fibrosis and long-term irreversible airways diseases. Thus, it is of paramount importance to treat their inflammation early and effectively.

Acknowledgments

The authors wish to thank Maureen Plourd-Sandoval for assistance in preparing this manuscript. Supported in part by Public Health Services Research Grants HL36577, AR41256, HL 37260, and General Clinical Research Center Grant 5 MO1 RR00051 from the Division of Research Resources, and an American Lung Association Asthma Research Center Grant

Address for correspondence:

Stanley J Szefler, MD
National Jewish Medical and Research Center
1400 Jackson St., Rm. J209
Denver, CO 80206
USA
Tel. +1 303 398-1193
Fax +1 303 270-2189
E-mail szeflers@njc.org

References

1. National Asthma Education and Prevention Program Expert Panel Report 2: Guidelines for the Diagnosis and Management of Asthma. 1997. National Institutes of Health, National Heart, Lung and Blood Institute, Pub. No. 97–4051.

2. Schwiebert LM, Beck LA, Stellato C, Bickel CA, Bochner BS, Schleimer RP, Schwiebert LA. Glucocorticosteroid inhibition of cytokine production: Relevance to antiallergic actions. J Allergy Clin Immunol 1996; 97:143.

3. de Benedictis FM, Canny GJ, Levison H. The role of corticosteroids in respiratory diseases of children. Pediatr Pulmonol 1996; 22:44.

4. Carmichael J, Paterson IC, Diaz P, Crompton GK, Kay AB, Grant IW. Corticosteroid resistance in chronic asthma. Br Med J (Clin Res Ed) 1981; 282: 1419.

5. Kamada AK, Leung DYM, Gleason MC, Hill MR, Szefler SJ. High-dose systemic glucocorticoid therapy in the treatment of severe asthma: A case of resistance and patterns of response. J Allergy Clin Immunol 1992; 90:685.

6. Lee TH, Brattsand R, Leung DYM. Corticosteroid action and resistance in asthma. Am J Respir Cell Mol Biol Suppl 1996; 154:S1.

7. Barnes PJ. Efficacy of inhaled corticosteroids in asthma. J Allergy Clin Immunol 1998; 102:531.

8. Chan MT, Leung DYM, Szefler SJ, Spahn JD. Difficult-to-control asthma: Clinical characteristics of steroid-insensitive asthma. J Allergy Clin Immunol 1998; 101:594.

9. Leung DYM, Szefler SJ. Corticosteroid insensitive asthma. Immunol Allergy Clin N Am 1999; in press.

10. Corrigan CJ, Brown PH, Barnes NC, Szefler SJ, Tsai JJ, Frew AJ, Kay AB. Glucocorticoid resistance in chronic asthma. Glucocorticoid pharmacokinetics, glucocorticoid receptor characteristics, and inhibition of peripheral blood T cell proliferation by glucocorticoids in vitro. Am Rev Respir Dis 1991; 144:1016.

11. Alvarez J, Surs W, Leung DYM, Iklé D, Gelfand EW, Szefler SJ. Steroid-resistant asthma: Immunologic and pharmacologic features. J Allergy Clin Immunol 1992; 89:714.

12. Corrigan CJ, Brown PH, Barnes NC, Tsai JJ, Frew AJ, Kay AB. Glucocorticoid resistance in chronic asthma. Peripheral blood T lymphocyte activation and comparison of the T lymphocyte inhibitory effects of glucocorticoids and cyclosporin A. Am Rev Respir Dis 1991; 144:1026.

13. Leung DYM, Martin RJ, Szefler SJ, Sher ER, Ying S, Kay AB, Hamid Q. Dysregulation of interleukin 4, interleukin 5, and interferon γ gene expression in steroid-resistant asthma. J Exp Med 1995; 181:33.

14. Sousa AR, Lane SJ, Atkinson BA, Poston RN, Lee TH. The effects of prednisolone on the cutaneous tuberculin response in patients with corticosteroid-resistant bronchial asthma. J Allergy Clin Immunol 1996; 97:698.

15. Lane SJ, Atkinson BA, Swaminathan R, Lee TH. Hypothalamic-pituitary-adrenal axis in corticosteroid-resistant bronchial asthma. Am J Respir Crit Care Med 1996; 153:557.

16. Lane SJ, Vaja S, Swaminathan R, Lee TH. Effects of prednisolone on bone turnover in patients with corticosteroid-resistant bronchial asthma. Clin Exp Allergy 1999; in press.

17. Sher ER, Leung DYM, Surs W, Kam JC, Zieg G, Kamada AK, Szefler SJ. Steroid-resistant asthma. Cellular mechanisms contributing to inadequate response to glucocorticoid therapy. J Clin Invest 1994; 93:33.

18. Adcock IM, Lane SJ, Brown CR, Peters MJ, Lee TH, Barnes PJ. Differences in binding of glucocorticoid receptor to DNA in steroid-resistant asthma. J Immunol 1995; 154:3500.

19. Leung DYM, Hamid Q, Vottero A, Szefler SJ, Surs W, Minshall E, Chrousos GP, Klemm DJ. Association of glucocorticoid insensitivity with increased expression of glucocorticoid receptor beta. J Exp Med 1997; 186:1567.

20. Hamid QA, Wenzel SE, Hauk PJ, Kamil AA, Chrousos GP, Szefler SJ, Leung DYM. Increased expression of glucocorticoid receptor beta in the airway cells of glucocorticoid insensitive asthma. Am J Respir Crit Care Med 1999; in press

21. Wenzel SE, Szefler SJ, Leung DYM, Sloan SI, Rex MD, Martin RJ. Bronchoscopic evaluation of severe asthma. Persistent inflammation associated with high dose glucocorticoids. Am J Respir Crit Care Med 1997; 156:737.

22. Fujimura M, Sakamoto S, Saito M, Miyake Y, Matsuda T. Effect of a thromboxane A2 receptor antagonist (AA-2414) on bronchial hyperresponsiveness to methacholine in subjects with asthma. J Allergy Clin Immunol 1991; 87:23.

23. Gavin LA, Wamboldt M, Brugman S, Roesler TA, Wamboldt F. Psychological and family characteristics of adolescents with vocal cord dysfunction. J Asthma 1998; 35:409.

24. Murray AB, Ferguson AC, Morrison BJ. The frequency and severity of cat allergy vs. dog allergy in atopic children. J Allergy Clin Immunol 1983; 72:145.

25. Nimmagadda SR, Szefler SJ, Spahn JD, Surs W, Leung DYM. Allergen exposure decreases glucocorticoid receptor binding affinity and steroid responsiveness in atopic asthmatics. Am J Respir Crit Care Med 1997; 155:87.

26. D'Alonzo GE, Smolensky MH, Feldman S, Gianotti LA, Emerson MB, Staudinger H, Steinijans VW. Twenty-four hour lung function in adult patients with asthma. Chronoptimized theophylline therapy once-daily dosing in the evening versus conventional twice-daily dosing. Am Rev Respir Dis 1990; 142:84.

27. Martin RJ, Cicutto LC, Ballard RD, Goldenheim PD, Cherniack RM. Circadian variations in theophylline concentrations and the treatment of nocturnal asthma. Am Rev Respir Dis 1989; 139:475.

28. Kossoy AF, Hill M, Lin FL, Szefler SJ. Are theophylline "levels" a reliable indicator of compliance? J Allergy Clin Immunol 1989; 84:60.

29. Spahn JD, Landwehr LP, Nimmagadda S, Surs W, Leung DYM, Szefler SJ. Effects of glucocorticoids on lymphocyte activation in patients with steroid-sensitive and steroid-resistant asthma. J Allergy Clin Immunol 1996; 98:1073.

30. Hill MR, Szefler SJ, Ball BD, Bartoszek M, Brenner AM. Monitoring glucocorticoid therapy: A pharmacokinetic approach. Clin Pharmacol Ther 1990; 48: 390.

31. Kamada AK, Spahn JD, Surs W, Brown E, Leung DYM, Szefler SJ. Coexistence of glucocorticoid receptor and pharmacokinetic abnormalities: Factors that contribute to a poor response to treatment with glucocorticoids in children with asthma. J Pediatr 1994; 124:984.

32. Spahn JD, Leung DYM, Surs W, Harbeck RJ, Nimmagadda SR, Szefler SJ. Reduced glucocorticoid binding affinity in asthma is related to ongoing allergic inflammation. Am J Respir Crit Care Med 1995; 151:1709.

33. Lanz MJ, Leung DYM, McCormick DR, Harbeck R, Szefler SJ, White CW. Comparison of exhaled nitric oxide, serum eosinophilic cationic protein, and soluble interleukin-2 receptor in exacerbations of pediatric asthma. Pediatr Pulmonol 1997; 24:305.

34. Ledford D, Apter A, Brenner AM, Rubin K, Prestwood K, Frieri M, Lukert B. Osteoporosis in the corticosteroid-treated patient with asthma. J Allergy Clin Immunol 1998; 102:353.

35. Bernstein DI, Bernstein IL, Bodenheimer SS, Pietrusko RG. An open study of auranofin in the treatment of steroid-dependent asthma. J Allergy Clin Immunol 1988; 81:6.

36. Jarjour N, McGill K, Busse WW, Gelfand EW. Alternative anti-inflammatory and immunomodulatory therapy. Szefler SJ, Leung DYM (Eds). Severe asthma: Pathogenesis and Clinical Management. New York: Marcel Dekker, Inc., 1996, p. 333.

37. Mazer BD, Gelfand EW. An open-label study of high-dose intravenous immunoglobulin in severe childhood asthma. J Allergy Clin Immunol 1991; 87:976.

38. Redington AE, Hardinge FM, Madden J, Holgate ST, Howarth PH. Cyclosporin A treatment and airways inflammation in corticosteroid-dependent asthma. Allergy 1998; 53:94.

39. Vrugt B, Wilson S, van Velzen E, Bron A, Shute JK, Holgate ST, Djukanovic R, Aalbers R. Effects of high dose intravenous immunoglobulin in two severe corticosteroid insensitive asthmatic patients. Thorax 1997; 52:662.

40. Hegele RG, Hogg JC. The pathology of asthma: An inflammatory disorder. Szefler SJ, Leung DYM (Eds). Severe asthma: Pathogenesis and clinical management. New York: Marcel Dekker, Inc., 1996, p. 61.

41. Minshall EM, Leung DYM, Martin RJ, Song YL, Cameron L, Ernst P, Hamid Q. Eosinophil-associated TGF-β1 mRNA expression and airways fibrosis in bronchial asthma. Am J Respir Cell Mol Biol 1997; 17:326.

Chlamydia pneumoniae and Bronchial Asthma

Luigi Allegra, Francesco Blasi*

Keywords: *Chlamydia pneumoniae*, asthma, chronic infection, severity

Chlamydia pneumoniae is an important cause of human respiratory tract diseases, and a possible role for *C. pneumoniae* in asthma has been recently hypothesized. In some patients the infection is associated with wheezing and asthma onset. *C. pneumoniae* is involved in about 10% of asthma exacerbations both in adults and children. Chronic *C. pneumoniae* infection is common in school-age children, and immune responses to *Chlamydia* are positively associated with frequency of asthma exacerbations. The immune response to chronic *C. pneumoniae* infection may interact with allergic inflammation to increase asthma symptoms. An association between previous *C. pneumoniae* infection and severe chronic asthma in adults has been proposed. We are part of a multinational study on the role of macrolide treatment in asthma, a randomized, double-blind, placebo-controlled trial of treatment with roxithromycin 150 mg b.d. for 6 weeks in subjects with asthma and IgG antibodies to *C. pneumoniae* $\geq$ 1:64 and/or IgA titers $\geq$ 1:16. Subjects were 18–60 years of age with a forced expiratory volume (FEV_1) 50–90% of predicted. During the 4-week run-in period, the subjects recorded PEFR and symptoms twice daily. Subjects were randomized to treatment if their symptom score was $\geq$ 2 for 7/14 days. In the screened population chronic infections with *C. pneumoniae* were associated with an increase in the severity of asthma. Treatment with roxithromycin led to an improvement in lung function and asthma symptoms in patients with serological evidence of infection with *C. pneumoniae*.

Chlamydia–Asthma Hypothesis

Chlamydia pneumoniae is an important cause of human respiratory tract diseases. It is involved in upper respiratory tract infections (pharyngitis, sinusitis, etc.), acute bronchitis, and exacerbations of chronic bronchitis [1–4].

Chlamydia pneumoniae is now known to be a relevant cause of community-acquired pneumonia, being involved in between 6% and 20% of cases [5]. Most recent reports rank this agent among the three most common etiologic agents, generally presenting a mild, and in some cases self-limiting, clinical course. This agent has been shown to cause severe forms of pneumonia, particularly in elderly patients, and in the presence of chronic cardiopulmonary diseases [6, 7]. A possible role for *Chlamydia pneumoniae* in asthma has been recently hypothesized. In several patients the infection is associated with wheezing and asthma onset [8, 9]. Hahn reported a dose-response relationship between specific antibody titers and wheezing prevalence [8]. He tested 365 adult outpatients with acute lower respiratory tract illnesses and identified 19 patients with acute *Chlamydia pneumoniae* infection diagnosed by serology and culture; 9 infected patients wheezed during the acute illness, 4 had exacerbations of previously diagnosed asthma, and 4 others had newly diagnosed asthma after illness.

The adjusted odds ratio (OR) for an MIF titer of 1:64 or greater and wheezing was 2.1 (1.1–4.2). Comparing 71 exposed cases (titer > 1:64) and 71 unexposed controls (titer < 1:16) with acute respiratory infections, Hahn also reported a highly significant association of antibody with the development of asthmatic bronchitis within 6 months after illness (OR 7.2, 2.2–23.4).

In a follow-up study in 1994, Hahn et al. [10] reported a significant association for *Chlamydia pneumoniae* seroreactivity (titer > 1:16) and pulmonary function-confirmed adult-onset asthma (100% of asthma cases versus 53% of nonwheezing controls with acute respiratory infections, $p < .001$). In 1994, Peters et al. [11] reported on 122 adult patients with acute respiratory illness (ARI) and well controls. They found that acute MIF antibody was present in 22% of 46 asthma exacerbations compared to 8% of nonasthma ARI ($p < .001$) and in 4% of matched controls without ARI ($p < .001$).

Other groups have demonstrated that *Chlamydia*

*   Institute of Respiratory Diseases, University of Milan, IRCCS Ospedale Maggiore Milano, Italy

pneumoniae causes asthma exacerbations. Allegra et al. [12] found that about 10% of all asthma exacerbations in adults were due to this pathogen. These results were later confirmed by Miyashita et al. [13], who found an incidence of about 9% of acute *Chlamydia pneumoniae* infection demonstrated by culture, serology, and PCR . Emre et al. [9] reported similar results in a pediatric population. Moreover, they demonstrated that the treatment with macrolide may improve the course of reactive airway disease.

A recent study [14] involving 108 children with asthma symptoms, aged 9–11 years, showed that chronic *Chlamydia pneumoniae* infection is common in school-age children, and that immune responses to *Chlamydia* are positively associated with frequency of asthma exacerbations. The authors suggest that the immune response to chronic *Chlamydia pneumoniae* infection may interact with allergic inflammation to increase asthma symptoms.

Furthermore, number of episodes reported by each child during the 13 months of the study was used to assess the possible relationship between asthma exacerbations and sIgA to *Chlamydia pneumoniae*.

A recent paper found an association between previous *Chlamydia pneumoniae* infection and severe chronic asthma [15]. In fact, in severe chronic asthma, antibody titers against *Chlamydia pneumoniae* suggesting previous infection were significantly more frequent than both in controls and in acute asthma with an odds ratio of 3.99 (95% CI 1.60–9.97). Moreover, Hahn [16] reported treatment results for 3 patients with severe, steroid-dependent asthma and anti-*Chlamydia pneumoniae* high IgG titers. All three patients were able to discontinue oral steroids after a macrolide treatment course. There is also *in vitro* evidence of a possible involvement of *Chlamydia pneumoniae* as a risk factor for immunoreactive disorders such as asthma. Epithelium ciliary activity was found to be blocked by *Chlamydia pneumoniae* but not by *Chlamydia trachomatis* 48 h after infection [17]. This could potentially be an important mechanism in increasing susceptibility to viral infections as well as increasing asthma severity by permitting a build up of mucus and inhaled foreign material such allergens. Another study has investigated the effect of *Chlamydia pneumoniae* infection on the human monocytic cell line Mono Mac 6. Typical inclusion formed within 48 h of infection, and this was associated with release of TNF-α, IL-1 β, and IL-6, along with the upregulation of the cell surface protein CD14, which is a receptor for LPS [18]. These cytokines play a key role in asthma pathogenesis and are highly expressed in bronchial epithelium. As these cytokines are implicated in the recruitment and activation of neutrophils, lymphocytes, and eosinophils, their release would have profound proinflammatory effects in the context of the on-going airway inflammation associated with asthma. Preliminary results support the use of prolonged course of antichlamydial therapy in some cases of adult-onset asthma [10, 16]. Clearly, as stated by Hahn [19] the danger of promiscuous overuse accompanies any recommendation for empiric antibiotic treatment based solely on uncontrolled clinical observation. There are as yet no controlled studies to help answer the question of the possible role of antibiotics in asthma, particularly in patients who are *Chlamydia pneumoniae* seroreactive.

The CARM Study

We are co-chairmen of a multinational study on the role of macrolide treatment in asthma. The CARM study (*Chlamydia pneumoniae*, Asthma, Roxithromycin, Multinational Study) is a multicenter study conducted in Australia, New Zealand, Italy, and Argentina. This randomized, double-blind, placebo-controlled trial of treatment with roxithromycin 150 mg b.d. for 6 weeks was conducted on subjects with asthma and IgG antibodies to *Chlamydia pneumoniae* $\geq$ 1:64 and/or IgA titers $\geq$ 1:16. Subjects were 18–60 years of age with an FEV_1 50–90% of predicted. During the 4-week run-in period, the subjects recorded PEFR and symptoms twice daily. Subjects were randomized to treatment if their symptom score was $\geq$ 2 for 7/14 days. We have examined the association between IgG and IgA titers to *Chlamydia pneumoniae* and the severity of asthma in the subjects who were screened in this study. By means of a logistic regression analysis, we compared the group with high titers of antibodies, i. e., IgG $\geq$ 1:64 and IgA $\geq$1:16, to the group without antibodies. Factors independently associated with the high titers of antibodies included age, male gender, and smoking. In comparison with low-dose inhaled steroids (< 800 µg/d of beclomethasone or budesonide), high titers of antibody were associated with treatment with moderate-dose inhaled steroids (> 800 µg $\leq$ 2000 µg/d beclomethasone or < 1600 µg of budesonide), treatment with high-dose inhaled steroids, and with

Table 1. Logistic regression comparing asthmatic subjects with anti-*C. pneumoniae* IgG ≥ 1:64 and IgA ≥ 1:16 ($n = 212$) with subjects with no antibodies ($n = 210$).

	Adjusted OR	95% CI	p
Age (per year)	1.02	1.00–1.04	0.09
Smoking (Pack years)	1.08	1.03–1.14	0.0015
No inhaled steroids*	2.76	1.38–5.53	0.0042
Moderate-dose inhaled steroids	3.96	2.09–7.52	0.0001
High-dose inhaled steroids	4.44	2.30–8.56	0.0001

*compared with low-dose inhaled steroids

Table 2. Relationship between dose of inhaled steroids and markers of severity.

	Not on inhaled steroids ($n = 130$)	Low-dose ($n = 128$)	Moderate-dose ($n = 181$)	High-dose ($n = 170$)
Daytime symptom score	1.89 (0.93)	1.74 (0.96)	1.89 (0.98)	2.21 (0.98)*
Nighttime symptom score	0.86 (0.77)	0.79 (0.77)	0.77 (0.69)	0.89 (0.95)
Hospitalized in the last 5 years (%)	10	9.4	14.4	30**

*$p = 0.0008$, **$p = 0.001$

not receiving any steroids (Table 1). In the screened population (619 subjects) the use of high-dose inhaled steroids was associated with an increase of 74% in the titer of IgG antibodies ($p = 0.035$) and an increase of 71% in the titer of IgA antibodies ($p = 0.0001$) when compared with the use of low-dose inhaled steroids. We also observed an inverse association between IgG antibodies and FEV_1 ($p = 0.043$). In this group, IgA antibodies were also associated with higher daytime symptom score ($p = 0.036$). It may appear surprising that the subjects who were not using inhaled steroids had higher titers of antibodies to *Chlamydia pneumoniae* than the subjects on low-dose inhaled steroids; but it should be noted that the subjects who were not using inhaled steroids had higher symptom scores than those on low-dose inhaled steroids (Table 2). The higher levels of antibodies in the subjects who were not using inhaled steroids is another reason for believing that our findings are not simply due to reactivation of infection of *Chlamydia pneumoniae* with the use of steroids. It raises the possibility that chronic infection with *Chlamydia pneumoniae* leads to an increase in the severity of asthma. Moreover, the preliminary results of the study show that treatment with roxithromycin led to an improvement in lung function and asthma symptoms in patients with serological evidence of infection with *Chlamydia pneumoniae*.

Conclusion

Confirmation of the hypothesis of *Chlamydia pneumoniae* involvement in asthma must await the final results of this study and of future studies, which are of high priority given the importance of the contribution of asthma to respiratory morbidity.

Address for correspondence:

Luigi Allegra, MD
Head, Istituto di Tisiologia e Malattie
dell'Apparato Respiratorio
Università degli Studi di Milano
Pad. Litta, IRCCS Ospedale Maggiore
di Milano
via F. Sforza, 35
I-20122 Milano
Italy
Tel. +39 2 5503-3782
Fax +39 2 5519-0332
E-mail lallegra@imiucca.csi.unimi.it

References

1. Grayston JT, Campbell LA, Kuo CC, Mordhorst CH, Saikku P, Thom DH. A new respiratory tract pathogen

Chlamydia pneumoniae strain TWAR. J Infect Dis 1990; 161:618–625.

2. Beaty CD, Grayston JT, Wang SP, Kuo CC, Reto CS, Martin TR. *Chlamydia pneumoniae*, strain TWAR, infection in patients with chronic obstructive pulmonary disease. Am Rev Respir Dis 1991; 144:1408–1410.

3. Blasi F, Legnani D, Lombardo VM, Negretto GG, Magliano E, Pozzoli R, Chiodo S, Fasoli A, Allegra L. *Chlamydia pneumoniae* infection in acute exacerbations of COPD. Eur Resp J 1993; 6:19–22.

4. von Hertzen L, Alakarppa H, Koskinen R, Liippo K, Surcel HM, Leinonen M, Saikku P. *Chlamydia pneumoniae* infection in patients with chronic obstructive pulmonary disease. Epidemiology & Infection 1997; 118:155–164.

5. Almirall J, Moratò I, Riera F, Verdaguer A, Priu R, Coll P, Vidal J, Murgui L, Vallas F, Catalan F, Balanzo X. Incidence of community-acquired pneumonia and *Chlamydia pneumoniae* infection: A prospective multicenter study. Eur Respir J 1993; 6:14–18.

6. Cosentini R, Blasi F, Raccanelli R, Rossi S, Arosio C, Tarsia P, Randazzo A, Allegra L.. Severe community-acquired pneumonia: A possible role for *Chlamydia pneumoniae*. Respiration !996; 63:61–65.

7. Pacheco A, Gonzales SJ, Aroncena C. Community-acquired pneumonia caused by *Chlamydia pneumoniae* strain TWAR in chronic cardiopulmonary disease in the elderly. Respiration 1991; 58:316–320.

8. Hahn DL, Dodge RW, Golubjatnikov R. Association of *Chlamydia pneumoniae* (strain TWAR) infection with wheezing, asthmatic bronchitis, and adult-onset asthma. JAMA 1991; 266:225–230.

9. Emre U, Roblin PM, Gelling M, Dumornay W, Rao M, Hammerschlag MR, Schacter J. The association of *Chlamydia pneumoniae* infection and reactive airway disease in children. Arch Pediatr Adolesc Med 1994; 148:727–732.

10. Hahn DL, Golubjatnikov R. Asthma and chlamydial infection: A case series. J Fam Pract 1994; 38:589–595.

11. Peters BS, Thomas B, Marshall B. The role of *Chlamydia pneumoniae* in acute exacerbations of asthma. Am J Respir Crit Care Med 1994; 149(part 2 of 2 parts):A341.

12. Allegra L, Blasi F, Centanni S, Cosentini R, Denti F, Raccanelli R, Tarsia P, Valenti V. Acute exacerbations of asthma in adults: Role of *Chlamydia pneumoniae* infection. Eur Respir J 1994; 7:2165–2168.

13. Miyashita N, Kubota Y, Nakajima M, Niki Y, Kawane H, Matsushima T. *Chlamydia pneumoniae* and exacerbations of asthma in adults. Ann Allergy Asthma Immunol 1998; 80:405–409.

14. Cunningham AF, Johnston SL, Julious SA, Lampe FC, Ward ME. Chronic *Chlamydia pneumoniae* infection and asthma exacerbations in children. Eur Respir J 1998; 11:345–349.

15. Cook PJ, Davies P, Tunnicliffe W, Ayres JG, Honeybourne D, Wise R. *Chlamydia pneumoniae* and asthma. Thorax 1998; 53:254–259.

16. Hahn D, Bukstein D, Luskin A, Zeitz H. Evidence for *Chlamydia pneumoniae* infection in steroid-dependent asthma. Ann Allergy Asthma Immunol 1998; 80:45–49.

17. Shemer-Avni Y, Lieberman D. Chlamydia pneumoniae induced ciliostasis in ciliated bronchial epithelial cells. J Infect Dis 1995; 171:1274–1278.

18. Heinemann M, Susa M, Simnacher U, Marre R, Essig A. Growth of Chlamydia pneumoniae induces cytokine production and expression of CD14 in a human monocytic cell line. Infect Immun 1996; 64:4872–4875.

19. Hahn DL. Acute asthmatic bronchitis: A new twist to an old problem. J Fam Pract 1994; 39:431–435.

Future Perspectives on Asthma Treatment

Thomas B Casale*

Keywords: Asthma, therapy, anti-cytokines, DNA

In recent years, the importance of inflammation has become apparent in the pathogenesis of asthma. Furthermore, much information has been forthcoming on the interactions between the immune and neurogenic systems in mediating the pathophysiologic manifestations of asthma. With this new insight has come an ever expanding list of therapeutic options aimed at controlling the underlying process of asthmatic inflammation. Strategies aimed at shifting the milieu of cytokines and helper T lymphocytes to one which inhibits allergic inflammation appear promising as newer therapeutic options. Indeed, studies in animal models have shown the potential therapeutic benefits of DNA and directed cytokine therapies aimed at the earliest stages of the allergic inflammatory cascade. Inhibitors of the production or effects of IgE have demonstrated efficacy in both animal models and human asthma. Strategies designed to inhibit the migration of inflammatory cells into the airways are also being examined. Specific antagonists to inflammatory mediators, such as LTD_4, clearly have proved beneficial in subsets of patients. The expanded utility of these antagonists in selected patients is undergoing clinical evaluation. Finally, selected phosphodiesterase antagonists and modulators of neurogenic pathways also hold promise. For example, early studies with muscarinic receptor subtype blockers have demonstrated clinical efficacy in both COPD and asthma. This review focuses on these newer therapeutic strategies for asthma outlining both the rationale for their development, effects *in vivo*, and potential for treating patients with asthma.

Introduction

Asthma is characterized by airway obstruction that is usually reversible either spontaneously or with treatment, airway inflammation, and airway hyperresponsiveness to a variety of stimulants. Recent studies have suggested that these are not independent events. Indeed, many of the mediators and pathways responsible for airway inflammation ultimately influence the development of airway hyperresponsiveness and airway obstruction. Similarly, the neurogenic pathways important in the development of airway hyperresponsiveness can also facilitate airway inflammation and airway obstruction.

In genetically susceptible atopic individuals, inhalation of an allergen to which they are sensitized results in a chain of biochemical events leading to the clinical features of asthma (Figure 1). Allergen in the context of an antigen presenting cell interacts with CD4 lymphocytes leading to the production and release of cytokines important in allergic inflammation. Interleukins (IL)-4 and -13 are important for IgE synthesis and mast cell growth and differentiation. IL-5 plays a critical role in the differentiation, recruitment and activation of eosinophils. Both mast cells and eosinophils, when stimulated, release multiple mediators. These mediators are capable of inducing bronchoconstriction, vascular permeability or edema, mucus secretion, airway hyperresponsiveness and inflammation. In addition, these mediators can interact with nerve fibers in the airways causing the release of neurotransmitters and neuropeptides that can contribute to the development of airway hyperresponsiveness as well as propagate airway inflammation and airway obstruction.

The therapy of asthma is evolving into an exciting field. In the past, asthma therapy was directed towards treating bronchoconstriction. Recently, emphasis has been placed on the importance of controlling inflammation, especially with corticosteroids. However, we now know considerably more about the pathogenesis of allergic inflammation in asthma. Based on this knowledge, novel therapies aimed at blocking specific molecules or pathways that are thought to be important in the pathogenesis of asthma have been developed. This review will focus upon some of the newer therapeutic strategies aimed at reducing allergic inflammation in asthma.

---

* Director, Nebraska Medical Research Institute; Clinical Professor, Creighton University, USA; Adjunct Professor, University of Nebraska Medical Center, USA

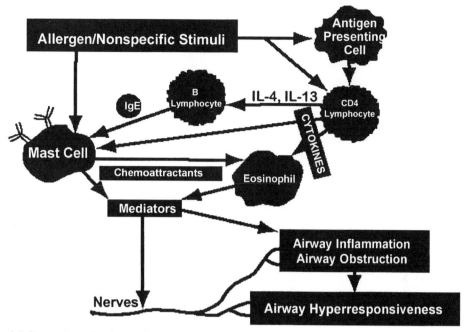

Figure 1. Inflammation and asthma pathogenesis. Pathways leading to the development of the major features of asthma are shown.

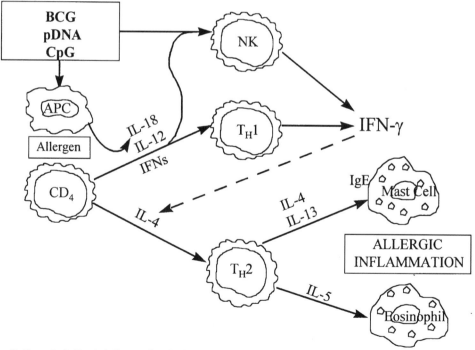

Figure 2. Control of allergic inflammation. Pathways leading to the development and control of allergic inflammation are shown. Dashed line indicates an inhibitory effect.

Th2 Directed Therapies

Allergic inflammation in asthma is characterized by increased numbers of activated T helper (Th) lymphocytes, eosinophils, and mast cells which express a Th2 profile of cytokines. Experimental data has shown a strong correlation between the levels of these cytokines, CD4[+] T cells and disease severity. Thus, one strategy to treat allergic inflammation and asthma is to shift the inflammatory paradigm from Th2 to Th1 prominence [1] (Figure 2). The production of interferon-γ from Th1 cells and NK cells could then inhibit the effects of IL-4 and the development of Th2 cells. This ultimately would result in a decrease in cytokines necessary for the promotion of allergic inflammation, including IL-4, IL-5, and IL-13.

IL-12 is important in the differentiation of CD4 T cells into Th1 cells. IL-12 is primarily produced by activated monocytes/macrophages and dendritic cells. IL-12 is also capable of inducing interferon-γ production from Th1 cells and NK cells. Recent studies in murine models of allergic asthma have shown that IL-12 has the capacity to decrease allergic inflammation by favoring the development of a Th1 response [2, 3]. Recombinant IL-12 given at the time of antigen challenge prevented the development of antigen-induced eosinophil infiltration into the mouse trachea in a dose-dependent manner. Recombinant IL-12 also suppressed IL-5 levels and increased interferon-γ levels in bronchoalveolar lavage fluids of mice after antigen inhalation. Furthermore, pretreatment with anti-interferon-γ monoclonal antibody prevented the IL-12 inhibition of antigen-induced eosinophil infiltration into the tracheas of the mice [2]. Other studies have indicated that IL-12 administration is capable of inhibiting airway hyperresponsiveness and antigen-induced allergic responses in a dose-dependent manner [3]. Taken together, these studies indicated that IL-12 may have a role in modulating allergic airway inflammation *in vivo*.

To improve upon and extend the observations using IL-12, Kim and colleagues developed an ovalbumin-IL-12 fusion protein [4]. They showed that the ovalbumin-IL-12 fusion protein induced an ovalbumin-specific, Th1-dominated immune response characterized by enhanced ovalbumin-specific interferon-γ production. Furthermore, in a setting of preexisting or ongoing immunity characterized by high IL-4 levels and IgE synthesis, the ovalbumin-IL-12 fusion protein greatly reduced ovalbumin specific IgE production, increased ovalbumin specific IgG 2a production, and greatly enhanced Th1 dominant cytokine synthesis in an antigen-specific fashion. These exciting results suggest that antigen-specific IL-12 fusion proteins may be beneficial in the treatment of diseases caused by undesired Th2-dominated responses. It is conceivable that one could inoculate at risk individuals with common antigens in combination with IL-12 to prevent and treat allergen-induced symptoms. This has much appeal since the therapy would be allergen-specific and would shift the paradigm of immune response to the Th1 phenotype.

Another strategy to influence allergic inflammation is to stimulate antigen presenting cells so that they produce cytokines necessary for the stimulation and production of Th1 cells. Several naturally occurring bacterial products such as BCG or plasmid DNA or specific immunostimulatory sequences of bacterial DNA might accomplish these goals. These agents cause antigen presenting cells to release cytokines including IL-12, IL-18, and interferon-γ which can then enhance the development of Th1 cells and stimulate NK cells to produce more interferon-γ.

Naked plasmid DNA encoding a particular antigen injected into animals caused a strong Th1-biased response with the production of high titers of IgG2 antibodies and the expansion of Th1 cells. This may provide a novel method of immunotherapy for the treatment of allergic diseases and allergic inflammation important in asthma. Indeed, studies have demonstrated that parenteral administration of plasmid DNA encoding housedust mite antigen prior to inhalation challenge of housedust mite-sensitized mice prevented IgE production and the development of increased airway responses [5].

Many recent studies have shown that bacterial, but not vertebrae, DNA causes activation of B cells and NK cells and the secretion of Th1 cytokines [6–8]. These effects appear to result from the presence of unmethylated CpG dinucleotides in particular base contexts and can be mimicked with synthetic oligonucleotides. Cellular activation by immunostimulatory DNA sequences, such as CpG, requires cellular uptake by adsorptive endocytosis. This process ultimately leads to the rapid generation of reactive oxygen species and nuclear factor-κB activation with subsequent cytokine expression. These immunostimulatory DNA sequences have been shown to induce the production of interferons, IL-12 and IL-18 by antigen presenting cells. All of these cytokines produce an initial burst of interfer-

192

on-γ by activating NK cells in an antigen-independent fashion, and they promote the differentiation of CD4+ T cells to Th1 cells. This ultimately leads to a second burst of interferon-γ production which is antigen-specific.

Knowledge of this process has lead several laboratories to conduct *in vivo* experiments with immunostimulatory DNA sequences in an attempt to alter allergic inflammation. Kline [7] and colleagues examined the effects of CpG motif oligonucleotides in a murine model of asthma. They were able to show that airway eosinophilia, Th2 cytokine induction, IgE production, and bronchial hyperreactivity were prevented by co-administration of CpG oligodeoxynucleotides (ODN) with the antigen. Also, in a previously sensitized mouse, CpG ODN was found to prevent allergen-induced inflammation. Broide [8] and colleagues using a mouse model of allergen-induced airway hyperresponsiveness also demonstrated that a CpG DNA motif significantly inhibited airway eosinophilia and reduced responsiveness to inhaled methacholine. In their studies, the immunostimulatory DNA sequences not only inhibited eosinophilia found in the airway and lung parenchyma, but also in the blood, suggesting that the immunostimulatory DNA sequences may have an effect on bone marrow production of airway eosinophils. These changes were accompanied by an inhibition of IL-5 generation and an increase in allergen-specific interferon-γ production with a redirection of the immune system response towards the Th1 phenotype. These data suggest that systemic or mucosal administration of immunostimulatory DNA sequences before allergen exposure could provide a novel form of active immunotherapy in allergic diseases. Since these therapies may alter the underlying immune process, they could potentially provide a cure for allergic diseases rather than just symptomatic relief. However, human studies are lacking, and thus, the efficacy, safety and timing of administration of these therapies still needs to be determined.

IL-4 Inhibition

Due to the prominence of IL-4 in the induction of Th2-like responses, another therapeutic approach is to neutralize IL-4 through the use of monoclonal antibodies, antagonists, or soluble IL-4 receptors. Of these approaches, soluble IL-4 receptors have been developed and used both in animal models and in humans. Mice sensitized to ovalbumin and treated with soluble IL-4 were shown to have a reduction in total IgE, frequency of positive skin tests, and airway hyperresponsiveness [9]. In a recent preliminary study of soluble IL-4 receptors in patients with moderate asthma, 25 patients received one single nebulization of the IL-4 receptor or placebo. IL-4 receptor administration was shown to be safe and without drug related toxicity. Mild favorable effects were noted on the pulmonary functions and asthma scores [10]. It was found that the IL-4 receptors' half-life was prolonged, lasting up to eight days, which could prove to be very beneficial in asthma therapeutic trials. Further human studies are needed to determine the relative efficacy and safety of soluble IL-4 receptors versus other agents.

Anti-IgE

Because IgE plays a central role in the cascade of biochemical events that result in allergic reactions, decreasing the total serum IgE in atopic patients would be expected to decrease available amounts of antigen-specific IgE to bind to and sensitize tissue mast cells. This reduction in available IgE would therefore reduce IgE-mediated symptoms and improve control of allergic diseases and asthma.

A recombinant humanized monoclonal anti-IgE antibody (rhuMAb-E25) has been developed and tested for the therapy of both allergic rhinitis and asthma. This antibody is specific for a unique epitope on human high affinity IgE receptors (FCεR1), thereby blocking the binding of IgE to mast cells and inhibiting mediator release. Administration of this antibody has been proven *in vivo* to dose-responsively decrease free IgE in the circulation [11]. Furthermore, administration of rhuMAb-E25 to asthmatics inhibited both the early and late responses [12]. In patients with moderate to severe asthma, clinical trials indicated that rhuMAb-E25 was capable of significantly improving symptoms' scores, peak expiratory flow rates, rescue use of β-agonists, and total dosage required of inhaled and/or oral corticosteroids [13, 14].

Thus, there are many ways by which one could shift either the paradigm of Th2 responses to Th1 responses or decrease the production or effect of IgE in mediating allergic inflammatory responses in the airways. Future clinical trials will ultimately prove their therapeutic potential for asthma.

Anti-IL-5

One could also target specific cytokines further downstream in the cascade of allergic inflammation that are thought to be important in the pathogenesis of asthma. In this regard, IL-5 may be an important target. IL-5 levels have been shown to be increased in patients with symptomatic asthma and associated with eosinophilic inflammation. IL-5 has also been proven to be important in eosinophil differentiation, survival, activation and chemotaxis. Thus, anti-IL-5 has potential as an asthma therapy.

Ovalbumin sensitized rodents have been shown to have increased levels of bronchoalveolar lavage eosinophils subsequent to antigen challenge or IL-5 administration. In sensitized animals treated with anti-IL-5, lung eosinophil numbers were markedly decreased compared with control antibody treatment. In addition, the development of hyperreactivity to histamine and arecoline after ovalbumin challenge was completely inhibited [15]. Thus, this line of investigation has shown that IL-5 is involved in airway eosinophilia and the development of airway hyperreactivity in certain animal models of asthma. Recently, a preliminary study of a humanized IL-5 monoclonal antibody (SB-240563) given to patients with asthma was reported in abstract form [16]. The investigators found that a single injection of SB-240563 was well tolerated and, though it did not modify the late asthmatic response to allergen challenge, produced reductions in both blood and sputum eosinophils indicating that the molecule is pharmacologically active. These data suggested that further clinical investigation with this approach might be warranted. Overall, the future of anti-IL-5 therapy awaits additional clinical trials with dose-response experiments.

Anti-Adhesion Molecule Strategies

The development of airway inflammation involves the stimulated migration of inflammatory cells out of the vasculature and into the airways towards a chemotactic gradient. This process involves the expression of adhesion molecules on inflammatory cells, endothelium and lung cells. Thus, inhibitors of chemotaxis and/or adhesion molecules have potential as therapeutic agents for asthma. Early studies with anti-endothelial leukocyte adhesion molecule (ELAM) monoclonal antibodies in a primate model of asthma demonstrated a decrease in both the influx of inflammatory cells into the airways and airway responsiveness [17].

Since these early experiments, several investigators have examined the therapeutic potential of various inhibitors to adhesion molecules. Selectin antagonists that are capable of being delivered by infusion or inhalation have been shown to inhibit early and late asthmatic responses in animal models. These agents have also been shown to reduce cell infiltration and block the development of airway hyperresponsiveness, and they can be given either prior to or after antigen challenge.

Both eosinophils and T lymphocytes express very late antigen 4 (VLA-4), and this molecule has been demonstrated to be important in adhesion of these cells to VCAM-1 on endothelial cells. Abraham and colleagues have shown that a small peptide inhibitor of VLA-4 is capable of significantly decreasing the early antigen-induced airway response and almost completely blocking the late phase airway response in allergic sheep. Moreover, 24 hours after antigen challenge, airway hyperresponsiveness to inhaled carbachol was not observed when the animals were treated with the small molecule VLA-4 inhibitor. Analysis of biopsy specimens taken 24 hours after challenge indicated that the total number of VLA-4 positive cells (lymphocytes, eosinophils, and metachromatic-staining cells) in the animals treated with the VLA-4 inhibitor did not increase as opposed to the control group [18].

Overall, these results support the use of specific antagonists or blockers of critical adhesion molecules necessary for the development of inflammation. Clearly, further research in humans must be done to determine the clinical efficacy as well as the potential risks factors from blocking adhesion molecules that may also be important in host defense mechanisms.

Mediators as Targets

Antagonists of specific mediators that are released from mast cells and eosinophils also have potential for the therapy of asthma. Histamine is released from mast cells in high quantities. Antihistamines have been shown to have a marginal beneficial effect on lung functions and symptoms in patients with asthma. However, they have not been extremely effective, and thus, it is unlikely that H1 antagonists could play a major role in the therapy of asthma.

Thromboxane A2 antagonists have also been studied. These agents have shown marginal efficacy for asthma as well, but overall the response rate is not significant enough to envision them as very useful therapeutic interventions.

Platelet activating factor (PAF) was originally thought to play a major role in the pathogenesis of allergic inflammation and asthma. However, PAF antagonists have not uniformly been shown to be efficacious for the management of asthma. Thus, it is unlikely that PAF plays a significant role in asthma and that PAF antagonists would be utilized for asthma therapy.

Bradykinin has a number of biologic effects that could contribute to the pathogenesis of asthma. In limited studies with bradykinin$_2$ receptor antagonists, only marginal effects have been noted for asthma. It is not clear whether these agents would ever play a significant role in the therapy of asthma. Tryptase is a serum protease that is contained in the secretory granules of mast cells. Tryptase has a number of biologic activities that could contribute to the pathogenesis of asthma. Tryptase has been found to increase airway hyperresponsiveness, cause the production of kinins, degrade the endogenous bronchodilator vasoactive intestinal peptide, activate mast cells and eosinophils, be a weak granulocyte chemoattractant, and have the potential to be a growth factor for fibroblasts. Furthermore, elevated levels of tryptase have been found in respiratory diseases. The abundance of this enzyme in mast cells in conjunction with its ability to mediate many important pathophysiologic events in asthma makes it an intriguing target for the therapy of asthma.

APC-366 is a tryptase antagonist that has been studied both in animal models of asthma and in humans. In a sheep model of asthma, APC-366 given prophylactically has been shown to reduce early and late asthmatic responses and the post challenge-induced airway hyperresponsiveness. Furthermore, APC-366 showed antiinflammatory activity by significantly inhibiting post antigen-induced bronchoalveolar lavage albumin and tissue eosinophilia when compared with control trials [19]. These results suggested that mast cell tryptase plays an important role in airway responses, including airway inflammation, to inhaled antigen. Thus, further studies were carried out in human volunteers. In Phase I studies, no adverse events were reported in over 100 subjects. In early Phase II studies, APC-366 was found to have a slight protective role against the early and late antigen-induced airway responses. Furthermore, there was also some protection noted in the development of bronchial hyperresponsiveness subsequent to antigen challenge [20]. The role of this and other tryptase antagonists in the therapy of asthma will be interesting to explore with future clinical trials.

Leukotrienes have been shown to be important molecules in asthma because they are produced by key effector cells, they are released during spontaneous and induced asthma, and they have potent pro-asthma effects. Leukotriene-mediated effects include bronchoconstriction, mucus secretion, the induction of vascular permeability or edema, the induction of airway hyperresponsiveness, and inflammation. Cysteinyl leukotrienes, and especially leukotriene B$_4$, have been shown to have chemotactic activity. Leukotriene antagonists and 5-lipoxygenase inhibitors have been shown to block bronchoconstriction due to various stimuli, to induce acute bronchodilation in asthmatics that is additive to β-agonists, to block allergen-induced early and late asthmatic airway responses and the consequent development of airway hyperresponsiveness, and to improve FEV$_1$ and symptoms when given chronically. Recent studies have been aimed at developing new roles for anti-leukotrienes in the therapy of asthma. Examples include the use of LTD$_4$ antagonists in children as young as age 2. Also, because they induce bronchodilation that is additive to β-agonists, they are being examined for the therapy of acute bronchospasm in the emergency room setting. Finally, several studies have indicated that they may have steroid-sparing effects [21]. Thus, in the percentage of people who do respond to these agents, newer ways of using them in the treatment of asthma will likely be forthcoming.

Heparin is a proteoglycan contained in mast cell granules. Upon mast cell degranulation, heparin is released in high quantities. Heparin has a number of effects that could be beneficial for asthma including: inhibition of complement-mediated activities; neutralization of eosinophil mediators through charge interactions; inhibition of antigen-induced airway contraction (both early and late asthmatic responses), hyperresponsiveness and eosinophilia; and inhibition of smooth muscle hyperplasia and hypertrophy. Although there are not many studies utilizing heparin as a therapy for asthma, an intriguing report in the *New England Journal of Medicine* in 1993 showed that pretreatment with aerosolized heparin was more effective than cromolyn sodium in blocking exercise-induced changes in specific airway conductance [22]. The use of low molecular weight heparins that do not significantly affect clotting times might be a novel way to treat asthma. Clearly, further studies are needed.

Phosphodiesterase Inhibitors

The nonspecific phosphodiesterase inhibitor, theophylline, is a long established treatment for asthma. It is thought that theophylline works by inhibiting the phosphodiesterase enzyme. Inhibition of phosphodiesterase results in increased cyclic AMP and cyclic GMP. These cyclic nucleotides can inhibit inflammatory cell chemotaxis and activation and relax smooth muscle. Recently, it has been shown that the phosphodiesterase enzyme exists in many forms comprising more than seven different families. The phosphodiesterase (PDE) 3 and 4 isoenzymes are most important for asthma because they are present in key inflammatory cells and airway smooth muscle. Inhibition of PDE 3 and 4 isoenzymes has been demonstrated in various animal models to inhibit many important inflammatory events including: The release of cytokines from T lymphocytes; the release of mediators from mast cells and eosinophils; the infiltration of inflammatory cells; and the effects of mediators in promoting inflammatory changes such as edema [23]. There is also evidence that these agents may have direct bronchodilatory effects and enhance nonadrenergic/noncholinergic nervous system-induced airway relaxation.

In humans, limited studies have been conducted with selective PDE inhibitors because they have been reported to produce nausea and vomiting. A recent study examined the effects of CDP840, a selective inhibitor of PDE4, on allergen-induced responses in asthmatic subjects [24]. CDP840 was fairly well tolerated, with no patients reporting nausea. CDP840 did not lead to changes in baseline airway function. However, the late asthmatic response to allergen was inhibited by 30% when this agent was dosed prior to allergen challenge. The early asthmatic response was not affected. Based on these early studies it would be reasonable to examine this and other PDE inhibitors for their therapeutic potential in asthma. These agents could conceivably provide a more specific means to inhibit the inflammatory cascade and promote bron-chodilation than the nonspecific PDE inhibitor, theophylline.

Neurogenic Pathway Agents

As indicated previously, neurogenic pathways must be considered when discussing airway inflammation and the pathogenesis of asthma [25]. Release of mast cell and eosinophil mediators can either directly stimulate or lower the threshold for stimulation of afferent fibers in and around the airway epithelium. Once stimulated, these fibers release acetylcholine through vagal reflex pathways. Acetylcholine acts on one of three receptors in human airways. Stimulation of M1 muscarinic receptors located primarily on efferent nerves facilitates the release of acetylcholine by neurons. Released acetylcholine stimulates M3 muscarinic receptors on airway smooth muscle and mucous glands promoting airway smooth muscle contraction and mucus release, respectively. M2 receptors are autoreceptors that when stimulated inhibit the release of acetylcholine by efferent nerve fibers. Coincident with the release of acetylcholine through vagal reflex pathways, afferent nerve stimulation may also result in a "short circuited" reflex loop release of neuropeptides. Released neurokinin A stimulates NK2 receptors on airway smooth muscle leading to contraction. Released substance P stimulates NK1 receptors, and this results in the promotion of airway inflammation, edema, and mucus production.

Based on this knowledge, many new classes of agents are being investigated that might favorably affect these nervous pathways [26]. Specific NK1 and NK2 antagonists might be expected to inhibit mucus release, edema, inflammation, and bronchoconstriction. In humans, early studies have indicated that these agents can prevent bradykinin-induced cough and airway responses [27]. These agents are also being investigated as chronic therapy for asthma because of the prominence of the role of various neuropeptides in the pathogenesis of asthma.

An intriguing prospect in the therapy of asthma has resulted from our knowledge of muscarinic receptor subtypes. Anticholinergics, such as atropine and ipratropium bromide, block all muscarinic receptors nonspecifically. This may be problematic since blocking M2 receptors results in increased acetylcholine release, thereby causing the loss of a putative protective mechanism. To improve the therapeutic effectiveness of anticholinergics one would like to have agents with receptor specificity. Specifically, a desirable drug would interact with muscarinic receptors in the following way: M3 > M1 > M2.

Tiotropium bromide is a long acting anticholinergic drug that has some of the desirable features mentioned above. Although it binds with relatively equal affinity to all three muscarinic receptors, the dissociation kinetics of tiotropium bromide results in a favorable therapeutic ratio. Tiotropium dissociates much more rapidly from M2 receptors versus M1 and M3 receptors. Indeed, the dissociation of tiotropium from M3 receptors is very slow. Thus, tiotropium has the desirable receptor subtype selectivity through kinetic mechanisms. Tiotropium bromide has been shown to produce long lasting bronchodilation (greater than 24 hours) and be protective against the bronchoconstricting effects of methacholine for 48 hours [28]. These bronchoprotective effects have been shown to be both dose- and time-dependent. Overall, in early studies tiotropium has been well tolerated.

Tiotropium and agents like it might have some advantages over long acting β-agonists since they can be dosed less frequently and may have a better side effect profile because they are devoid of adrenergic side effects. Tiotropium could prove useful for the management of nocturnal symptoms. Further studies are needed to answer whether tolerance will develop after long term use, but this is unlikely since these agents are antagonists rather than agonists. Also, one would like to know whether this class of drugs would have any antiinflammatory or disease modifying effects. It is also not clear what types of patients are most likely to benefit from these types of agents. Finally, it remains to be determined if these agents have additive effects to other anti-asthmatic agents such as those shown with the combination of long acting β-agonists and inhaled corticosteroids. Nonetheless, the use of receptor specific muscarinic agents is indeed intriguing.

Conclusion

There are many other potential therapies for asthma that are being investigated including respirable anti-oligonucleotides and nonglucocorticoid inhibitors of transcription factors. Where these and the agents discussed above will fit into the therapy of asthma is unclear. All of these agents may prove helpful as diagnostic tools and in defining the pathogenesis of asthma. Ultimately, better therapeutic options should decrease symptoms and improve quality of life; improve the course of asthma; reverse pathogenic and physiologic changes; have low side effects; and be cost effective. It is unlikely that the agents discussed above will fit all of those characteristics, but many will fulfill several.

In conclusion, based on our expanding knowledge of the pathogenesis of asthma and strategies to control inflammation, many future therapies will be evaluated as potential treatments for asthma. Because of the heterogeneous nature of asthma, specific agents will probably work best for selected types of patients. Ubiquitous treatments will be difficult to develop and most likely will involve agents that target the earliest stages of asthmatic inflammation.

Acknowledgment

The author gratefully acknowledges the expert help of Victoria Sears in the preparation of this manuscript.

Address for correspondence:

Thomas B Casale, MD
Nebraska Medical Research Institute
401 East Gold Coast Road, Suite 124
Papillion, NE 68046-4796
USA
Tel. +1 402 596-9965
Fax +1 402 596-9915
E-mail casalet@nfinity.com

References

1. Huang S-K. Molecular modulation of allergic responses. J Allergy Clin Immunol 1998; 102:887–892.

2. Iwamoto I, Kumano K, Kasai M, Kurasawa K, Nakao A. Interleukin-12 prevents antigen-induced eosinophil recruitment into mouse airways. Am J Respir Crit Care Med 1996; 154;1257–1260.

3. Gavett SH, O'Hearn DJ, Li X, Huang S, Finkelman FD, Wills-Karp M. Interleukin 12 inhibits antigen-induced airway hyperresponsiveness, inflammation, and Th2 cytokine expression in mice. J Exp Med 1995; 182:1527–1536.

4. Kim TS, DeKruyff RH, Rupper R, Maecker HT, Levy S, Umetsu DT. An ovalbumin-IL-12 fusion protein is

more effective than ovalbumin plus free recombinant IL-12 in inducing a T helper cell type 1-dominated immune response and inhibiting antigen-specific IgE production. J Immunol 1997; 158:4137–4144.

5. Hsu CH, Chua KY, Tao MH, Lai YL, Wu HD, Huang SK, Hsieh KH. Immunoprophylaxis of allergen-induced immunoglobulin E synthesis and airway hyperresponsiveness *in vivo* by genetic immunization. Nature Med 1996; 2:540.

6. Krieg AM. The CpG Motif: Implications for clinical immunology. BioDrugs 1998; 10:341–346.

7. Kline JN, Waldschmidt TJ, Businga TR, Lemish JE, Weinstock JV, Thorne PS, Krieg AM. Modulation of airway inflammation by CpG oligodeoxynucleotides in a murine model of asthma. J Immunol 1998; 160: 2555–2559.

8. Broide D, Schwarze J, Tighe H, Gifford T, Nguyen M-D, Malek S, Van Uden J, Martin-Orozco E, Gelfand EW, Raz E. Immunostimulatory DNA sequences inhibit IL-5, eosinophilic inflammation, and airway hyperresponsiveness in mice. J Immunol 1998; 161: 7054–7062.

9. Renz H, Bradley K, Enssle K, Loader JE, Larsen GL, Gelfand EW. Prevention of the development of immediate hypersensitivity and airway hyperresponsiveness following *in vivo* treatment with soluble IL-4 receptor. Int Arch Allergy Immunol 1996; 109:167–176.

10. Borish LC, Nelson HS, Lanz M, Claussen LR, Martin DW, Garrison L. Phase I/II study of interleukin-4 receptor (IL-4R) in moderate asthma. J Allergy Clin Immunol 1998; 101:S8.

11. Casale TB, Bernstein IL, Busse WW, LaForce CF, Tinkelman DG, Stoltz RR, Dockhorn RJ, Reimann J, Su JQ, Fick RB, Jr, Adelman DC. Use of an anti-IgE humanized monoclonal antibody in ragweed-induced allergic rhinitis. J Allergy Clin Immunol 1997; 100: 110–121.

12. Fahy JV, Fleming HE, Wong HH, Liu JT, Su JQ, Reimann J, Fick RB, Jr, Boushey HA. The effect of an anti-IgE monoclonal antibody on the early- and late-phase responses to allergen inhalation in asthmatic subjects. Am J Respir Crit Care Med 1997; 155:1828– 1834.

13. Fick RB, Simon SJ, Su JQ, Zeiger R, and E25 Study Group. Anti-IgE (rhuMAb) treatment of symptoms of moderate-severe allergic asthma. Ann Allergy Asthma Immunol 1998; 80:80.

14. Metzger WJ, Fick RB and the E25 Asthma Study Group. Corticosteroid (CS) withdrawal in a study of recombinant humanized monoclonal antibody to IgE (rhuMAbE25). J Allergy Clin Immunol 1998; 101: S231.

15. Van Oosterhout AJM, Ladenius ARC, Savelkoul HFJ, Van Ark I, Delsman KC, Nijkamp FP. Effect of anti-IL-5 and IL-5 on airway hyperreactivity and eosinophils in guinea pigs. Am Rev Respir Dis 1993; 147: 548–552.

16. Leckie MJ, ten Brinke A, Lordan J, Khan J, Diamant Z, Walls CM, Cowley H, Hansel TT, Djukanovic R, Sterk PJ, Holgate ST, Barnes PJ. SB 240563, a humanized anti-IL-5 monoclonal antibody initial single dose safety and activity in patients with asthma. Am J Respir Crit Care Med 1999; 159:A624.

17. Gundel RH, Wegner CD, Torcellini CA, Clarke CC, Haynes N, Rothlein R, Smith CW, Letts LG. Endothelial leukocyte adhesion molecule-1 mediates antigen-induced acute airway inflammation and late-phase airway obstruction in monkeys. J Clin Invest 1991; 88:1407–1411.

18. Abraham WM, Ahmed A, Sielczak MW, Narita M, Arrhenius T, Elices MJ. Blockade of late-phase airway responses and airway hyperresponsiveness in allergic sheep with a small-molecule peptide inhibitor of VLA-4. Am J Respir Crit Care Med 1997; 156: 696–703.

19. Clark JM, Abraham WM, Fishman CE, Forteza R, Ahmed A, Cortes A, Warne RL, Moore WR, Tanaka RD. Tryptase inhibitors block allergen-induced airway and inflammatory responses in allergic sheep. Am J Respir Crit Care Med 1995; 152:2076–2083.

20. Krishna MT, Chauhan AJ, Little L, Sampson K, Mant TGK, Hawksworth R, Djukanovic R, Lee TH, Holgate ST. Effect of inhaled APC 366 on allergen-induced bronchoconstriction and airway hyperresponsiveness to histamine in atopic asthmatics. Am J Respir Crit Care Med 1998; 157:A456.

21. Tamaoki J, Kondo M, Sakai N. Leukotriene antagonist prevents exacerbation of asthma during reduction of high-dose inhaled corticosteroid. Am J Respir Crit Care Med 1997; 155:1235–1240.

22. Ahmed T, Garrigo J, Danta I. Preventing bronchoconstriction in exercise-induced asthma with inhaled heparin. N Engl J Med 1993; 329:90–95.

23. Torphy TJ. Phosphodiesterase isozymes. Am J Respir Crit Care Med 1998; 157:351–370.

24. Harbinson PL, MacLeod D, Hawksworth R, O'Toole S, Sullivan PJ, Heath P, Kilfeather S, Page CP, Costello J, Holgate ST, Lee TH. The effect of a novel orally active selective PDE4 isoenzyme inhibitor (CDP840) on allergen-induced responses in asthmatic subjects. Eur Respir J 1997; 10:1008–1014.

25. Casale TB, Baraniuk JN. Neurogenic control of inflammation and airway function. In E Middleton, Jr, CE Reed, EF Ellis, NF Adkinson, Jr, JW Yunginger (Eds), Allergy: Principles and practice, 5th edition. St. Louis, Missouri: Mosby-Yearbook Co. 1998, pp. 183–203.

26. Advenier C, Lagente V, Boichot E. The role of tachykinin receptor antagonists in the prevention of bron-

chial hyperresponsiveness, airway inflammation and cough. Eur Respir J 1997; 10:1892–1906.

27. Ichinose M, Nakajima N, Takahashi T, Yamauchi H, Inoue H, Takishima T. Protection against bradykinin-induced bronchoconstriction in asthmatic patients by

neurokinin receptor antagonist. Lancet 1992:1248–1251.

28. O'Connor BJ, Towse LJ, Barnes PJ. Prolonged effect of tiotropium bromide on methacholine-induced bronchoconstriction in asthma. Am J Respir Crit Care Med 1996; 154:876–880.

Asthma in a Critical Age: The Elderly

G Melillo, G Balzano*

Keywords: Pulmonary function, comorbidities, pathology, treatment, compliance

Elderly asthmatics can be categorized into two groups: One with long-standing or recurrent asthma in which the disease persists from youth into old age (early-onset asthma); the other in which asthma occurs *de novo* at age of 65 years or later (late-onset asthma). In our material the frequency of early-onset asthma was 62% and that of late-onset asthma was 38%, confirming that asthma may occur at any age. Diagnosis of asthma in the elderly may be complicated by many factors. One of most important problems is distinguishing asthma from COPD, particularly in current or former smokers. At this regard a functional parameter – the forced expiratory volume (FEV_1) percent increase of predicted value after an inhaled bronchodilator – is suggested as useful parameter for distinguishing the two diseases. The method of induced sputum has been used for comparing the cellularity of elderly and younger asthmatics. An increase of neutrophils and a decrease of eosinophils was observed in late-onset asthma compared with younger asthma. A coexisting disease with asthma was observed in 65% of the 129 cases examined. The pneumologic treatment of elderly asthmatics is complicated by alterations of pharmacokinetics, concomitant diseases, adverse effect of medications, and reduced compliance. Asthma in elderly requires an intense monitoring of the disease and an active involvement of patient, families and other care-givers in a comprehensive program.

Asthma is not uncommon disease in the elderly, and it occurs more frequently than is usually appreciated. In population studies the prevalence of the disease is generally estimated to be about 5–6% [1–4]. Mortality is considered to be still on the rise in old age, while it has leveled out or fallen in other age groups [5]. Moreover, ambulatory visits and hospitalization rates are higher in elderly asthmatics than for any other age group [6].

Only few studies with a limited number of patients have been done on asthma in the elderly [7]. A report was published in 1996 by the NAEPP Working Group with special emphasis on the diagnosis and management of asthma in the elderly [8].

One year ago we organized a multicenter investigation in order to supplement our knowledge about some problems and aspects of asthma to determine the best approach and treatment of the disease.

Method and Material

Over a period of 2 years 220 asthmatics aged ≥ 65 years were enrolled. Each patient satisfied the ATS definition of asthma. Particular attention was given to avoiding the possibility of including patients who often may mimic asthma on both clinical and functional aspects. When diagnosis was doubtful, the subject was excluded. A questionnaire concerning the different aspects of asthma was filled out by the doctor during the clinical consultations.

Characteristics and Problems of Asthma in the Elderly

Elderly asthmatics can be categorized into two groups: One with long-standing or recurrent asthma in which the disease persists or recurs from youth into old age (early-onset asthma); the other

* Foundation "S. Maugeri" Care and Research Institute, Telese Terme (BN), Italy. With the collaboration of: B. Foschino, R. Di Tullio (Bari), F. Milone (Palermo), C. Cristina (Bologna), C. Pomari (Bussolengo), D. Rossano (Sassuolo), Longhi R. (Rimini), R. Battiloro, E. Melillo (Telese Terme), R. Tazza, P. Ferranti (Terni), F. Strinati (Tabiano Terme), F. Sonaglioni (Ascoli Piceno), A. Aufiero (Eremo Cambiasca VB), R. Ariano (Bordighera), L. Tarantino (Salerno), M. Marvisi (Corte Maggiore), A. Meriggi (Montescano), M. Sivori, A. Scardamaglia (Genova), E. Gonnella (Potenza), A. Tranchida (Mazara del Vallo)

in which asthma occurs *de novo* at age of 65 years or later (late-onset asthma) [9].

The frequency of the two types of asthma in our subjects was 62% of early-onset and 38% of late-onset asthma. This frequency is not significantly different from that of Braman [9], who observed 48% of late-onset asthma in a pulmonary clinic, or from that of Burr et al. [10], who observed 40% of late-onset asthma in a general population. These findings confirm that the first appearance of asthma in old age is more common than is widely realized, and that it can develop even in 80- and 90-year-olds [11].

As with other diseases of the elderly, when examining asthma we must take in account some peculiarities of the elderly patient. These concern the general decrease of anatomo-functional reserve of different organs and apparatus, the atypical appearance of clinical presentation, multiple comorbidities, the increased iatrogenic risk, and the increased risk deriving from nonautosufficiency.

Concerning asthma, the main problems are the difficulty of diagnosis, the functional evaluation, the pathogenesis, and pathology of late-onset asthma, the pharmacological treatment and compliance to the therapy.

Many factors may complicate the diagnosis of asthma in the elderly (Table 1).

In no age group is the potential for diagnostic confusion greater than in the elderly. One of the most relevant problems in diagnosis is to distinguish asthma from COPD, especially in current or former smokers. As in asthma of other ages, the functional pulmonary tests (FPT), in addition to clinical history, may help differentiate. Pre/post bronchodilator spirometry is useful if there is a significant improvement in FEV_1 (FEV_1 increase of 12% and 200 ml or greater). But the method of cal-culating the bronchodilator response by using the percent change from baseline – which is currently used in the laboratories – is not helpful in some cases in separating asthma from COPD [12]. Moreover, this parameter is affected by the degree of baseline obstruction, and the patients with a lowest FEV_1 (as commonly observed in COPD) have a large percentage change compared with patients having a relatively high baseline FEV_1 as commonly seen in asthma [14].

In order to identify a functional parameter with discriminating capacity between asthma and COPD, we compared the post-bronchodilator reversibility by examining the modifications of FEV_1 as percentage increase from baseline and as percentage increase of predicated value.

Two groups of elderly patients were studied: one with asthma ($n = 220$), the other with COPD ($n = 111$) (Table 2). Each patient inhaled salbutamol (400 μg) from an MDI through a large volume spacer (Volumatic Glaxo), this avoiding the risk of incorrect inhalation technique that almost frequently occurs in elderly patients. A significant reversibility ($FEV_1 \geq 12\%$) was observed in both the groups (in 54% of the asthmatics and 30% of persons with COPD) when the bronchodilating response was expressed as a percentage increase in FEV_1 from baseline. However, if bronchodilating response was expressed as percentage increase of FEV_1 of predicted value, only 44.5% of asthmatics demonstrated a significant increase, while no COPD patient reached this increment.

These data suggest that an increase in $FEV_1 \geq 12\%$ of predicted value can be indicative of asthma. Nevertheless, the absence of such reversibility cannot exclude the diagnosis of asthma because the lack of reversibility may be due to an inflammatory component that does not respond within minutes to inhaled bronchodilators. In these cases a therapeutic trial with oral steroids is recommended.

Table 1. Factors complicating the diagnosis of asthma in the elderly.

- Nonspecific symptoms that may be referred to other diseases (i. e., COPD, congestive heart failure)
- Other diseases mimicking asthma symptoms (i. e., pulmonary embolism, gastroesophageal reflux, endobronchial obstruction, upper airway obstruction, etc.)
- Differential diagnosis with COPD often challenging
- Reduced perception of airway narrowing and related dyspnea with delayed request for medical assistance
- Unlikeliness of atopy in the elderly
- Assumption by patients that all symptoms are related to aging

Table 2. Postbronchodilator reversibility of airway obstruction in a group of elderly asthmatic and COPD patients.

	Asthma $n = 220$	COPD $n = 111$
FEV_1 percent increase from baseline	$n = 120$ (54.5%)	$n = 33$ (30%)
FEV_1 percent increase of predicted value	$n = 98$ (44.5%)	none

Pulmonary Function Tests

A measure of airway obstruction is required for the characterization of the severity of the disease, for the assessment of acute exacerbations, and for modulating the pharmacologic treatment. Spirometry with an accurate FEV_1 may be obtained in most elderly patients, while peak flow measurements (PEF) can be used for ambulatory monitoring even if PEF is less sensitive and specific than FEV_1. Measurement of diffusing capacity is also helpful in differentiating between asthma and emphysema in smokers and older patients. It is important to consider that normal values of FEV_1 and FVC decline with age [15]. The normal value of FEV_1/FVC is approximately 70% or 65% after age 70. Spirometry and PEF may sometimes be difficult to perform in the elderly, debilitated, or cognitive-impaired subjects. Because of these difficulties, the respiratory impedance measurement by forced oscillation technique is used in patients with cognitive or physical disabilities [16]. The results obtained with this technique correlate with spirometric indices such as FEV_1 and FVC and airway resistance as measured using body plethysmograph [17].

Pathogenesis and Pathophysiology

Pathogenesis of early-onset asthma does not differ significantly from that of younger subjects. Concerning the pathogenesis of late-onset asthma, some potential factor such as the dysfunction in the β_2-adrenoreceptor pathway [18] and downregulation of corticosteroid receptors have been suggested, but further investigations are required.

The pathology of asthma has been well documented in younger patients, while only very limited studies exist in asthma of the elderly. Sobona [19] described structural changes in the elderly similar to those observed in younger patients. Aoki et al. [20] examined the morphologic and morphometric characteristics of bronchial wall in lungs obtained at autopsy. The conclusion was that the morphometric findings of bronchial wall in elderly asthmatics were similar to those in their younger counterparts. Nevertheless, in these two studies the category of asthma, i. e., early or late-onset asthma, was not specified. Detailed studies of airway inflammation in asthma of elderly have probably been hampered by the fact that methods for this type of investigation were, until recently, invasive (endobronchial biopsy, bronchoalveolar lavage).

Presently, the method of induced sputum by ultrasonic nebulization of hypertonic solution is largely used for the study of airway inflammation. We used this method for evaluating the cellularity of elderly asthmatics, and we present here the preliminary results.

We examined the cellularity in induced sputum in three groups of asthmatics: group A, 7 F, mean age 68 ± 4.3 years, who develop asthma before the age of 65 years (early-onset asthma); group B, 10 F, mean age 70.6 ± 4.7 years who developed asthma after the age of 65 years (late-onset asthma): and group C, 9 F, mean age 42 ± 14.9 years, younger asthmatics (Table 3).

A increase of neutrophils ($p < 0.01$) and a decrease of eosinophils ($p < 0.05$) was observed in late-onset asthma compared to younger asthmatics. Also, elderly persons with early-onset asthma showed a tendency toward an increase in percentage of neutrophils, though without statistical significance ($p > 0.05$).

These data show that late-onset asthma, though possessing an eosinophil percentage (5.1 ± 10.2) in the range of asthmatics, tends to have a percent of neutrophils (56.6 ± 14.7) approaching that of COPD.

Comorbid Conditions in Elderly Asthmatics

Table 4 summarizes the medical conditions that may coexist in the elderly asthmatics and that can potentially influence or complicate asthma and its management.

Table 3. Inflammatory cells in induced sputum of asthmatics.

	A. Early onset	B. Late onset	C. Younger
Eosinophils % NSC	13.6 ± 15.8	5.1 ± 10.2*	15.2 ± 14.3*
Neutrophils % NSC	51.1 ± 22.6	56.6 ± 14.7**	37.7 ± 11.1**

* $p < 0.05$ Mann-Whitney v. test, ** $p < 0.01$; NSC = nonsquamous cells

Table 4. Coexisting diseases with asthma in the elderly. Number of patients evaluated: 197. Coexisting diseases in 129 (66%).

Disease	%
Hypertension	41%
Arrhythmias	7%
Coronary artery disease	7%
Previous myocardial infarction	3%
Congestive heart failure	2%
Arthritis	16%
Diabetes	14%
Gastro-esophageal reflux	10%
Osteoporosis	10%
Visual impairment	8%
Stroke	2%
Tremor	2%
Parkinson's	2%
Obesity	5%
Hypothyroidism	5%

The list is not complete, since it includes only the most frequent and important diseases. The most prevalent comorbid conditions are cardiovascular diseases, which together are present in 60% of cases.

Pharmacological Treatment

The treatment of an elderly asthmatic is complicated by concomitant disease and pharmacological interactions. Although there are biological changes of aging that influence respiratory function, by far the most common reason for altering the approach of respiratory care in the older patient is the presence of other diseases or drugs that interact with asthma treatment [21].

The risk of drug interactions increases with age and number of medications. Among the various factor that may complicate the pharmacological treatment of asthma in the elderly the most important are indicated in Table 5.

Because of the age-related physiologic changes in homeostatic mechanisms and supervening disease, the elderly tend to be less tolerant of many drugs, some of which may also adversely interact with the disease. There is an increased potential for drug-disease interactions because elderly patients

Table 5. Factors complicating the pharmacological treatment of asthma in the elderly.

– Alterations of pharmacokinetics
– Comorbid conditions
– Adverse effects of medications
– Reduced compliance

Table 6. Adverse effects of medications in elderly asthmatics.

Antiasthmatic drug	Effects
– High doses of β_2-agonist	– Tachyarrhythmia, angina
– β_2 + diuretics	– Arrhythmias by hypokalemia, hypomagnesiemia
– Anticholinergics	– Mucosal dryness, blurred vision and acute angle-closure glaucoma if administered in the eye
– Theophylline	– Tachyarrythmias, gastrointestinal symptoms, insomnia and seizures, etc.
– Systemic steroids	– Sodium retention, aggravation of congestive heart failure, decrease of serum potassium, hypertension, acceleration of osteoporosis

Drugs for coexisting diseases	Effects
– β-adrenergic blocking agents (even if applied topically for glaucoma)	– Exacerbate asthma, decrease response to β_2-agonists
– Nonsteroidal antiinflammatory drugs (NSAIDs) even in eyedrops	– Exacerbate asthma
– No-sparing K diuretics especially if used with β_2-agonists, digitalis and steroids	– Cardiac dysrhythmias by hypokalemia
– Some antiarrhythmic agents (edrophonium, adenosine, sotalol)	– Provoke bronchoconstriction

tend to receive overall more medications for co-morbid conditions [8].

The mechanism of interaction may be pharmacological (β-blockers) or due to intolerance (Aspirin) or alterations of bioavailability or clearance of a drug (theophylline) [23]. Adverse effects may be due either to the antiasthmatic drugs as to various drugs for coexisting disease (see Table 6).

A complicated situation is present when asthma and other diseases coexist, since the treatment of asthma may complicate the management of other diseases and, conversely, medications of concurrent diseases may aggravate asthma. Consequently, elderly asthmatics should be evaluated for concomitant disorders and monitored for adverse drug-related side effects or interactions [22].

Compliance

Noncompliance with treatment often complicates the course of therapy. The main causes of noncompliance in our cases were the lack of understanding of the purpose of the medications prescribed, forgetfulness, a medical regimen with multiple drugs, cognitive impairment, anxiety, and depression. Compliance problems depend not only on the patient, but also on the patient's family. A patient educational program, specifically designed for the elderly, is an important part for maximizing compliance no matter what medication is prescribed. Considering that asthma in the elderly is frequently underperceived by the patient, underdiagnosed, and, consequently, undertreated by the physician [23], treatment requires the active involvement of the patient, his or her family, and other caregivers in a comprehensive program to assure that appropriate therapy is prescribed and regularly taken.

Address for correspondence:

Prof. Gaetano Melillo
Foundation "S. Maugeri"
Occupational & Rehabilitative Medicine
Medical Center
Via Bagui Vecchi
I-82037 Telese Terne
Italy
Tel. +39 0824 909-111, ext. 351
Fax +39 0824 909-614
E-mail pneumotel@fsm.it

References

1. Speizer FE. Epidemiology and mortality patterns in asthma. In Weiss EB (Ed), Status asthmaticus. Baltimore: University Park Press 1978, pp. 13–18.

2. Burr M, Charles T, Roy KL, et al. Asthma in the elderly. An epidemiologic survey. Br Med J 1979; 1:1041–1044.

3. National Center for Health Statistics. National Health Interview Service 1989.

4. Enright PL, Ward BI, Tracy RP, et al. Cardiovascular Health Study Research Group: Asthma and its association with Cardiovascular disease in the elderly. J Asthma 1996; 33:45–53.

5. Campbell MJ, Cogman GR, Holgate ST. Age-specific trends in asthma mortality in England and Wales 1983–95: Result of an observation study. BMJ 1997; 314:1439–1441.

6. Weiss KB, Gergen PJ, Wagner DK. Breathing better or wheezing worse? The changing epidemiology of asthma morbidity and mortality. Am Rev Publ Health 1991; 14:491–513.

7. Weiner P, Magadle R, Waizman J, et al. Characteristics of asthma in the elderly. Eur Respir J 1998; 12:564–568.

8. NAEPP Working Group Report. Considerations for diagnosing and managing asthma in the elderly. NH Publication No. 963662, February 1995.

9. Braman SS, Kaemmerlen JT, Davis GM. Asthma in the elderly. A comparison between patients with recently acquired and long-standing disease. Am Rev Respir Dis. 1991; 143:336–340.

10. Burr ML, Charles T, Roy K, et al. Characteristics of asthma among elderly adults in a sample of general population. Chest 1991; 100:935.

11. Braman SS. Asthma in the elderly patient. Clin Chest Med 1993; 14:413–422.

12. Melillo G. Asthma in the elderly. ACI Int 1996; 8/5–6:161–163.

13. Celli BR. Standards for the optimal management of COPD. Chest 1998; 113–4:283s.

14. Enright PL, Rodarte JL. Physiology of aging lung. In RA Barbee, JW Bloom (Eds), Asthma in the elderly. New York: Marcel Dekker 1997, p. 69–92.

15. Burrows B, Clin MG, Kudson RJ, et al. A descriptive analysis of the growth and decline of the FVC and FEV$_1$. Chest 1983; 83:714–724.

16. Corvalhaes-Neto N, Lorino H, Gallinari C, et al. Cognitive function and assessment of lung function in the elderly. Am J Respir Care Med 1995; 152:1611–15.

17. Chalker RB, Cell RR. Special considerations in the elderly patients. Clinics in Chest Medicine 1993; 143:437–452.

18. Connolly MJ, Crowley JJ, Nielson CP, et al. Periph-

eral mononuclear leucocyte β-adrenoreceptor and specific bronchial responsiveness to methacoline in young and elderly normal subjects and asthmatic patients. Thorax 1994; 49:26–32.

19. Sobona RE. Pathology of asthma in the elderly. In RR Barbee, JW Bloom (Eds), Asthma in the elderly. New York: Marcel Dekker Inc. 1997, pp. 53–67.

20. Aoki K, Ohtsubok, Yoshimura K, et al. Histological evaluation of bronchial tissue from elderly individuals with bronchial asthma. Jap J Thoracic Dis 1995; 33(12):1421–1429.

21. Dow L. Asthma in older people. Clin and Exp Allergy 1998; 28(55):195–202.

22. Gong H. Coexisting conditions that complicate asthma management in the elderly. In RA Barbee, JW Bloom (Eds), Asthma in the elderly. New York: Marcel Dekker 1997, pp. 219–285.

23. Parameswara K, Hildreth D, Chada D, et al. Asthma in the elderly: Underperceived, underdiagnosed and undertreated: A community survey. Respir Med 1998; 92(3):573–577.

The Epidemiology and Natural History of Asthma in the Elderly

Robert A Barbee*

Keywords: Asthma, elderly, natural history, epidemiology

After many years in which the major emphasis of epidemiologic asthma studies has been on childhood disease, increasing attention is now focused on older patients. As has been true of younger asthmatics, both the prevalence and mortality in the elderly has greatly increased in recent years. In contrast to children, for which heredity and atopy are factors in the onset of disease, risk factors for adult disease are less clear. Most studies have implicated childhood respiratory disease. Atopy, bronchial hyperresponsiveness and cigarette consumption have also been correlated with adult onset.

The most difficult problem in studies of asthma in the elderly is the variation in criteria by which an asthma diagnosis has been made. Lifelong moderate or severe disease may have only minimal reversibility possibly secondary to airway remodeling. Patients with COPD who demonstrate significant reversibility may be said to have asthma in addition to chronic bronchitis and/or emphysema. Finally, some older asthmatics with recent onset disease have more classical asthma, but with less clinical allergy. Given the extensive variability in clinical and physiologic presentation of older asthmatics and the limitations of the current data bases additional longitudinal studies of older subjects with well characterized asthma will be necessary to provide answers to the many questions that remain concerning their natural history.

Introduction

In contrast to the many reports which describe the epidemiology and course of childhood asthma into adulthood, only a small number of studies have followed the course of adult asthma. Similarly, epidemiologic studies in older populations have been difficult to carry out, in large measure because of the difficulty in distinguishing asthma from chronic obstructive lung disease and other pulmonary and non pulmonary causes of wheezing and airflow obstruction in this population. Despite these limitations, a number of studies have provided both epidemiologic and natural history data on older patients with asthma. The review which follows summarizes much of the data that has been obtained from both young and older populations. When the subjects involved are children or young adults, an attempt will be made to relate the findings to the older patient with asthma, and the special epidemiological problems that exist in the elderly.

Remissions and Relapses

One of the most difficult variables to account for in longitudinal asthma studies is that of remissions and relapses. In the 1960s a number of investigators addressed this problem, starting with asthma in childhood [1]. Depending upon the individual study, between 40 and 50% of childhood asthmatics enjoyed a remission of their disease during their early teen years. However, a significant percentage had relapsed by age 21. When studied again at age 28, almost a third of those who were asymptomatic at 21 were again wheezing, seven years later [2]. Because, in many cases, their disease had been quite mild when they were children, the authors speculated that many of these relapsed subjects were thought to have adult onset disease. Of particular significance in this study was the fact that 95% of subjects who had persistent, or more severe childhood asthma continued to have their disease over 20 years later. Many of them were not under treatment, and demonstrated persistent airflow obstruction. In another longitudinal study of childhood asthma it was reported that 76% had

* Pulmonary/Critical Care Section, Department of Medicine, University of Arizona, Tucson, AR, USA

continuing symptoms 15 years later, but only 19% were under treatment. A third study indicated that only 30% of children with asthma achieve permanent remission [3].

In addition to severity, remission and relapse rates appear to correlate with age. A report from the Tucson community study indicated that among asthmatics between ages 10 and 19, 65% would deny the presence of symptoms nine years later. By contrast, only 6% of those between 40 and 49 years experienced remissions during the follow up period. In addition to this age difference, most remissions were among those with mild disease. Age and disease severity were also related to asthma relapse rates. For the entire study population, from childhood through the eighth decade, the relapse rate was 38%. Although they occurred during each decade of life, relapses were especially common among the elderly. Between 60 and 69, eight of twelve who denied symptoms on the initial survey had active disease nine years later [4].

Taken together, these reports make it clear that a majority of those with moderate or severe childhood disease have either continuing symptoms in adulthood or have a high incidence of recurrent disease later in life. Because airway remodeling and the loss of reversibility which accompanies it is felt to be the result of continuing airway inflammation over many years these studies of untreated childhood asthma are of special interest. Without a significant change in their course, young adults with 20 year asthma histories may present many years later with irreversible "fixed" disease. At that point the differential diagnosis between asthma and COPD may be difficult, if not impossible.

Prevalence, Morbidity, and Mortality

A major objective of large epidemiologic asthma studies is the determination of disease prevalence, morbidity, and mortality. To achieve these goals it is necessary to have diagnostic tools available which ensure both sensitivity and specificity in identifying subjects with asthma. In most studies, subjects with asthma are identified by questionnaire responses indicating the presence of symptoms which are typical of those with asthma. Most questionnaires also ask whether a physician or other clinician has made a specific diagnosis of

asthma, and whether symptoms have been present within the past year. Utilizing these and other tools it has been possible to achieve a high rate of sensitivity in regard to asthma prevalence. Those with asthma are identified over 90% of the time, especially in older children and young adults, populations in which the differential diagnosis of asthma is more straight forward. Unfortunately, it is more difficult to achieve high levels of specificity in epidemiologic asthma studies. That is, the exclusion of those with symptoms which are found in asthma, but do not have the disease [5]. This is especially difficult in very young children and older adults. Wheezing syndromes in children under age three may of may not indicate the likelihood of future asthma [6]. Older adults, as noted earlier, may have a variety of pulmonary and nonpulmonary entities in which wheezing and chest tightness are common symptoms. Differentiation between asthma and COPD may be especially difficult. Even the addition of methacholine challenge tests fails to eliminate the overlap between these two entities [7].

Despite these limitations, a number of reports have provided estimates of asthma prevalence in many parts of the world. One of the first to specifically examine the prevalence of asthma in the older adult was reported from Australia in 1969. In a survey of 11,000 asthma sufferers, only 15% dated the onset of their disease between age 45 and 59. Less than 3% had their initial diagnosis made after age 60 [8]. Subsequently, a report from Tucson suggested that both the prevalence and incidence of asthma in the elderly was much higher than previously reported. During a four year follow up, the prevalence of asthma in those over age 60 in both males and females, was over 6.0% [9]. A similar finding was reported from Wales, where the prevalence in the older population was 6.5% [10]. More recent data from the 1995 National Health Interview Survey in the US [11] reported an overall prevalence of asthma of 56.8 per 1,000 population. The highest rate, 74.9/1000 occurred in those under age 18. In the 45–64 year age group the rate was 51.6 and for age 65 and above, 39.8. From a number of international reports it is clear that the prevalence of asthma varies greatly from one country to another, and from one geographic area to another, often depending upon climatic conditions. Countries with the highest prevalence rates include the United Kingdom, New Zealand, Australia, and Ireland. Among the lowest are Indonesia, Albania, Romania, and Georgia.

In most parts of the world recent studies of prevalence and the incidence of new disease have found a significant increase in asthma compared to studies carried out 15 to 20 years previously. While it has been asserted by some that a major portion of this increase is secondary to an increase in asthma awareness and changes in disease labeling by physicians, it is generally agreed that at least a portion of the increase is real. The exact cause for the increase in unclear, but most authors attribute it to a combination of increased allergen exposure in the environment and an overall deterioration in the quality of the air we breathe. Utilizing data from the US, it is estimated that since 1980, the overall increase in prevalence has been 75%. The biggest increase has been in children under age 4, but all age groups, including the elderly have contributed to the increase [11]. Female prevalence has increased more than male, and blacks have had a greater increase than whites.

Many of the factors that serve to confound the validity of asthma prevalence data also impact on the determination of morbidity and mortality. Morbidity is usually defined by the effect a disease has on quality of life, including hospitalizations and both direct and indirect costs related to the disease. Unfortunately, changes in disease labeling at the time of hospital discharge, increased use of emergency rooms, and other factors unrelated to asthma severity itself may alter morbidity data. Despite these difficulties, a report in 1987 from the US National Health Interview Study was able to document an increase in hospitalizations during the period from 1965 to 1983 [2]. The increase was greater in children, but was also seen in adults. Data for older asthma patients is extremely difficult to validate. If a high percentage of elderly patients with airways obstructive disease have multiple disease labels, including both asthma and COPD, an exacerbation of one might well be labeled the other at the time of hospital discharge. The most recent data from the US would indicate that the overall rate of hospitalizations for asthma in the last few years has actually decreased, although childhood asthma hospitalizations have continued to increase.

Prior to the 1960s asthma mortality was unusual, and declining on a yearly basis. Worldwide it was estimated that in most age groups a diagnosis of asthma as a cause of death was less than two per million [13]. Since the 1960s, increases in asthma mortality have taken two forms. The first was episodic, occurring first in England during the 1960s and subsequently, in New Zealand in the 1970s. At the time, both were attributed to the introduction of new asthma therapy, and its possible misuse, or overuse. In neither instance was the association convincingly proven. More troubling has been the gradual and progressive increase in asthma deaths that have occurred throughout the world over a number of years. If, as has been stated previously, both asthma prevalence and morbidity have increased, it would be expected that mortality would also increase. The question is whether this increase has been greater than can be accounted for by an increase in prevalence. On the one hand, investigators have examined whether treatment factors have played a role. It has been suggested that more effective treatment of asthma symptoms has led patients to have a false sense of security, and allowing themselves to be exposed to life threatening triggers. The fact that a large number of asthma deaths occur at home might imply that both clinician and patient may be underestimating the severity of the disease. The fact that asthma death rates are increased among socio-economically deprived populations suggests that lack of access to care may play a role.

Of particular importance in the assessment of asthma mortality among older adults is the accuracy of death certificate diagnoses. It has been estimated that under age 35, death certificate diagnoses of asthma are 95% accurate, but over age 75, accuracy decreases to less than 35% [13]. Several other reports have emphasized that the differentiation between an asthma and COPD death in older individuals is not only difficult, but in the presence of both diseases simultaneously, virtually impossible. Whether this difficulty in death certificate diagnoses increases or decreases the asthma mortality rate has been debated in the literature, without a definitive conclusion. However, it is clear that overall, asthma deaths have increased significantly in most parts of the world. How evenly this increase has been spread throughout the age ranges is unclear. The largest reported increases have been in children. Because of the diagnostic problems which are inherent in the older individual, it is not possible to determine the extent to which deaths in older asthma patients have increased.

Risk Factors for Adult Onset Asthma

The relationship between childhood asthma and a combination of heredity and allergen exposure is well known. Factors that relate to adult onset asthma are much less clear. For years it has been known that a history of respiratory disease in childhood is related to the onset of wheezing as an adult [14]. The presumption was that airways that are damaged during childhood are more susceptible to disease later on. A number of investigators have attempted to identify other factors that are related to the onset of asthma during adulthood in the absence of a history of childhood respiratory disease. A common factor in many studies is the presence of bronchial hyper-responsiveness prior to the onset of overt asthma [15]. In younger adults, atopy has been found to be a major co-factor. Over the age of 40, it appears to be much less important. Reports from studies that have measured spirometry longitudinally have described a fall in the first second forced expiratory volume (FEV_1) prior to the onset of clinical asthma. In all reports, when a smoking history is present, it tends to overshadow both atopy and other factors as a contributing factor in adult onset asthma.

Despite the fact that markers of clinical allergy are much less evident in the older individual, those with asthma appear to have elevated levels of IgE when levels are corrected for age. Those with levels in the lowest quartile for their age rarely had asthma. This correlation has been confirmed in a number of reports. A question that is not answered in these studies is whether these are truly risk factors for the development of asthma, or signs that subclinical asthma has been present for some time prior to an asthma diagnosis being made.

Asthma Versus COPD: A Diagnostic Dilemma in the Elderly

The term asthma has been in the medical lexicon for over 2,000 years. Chronic Obstructive Pulmonary Disease (COPD) was unknown to medicine until 30 to 40 years ago. When British and American investigators examined the features of chronic bronchitis, the British term for progressive airways obstruction, and the more common American term, emphysema, they concluded that a majority of patients had features which were common to both. Only a minority of patients had a pure form of either entity. From this mixture of emphysema and chronic bronchitis the term COPD emerged. Initial-

ly it was characterized as a chronic obstructive disease resulting from cigarette consumption that was unresponsive to therapy, and inevitably progressed to death. since that time, a number of modifications have been made in its clinical description. Those with the same tobacco background, but with at least some evidence of reversibility in response to therapy were labeled COPD with an asthmatic component. For some patients, stable lung function could be achieved with a much better prognosis than had been imagined initially. Even those with fixed obstruction were found to be capable of increasing their FEV_1 by 15% or more after a bronchodilator on an occasional test. At the same time, reports appeared that described older asthma patients with little reversibility, and a relatively fixed airflow obstruction. Although the pathology of the airway might be quite different, the clinical picture often presented considerable overlap, and not a little confusion. A 1986 report from Tucson indicated that among new asthma diagnoses in patients over age 40, only 29% did not have either a prior or concomitant diagnosis of either chronic bronchitis or emphysema. Many such subjects could not be distinguished on the basis of allergic background or evidence of current atopy [16]. The only clear distinguishing historical feature was the extent of previous tobacco consumption.

Despite this diagnostic confusion, asthma diagnoses are increasingly being made in the older population. In one report, new asthma diagnoses were made in 40 subjects during a longitudinal study. The average age was 70.8 years. For a majority of the forty, the onset of a new wheezing complaint was correlated with the asthma diagnosis. A prior diagnosis of chronic bronchitis and a history of childhood respiratory disease was common. Smoking histories were not different among those with asthma compared to nonasthmatic controls [17].

The Prognosis of Asthma in the Elderly

A limited number of studies have attempted the arduous talk of identifying a population of older subjects with asthma and collected longitudinal physiological and mortality data. From Tucson, a variety of factors were used to separate the community study population into two airways obstructive groups. In the first group were those with a high prevalence of atopy, limited smoking histories, and physician confirmed histories of asthma. Many also had a concomitant diagnosis of chronic bronchitis or emphysema. The second group consisted of nonatopic smokers, some of whom had no prior airway obstructive diagnosis. Both groups had a similar degree of airway obstruction, with FEV_1 values of less than 65% predicted. During a ten year follow-up period, the FEV_1 decline in group two was 70 ml per year compared to 5 ml in group one. The death rate in group one was less than predicted for age, with no death attributed to a respiratory cause. By contrast, the death rate in group two was 60%, a majority of which were attributed to an airway obstructive disease [18]. In this study, asthma, by itself, or combined with simple chronic bronchitis was not associated with an increased mortality, while the prognosis of the more insidious emphysematous disease was more typical of COPD as it was initially described.

In addition to this report, a number of investigators have conducted longitudinal follow-up studies, comparing the course and prognosis of adults with asthma to that of normal controls. In each study, the yearly decline in FEV_1 was greater in asthmatics than age matched normal controls. When a diagnosis of chronic bronchitis was present, in addition to asthma, the decline in pulmonary function and subsequent mortality was greatest. Because all studies included subjects with at least some smoking history, it is not possible to assess the outcome of nonsmoking adults with asthma. Cough and sputum were common symptoms in those with a smoking history. When subjects were divided into allergic and nonallergic categories, the latter was associated with a more rapid decline in pulmonary function. In virtually all studies that have compared asthmatics with normal controls, the mortality in the asthma populations was greater [19, 20, 21, 22].

Missing from all reported studies is information which would relate physiologic decline and mortality to disease management. As a result, the effect of management is entirely unknown. When this uncertainty is combined with the uncertainty of diagnostic labeling between asthma and COPD, it is clear that firm conclusions concerning mortality are only tentative.

Perhaps the most often quoted study is that reported from Australia in 1987. Over an 18 year period in Busselton, West Australia, 92 asthmatic subjects aged 22 to 69 were repeatedly assessed. Compared to a rate of FEV_1 decline of 35 ml/year in their normal controls, subjects with asthma had a decline of 50 ml/year. Asthmatics also had a lower baseline FEV_1. Unfortunately, only 22 nonsmoking males with asthma were included, four each in the two decades between age 45 and 64. Constructing regression slopes with so few subjects limits the capacity to generalize from their data [22].

If, as is implied by the studies discussed above, a majority of patients with asthma experience a gradual decline in pulmonary function, a significant number have a course which is either much more favorable, or severe. As an example of a more favorable outcome, a 1997 report described 181 young adults with asthma who were studied in the 1960s, then retested 25 years later. At the time of their retesting, 21% no longer had bronchial hyperresponsiveness, 25% had normal FEV_1s and 40% had no pulmonary symptoms. Eleven per cent of the original 181 subjects had neither BHR, abnormal FEV_1, or symptoms. In the absence of any of those criteria, the authors concluded that they no longer had asthma [23]. Among the several factors which were associated with this outcome were mild initial disease and early therapeutic intervention. Both this study, and one reported earlier suggest that if one is symptom free for a long enough period, the BHR which characterizes asthma may no longer be present.

At the other end of the spectrum, several recent reports have emphasized the development of irreversible obstruction in older patients with continuing asthma of long duration. They are unresponsive to intensive therapy and in most respects are indistinguishable from what has commonly been called end stage COPD [24, 25].

Summary

The natural history of asthma in the elderly is largely unknown. In part this is because the longitudinal studies which would provide the definitive data base have not been done. Perhaps more importantly, there is no single or typical history which would be applicable for a majority of older individuals with asthma. For some older patients, asthma has been a lifelong affliction with progressive airflow obstruction, which becomes less and less responsive to therapy. For others it is a recent onset of wheezing following a long history of upper respiratory allergic symptoms. Still others have had a chronic cough for some time which is now accompanied by a wheeze. Finally, there are probably a few patients with the recent onset of wheezing and shortness of breath from illnesses which are not of pulmonary origin. Whether the diagnostic labels which are attached to elderly individuals with airway obstructive disease will ever allow us to distinguish the several disease entities remains uncertain.

Address for correspondence:

Robert A Barbee, MD
P.O. Box 245030
1501 N. Campbell Avenue
Tucson, AR 85724
USA
Tel. +1 520 626-6115
Fax +1 520 626-6970
E-mail rbarbee@resp-sci.arizona.edu

References

1. Williams H, McNicol K. Prevalence, natural history, and relationship of wheezy bronchitis and asthma in children. An epidemiological study. Br Med J 1969; 8:321–325.

2. Kelly WJ, Hudson I, Phelan PD, Pain MC, Olinsky A. Childhood asthma in adult life: A further study at 28 years of age. Br Med J 1987; 294:1059–62.

3. Roorda RJ, Gerritsen J, van Aalderen WMC, Schouten JP, Veltman JC, Weiss ST, et al. Follow-up of asthma from childhood to adulthood: Influence of potential childhood risk factors on the outcome of pulmonary function and bronchial responsiveness in adulthood. J Allergy Clin Immunol 1994; 93:575–84.

4. Bronnimann S, Burrows B. A prospective study of the natural history of asthma – Remission and relapse rates. CHEST 1986; 90:480–484.

5. Toren K, Brisman J, Jarvholm B. Asthma and asthma-like symptoms in adults assessed by questionnaires. Chest 1993; 104:600–8.

6. Martinez FD, Wright AL, Taussig, LM, Holberg CJ, Halonen J, Morgan WJ. Asthma and wheezing in the first six years of life. N Engl J Med 1995; 323(3):133–138.

7. Peat JK, Woolcock AJ. Sensitivity to common allergens: Relation to respiratory symptoms and bronchial hyperresponsiveness in children from three different climatic areas of Australia. Clin Exp Allergy 1991; 21:573–581.

8. Ford RM. Etiology of asthma: A review of 11,551 cases (1958 to 1968). Med J Aust 1969; 1:628–631.

9. Dodge R, Burrows B. The prevalence and incidence of asthma and asthma-like symptoms in a general po-

pulation sample. Ann Rev Respir Dis 1980; 122:567–575.

10. Burney PG, Britton JR, Chinn S, Tattersfiled AE, Papacosta AO, Kelson MC, Anderson F, Corfield DR. Descriptive epidemiology of bronchial reactivity in an adult population: Results from a community study. Thorax 1987; 42:38–44.

11. National Institutes of Health, National Heart, Lung, and Blood Institute. Data Fact Sheet, January, 1999.

12. National Health Interview Survey. National Center for Health Statistics, 1989.

13. Sears MR, Rea HH, deBoar G, et al. Accuracy of certification of deaths due to asthma: A national study. Am J Epidemiol 1986; 124:1004–1011.

14. Burrows B, Knudson RJ, Lebowitz MD. The relationship of childhood respiratory illness to adult obstructive airway disease. Am Rev Respir Dis 1977; 115:751–760.

15. Bodner CH, Ross S, Little J, Douglas JG, Legge JS, Friend JA, et al. Risk factors for adult onset wheeze: A case control study. Am J Respir Crit Care Med 1998; 157:35–42.

16. Dodge R, Cline MG, Burrows B. Comparisons of asthma, emphysema, and chronic bronchitis diagnoses in a general population sample. Am Rev Respir Dis 1986; 133:981–986.

17. Burrows B, Lebowitz M, Barbee R, Cline M. Findings before diagnosis of asthma among the elderly in a longitudinal study of a general population sample. J All Clin Immunol 1991; 88:870–877.

18. Burrows B, Bloow JW, Traver GA, Cline MG. The course and prognosis of different forms of chronic airways obstruction in a sample from the general population. N Engl J Med 1987; 317:1309–1314.

19. Peat JK, Woolcock AJ, Cullen K. Rate of decline of lung function in subjects with asthma. Eur J Respir Dis 1987; 70:171–179.

20. Schachter EN, Doyle CA, Beck GJ. A prospective study of asthma in a rural community. Chest 1984; 85:623–630.

21. Almind M, Viskum K, Evald T, Dirksen A, Kok-Jensen A. Seven-year follow-up study of 343 adults with bronchial asthma. Dan Med Bull 1992; 39:561– 565.

22. Woolcock AJ, Peat JK, Salome CM, Yan K, Anderson SD, Schoeffel RE, et al. Prevalence of bronchial hyperresponsiveness and asthma in a rural adult population. Thorax 1987; 42:316–68.

23. Manhuysen CIM, Vonk JM, Koeter GH, et al. Adult patients may outgrow their asthma: A 25-year follow-up study. Am J Respir Crit Care Med 1997; 155:1267–1272.

24. Braman SS, Kaemmerlen JT, Davis SM. Asthma in the elderly: A comparison between patients with recently acquired and long standing disease. Am Rev Resp Dis 1991; 143:336–340.

25. Brown PJ, Greville HW, Finucane KE. Asthma and irreversible airflow obstruction. Thorax. 1984; 39:131–136.

Epidemiology of Asthma in Children

Carlos E Baena-Cagnani*, Hugo E Neffen**, Sandra E Gurné***, M Cristina Minervini*

Keywords: Epidemiology, wheezing, asthma, prevalence, ISAAC, Argentina

In the last decades, an enormous interest in asthma has arisen along with the number of consultations, hospital admissions, and antiasthmatic prescriptions. At the same time, there has been an increase in asthma mortality in various parts of the world. In order to evaluate the magnitude of the problem, epidemiological studies have been conducted. Among them, the European Community Respiratory Health Survey (ECRHS) and the International Study of Asthma and Allergies in Children (ISAAC) have provided very valuable information on the prevalence and severity of asthma, wheezing, and other allergic diseases (e. g., atopic dermatitis and allergic rhinitis). Current data show a large geographic variety in the asthma prevalence in different parts of the world. Nevertheless, asthma has become a world-wide public health problem, and there is evidence that the trend in the spreading prevalence of asthma is rising now even in countries in which it has been low.

In the last 20 years, a remarkable interest in asthma has arisen. The increase in the number of admissions to hospitals, consultations, and prescriptions for asthma drugs have raised the interest in asthma.

At the same time, there has been an increase in asthma mortality in different parts of the world [1]. Asthma mortality has also been studied in different Latin American countries, showing a great variety in mortality rates [2]. This particular aspect of asthma epidemiology has created a great concern among researchers, and as a consequence a great effort has been carried out in order to gain insight into asthma prevalence in both adults and children, and to evaluate whether prevalence has indeed risen in the last decades. Furthermore, different aspects of morbidity such as severity, hospitalization rate, emergency-room visits, among others, have also been studied.

Worldwide Asthma Prevalence

Until recently, the worldwide epidemiology of asthma had not been well established for many reasons. The lack of a clear definition of asthma, particularly in preschool children, and the lack of international questionnaires permitting comparison have hindered our understanding of asthma epidemiology. However, two major systematic research protocols have now been conducted to study the prevalence of asthma in both adults and children:
- the European Community Respiratory Health Survey (ECRHS),
- the International Study of Asthma and Allergies in Children (ISAAC). This study was conducted on two groups of children, one 6–7 years old and the second 13–14 years old. It is more feasible to establish the diagnosis of asthma in these children than in younger ones.

The ECRHS has proved to be a very reliable tool for studying the prevalence of asthma in adults aged 22 to 40 [3]. The prevalence of current asthma (symptoms or use of asthma medications in the last 12 months) in European countries ranged from lows of 2.0/2.1%, for example, in Tartu (Estonia), Athens (Greece), Erfurt (Germany), and Galdakao (Spain), to higher figures in Sweden and the United Kingdom. Inbetween lie the figures from different cities and countries showing great variety, for instance, in Germany (2.1% in Erfurt and 4.4% in Hamburg). This study thus shows a geographical variation in prevalence.

The ISAAC study has provided data on the worldwide prevalence of wheeze and asthma in children [4]. The prevalence of wheeze in the last 12 months ranged from 2.1% to 32.2% in the

*   Division of Allergy, Clinical Immunology and Respiratory Medicine, Department of Paediatrics, Infantile Hospital, Córdoba, Argentina
**   Allergy Unit, Children's Hospital, Santa Fe, Argentina
*** Centre for Research and Diagnostic in Immunology, San Roque Hospital, Córdoba, Argentina

13–14-year-old group and from 4.1% to 32.1% in the 6–7-year-old group. The highest prevalence of current asthma was reported in English-speaking countries such as UK, New Zealand, and Australia, while the lowest was found in Eastern Europe, Greece, China, India, and Ethiopia.

Data on asthma epidemiology in Latin America [5], and particularly in Argentina, has been scarce [6]. In addition, different questionnaires have been used, making comparisons among studies impossible. An epidemiological study using the ISAAC questionnaire was performed in Córdoba, Argentina, according to the original protocol [7]. A random sample of children aged 13–14 years was recruited through secondary school class registers and asked to complete the Spanish translation of the ISAAC written questionnaire. The study was conducted on 3044 children in Córdoba, Argentina, during 1996–1997. The response rate was 95%. Results are shown in Table 1.

The prevalence of wheezing and asthma varies considerably in the different regions of the world [3]. Four prevalence ranges have been established: (1) <5%, (2) 5 to <10%, (3) 10 to <20%, and (4) ≥20%. The prevalence of wheezing in infants (22.8%) and asthma in the 13–14 years old group (11.2%) from Córdoba is high, although it is lower than in regions showing the highest prevalence (see Table 2). Our results are very similar to other data recently published from the Atlantic coast in Latin America [4]. Different environmental factors might explain the worldwide prevalence variations [8], among them indoor allergen exposure [9].

The majority of children with persistent severe asthma represent the smaller group [10]. Night awakenings and the number of attacks are good indicators of asthma severity. Sleep disturbances due to wheezing identifies and quantifies persistent

Table 2. Prevalence (%) among 13–14-year-olds of wheezing in previous year, and of wheezing four or more times per year, in representative countries participating in the ISAAC. Modified from [11].

Location	Wheeze in previous year	Wheeze > 4x/year
Australia (Adelaide)	29	12
UK (West Sussex)	29	37
New Zealand (Wellington)	28	8
Germany (Bochum)	20	4
Spain (Barcelona)	14	
Norway (Oslo)	13	
Hongkong	12	4
Argentina (Córdoba)	11	11
Singapore	10	2

wheezing. Despite the fact that 10.1% of children experienced night awakenings more than once a week, most of the asthmatics surveyed in this region are not severely affected (in agreement with other studies). A strong association between *ever having wheezed* and *ever having asthma* was found, suggesting an overlap between these two clinical situations of airway obstruction.

These results show that wheezing during childhood and asthma among adolescents are important public health problems in Argentina, in agreement with other ISAAC studies from other parts of the world.

Trends in Asthma Prevalence

There is evidence suggesting an increase in the prevalence of asthma [11]. This rising trend is found worldwide, particularly in children, as was recently suggested [12]. There are studies suggesting an increase in the prevalence of asthma, particularly in children. A study from Aberdeen in the UK has shown an increase in the prevalence of asthma, wheeze, and shortness of breath as well as allergic rhinitis and eczema in children in the years 1964 to 1989. The rise in the prevalence of wheeze, asthma, atopic dermatitis and hayfever was more than 50% in the period surveyed. [13]. Other studies from developed and developing countries have shown a similar trend, for instance, an increase in asthma prevalence has been found in both Australia and Taiwan [14, 15].

In the United States, it has been estimated that more than 10 million people have asthma, with the

Table 1. Prevalence of respiratory symptoms and indicators of severity. From [7].

Question	Total (%)	F (%)	M (%)
Ever wheeze	23.8	24.6	23.1
Current wheeze	11.2	12.2	10.5
1–3 attacks	47.7	44.8	50.1
4–11 attacks	10.7	12.0	9.6
≥12 attacks	5.0	4.4	5.4
Night awakenings			
Never	41.9	38.6	44.6
Once a week	19.8	20.8	18.8
> Once a week	10.1	11.5	8.8

prevalence rate increasing 29% from 1980 to 1987 [16]. More recently, the Centers for Disease Control and Prevention in Atlanta published a report on the status of asthma in the USA between 1960–1995. An increase of more than 75% in the prevalence rate of self-reported asthma was found for the years 1980 to 1994. This trend was found among all age groups, all races, and both sexes. In addition, an even greater rise was found in self-reported asthma among persons aged 5–35, particularly between 1987/1989 and 1993/1994. The most remarkable increase occurred among children aged 0–4 (160%) [17].

Risk Factors

If we consider asthma as a global public health problem, it is crucial to identify the risk associated with the development and natural history of asthma in order to design strategies for primary and secondary prevention. In this sense, epidemiological studies are the only way to measure the risk factors associated with asthma. Many studies conducted in the last 20 years have given substantial information about the nature of asthma, probable risk factors associated, and natural history [18]. Many risk factors likely associated with the development of asthma have been studied such as diet (including breastfeeding), maternal tobacco smoking, exposure to indoor allergens (particularly house dust mite) and other pollutants, race, gender, family size, and infections (Table 3).

Because of the rise in the prevalence of atopic diseases [13, 19, 20], an association between atopy and asthma was also studied. Epidemiological studies consistently show an association between atopy and asthma [21]. The association between atopy, asthma, and airway hyperresponsiveness (AHR) has also been shown using skin prick tests and total

and specific serum IgE levels as markers of atopy [22, 23]. Furthermore, the association between the size of positive skin prick tests and AHR to methacoline was shown in asthmatic and nonasthmatic patients [24].

Among other factors, indoor allergen sensitization, particularly to house dust mite allergens, is one of the major risk factors for the development of asthma. Early exposure to house dust mite allergens has been associated with early wheeze and persistent asthma later in life [25]. The Tucson cohort study showed that children with persistent wheezing were significantly more sensitized to aeroallergens than children who never wheeze [26], in agreement with another study also showing an association between atopy and diminished lung function in symptom-free patients [27].

House dust mite allergen levels in Córdoba and Santa Fe are very high [28] (1), and the frequency of asthmatic children sensitized to indoor allergens in Córdoba is similar to the prevalence of allergen sensitivity found in children from developed countries. This could explain, at least in part, the relatively high prevalence found in our study [9]. An association between asthma and other allergens such as *Alternaria*, grass, birch pollen, or cat, has also been found. Still, it is estimated that about 50% of all asthma cases can be attributed to atopy [29].

Infections early in life have been incriminated as a "protective" factor for the development of atopy [30]. There is evidence showing the influence of early respiratory infection on the behavior of Th1 and Th2 cells through the action of the cytokines IL-12 and INF-γ. Nevertheless, infections might "help" in the development of Th2 phenotype and consequently atopy. Infections inducing Th1 type response could result in the inhibition of atopic disorders in developing countries. In addition,

Table 3. Risk factors in asthma and wheeze in childhood.

– Genetic predisposition
– Atopy
– Infections
– Infant feeding
– Diet
– Parental smoking
– Air pollution
– Family structure
– Socioeconomic aspects

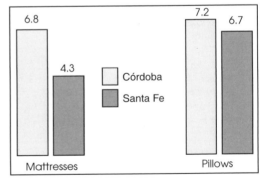

Figure 1. Group 1 mite-allergen levels (μg/g) in pillows and mattresses from Córdoba and Santa Fe, Argentina.

Helmintic infection could suppress allergic reactivity despite the induction of Th2 phenotype [31].

The role of diet in the rise of atopic diseases, particularly asthma, has also been studied. Since the major change in asthma prevalence seems to have taken place after the 1960's, diet is a major candidate as risk factor. Recently, a positive association between the prevalence of asthma and other atopic manifestations (allergic rhino-conjunctivitis and atopic dermatitis) and intake of *trans* fatty acid was established [32]. These *trans* fatty acids are part of the "Western" diet and could explain, at least in part, the rise in asthma prevalence in affluent areas.

Despite the fact that great insight has been gained into the relationship between allergen exposure and sensitization and the development of asthma, as well as with other "candidate" risk factors, more research should be done in order to gain insight into their impact on the "asthma epidemic." Preventive measures could be taken if the risk factors associated with this trend were better identified.

during infancy, among others. Nevertheless, more research should be conducted to elucidate this issue. Asthma is currently considered an important worldwide public health problem with a high incidence, high prevalence, an unacceptable mortality rate, and high impact on quality of life. It is a severe burden to the public health systems from a socioeconomic point of view in both high- and low-income countries.

Address for correspondence:

Carlos E Baena-Cagnani, MD
Division of Allergy, Clinical
Immunology and Respiratory Medicine.
Department of Paediatrics
Infantile Hospital
Lavalleja 3052
(5001) Córdoba
Argentina
Tel./fax + 54 351 470-3512
E-mail baena@powernet.com.ar

Concluding Remarks

The prevalence of asthma is very high in many parts of the world. An estimated 200,000,000 people suffer from asthma worldwide. Considering this figure, the socio-economic aspects, and the unacceptable mortality, asthma must be considered a global public health problem [33]. There is a rising trend in asthma that is alarming the international medical community. This phenomenon is more evident in children and has occurred since 1960. In addition, there is recent evidence showing that the rise is still continuing.

The prevalence of asthma varies greatly in different regions of the world, ranging from very high in English-speaking countries to very low in some regions of Eastern Europe, Asia, and Africa. North and Latin America lies somewhere in between these two groups. Moreover, differences in prevalence among different research centers in the same country have been verified.

Those factors associated with a rise in asthma prevalence particularly in children have not been fully recognized. Many hypotheses are now being tested, and there is evidence supporting the role of some risk factors associated with this trend, such as indoor allergen exposure, family size, infections

References

1. Pearce N, Beasley R, Burgess C, Crane J. Asthma epidemiology. Principles and methods. New York: Oxford University Press 1998.

2. Neffen H, Baena-Cagnani CE, Malka S, Solé D, Sepúlveda R, Caraballo L, Carabajal E, Rodríguez Gavaldá R, González Díaz S, Guggiare Chase J, Díaz C, Baluga J, Capriles Hullet A. Asthma mortality in Latin America. J Invest Allergol Clin Immunol 1997; 7:249–254.

3. European Community Respiratory Health Survey (ECRHS). Variation in the prevalence of respiratory symptoms, self-reported asthma attacks and use of asthma medications in the European Community Respiratory Health Survey (ECRHS). Eur Respir J 1996; 9:687–95.

4. ISAAC Steering Committee: Worldwide prevalence of Asthma symptoms: The International Study of Asthma and Allergy in children (ISAAC). Eur Respir J 1998; 350:1015–1020.

5. Carrasco E. Epidemiology of asthma in Latin America. Chest 1987; 91:93S–97S.

6. Bustos GJ, Baena-Cagnani CE, Minervini MC, Saranz R. Asma bronquial en niños y adolescentes. Actualización en diagnóstico y tratamiento. Arch Arg Ped 1994; 92:37–46.

7. Baena-Cagnani CE, Patiño CM, Cuello MN, Minervini MC, Fernández AM, Garip EA, Salvucci KD, San-

cho ML, Corelli S, Gómez RM. Prevalence and severity of asthma and wheezing in an adolescent population. Int Arch Allergy Immunol 1999; 118:245–246.

8. Sears MR. Epidemiology of childhood asthma. Lancet 1997; 350:1015–20.

9. Baena-Cagnani CE, Patiño CM. Mite allergy in Latin America. In Johansson SGO (Ed), Progress in allergy and clinical immunology, volume 3. Seattle: Hogrefe & Huber 1995, pp. 330–334.

10. Warner JO, Naspitz CK, Cropp GJA. Third International Consensus Statement on the Management of Childhood Asthma. Pediatr Pulmonol 1998; 25:1–17.

11. Sears MR. Descriptive epidemiology of asthma. Lancet 1997; 350 (suppl II): 1–4.

12. Woolcock AJ, Peat JK. Evidence for the increase in asthma worldwide. In Chadwick DJ, Cardew G (Eds), The rising trends in asthma. Ciba Foundation. Chichester: Wiley 1997, pp. 173–189.

13. Ninan TK, Russel G. Respiratory symptoms and atopy in Aberdeen schoolchildren; evidence from two services 25 years apart. Br Med J 1992; 304:1452–1456.

14. Peat JK, van der Berg RH, Green WF, Mellis CM, Leeder SR, Woolcock AJ. Changing prevalence of asthma in Australia children. Br Med J 1994; 308:1591–1596.

15. Hsie K-H, Tsai Y-T. Increasing prevalence of childhood allergic disease in Taipei, Taiwan, and the outcome. In Miyamoto T, Okuda M (Eds), Progress in allergy and clinical immunology, vol. 3. Seattle: Hogrefe & Huber 1992, pp. 223–225.

16. Guidelines for the diagnosis and management of asthma. National Asthma Education Program. US Department of Health and Human Services. National Heart Lung and Blood Institute. NIH. Publ No. 91–3042, 1991.

17. Centers for Disease Control and Prevention. CDC Surveillance Summaries. MMWR 1998; 47 (SS-1):1–27.

18. Woolcock AJ, Peat JK. Definition, classification, epidemiology and risk factors for asthma. In O'Byrne P, Thompson NC (Eds), Manual of asthma management. London: WB Saunders 1995, pp. 3–27.

19. Epidemiology: Prevalence of atopic diseases. European Allergy White Paper. UCB Institute of Allergy. Braine-l'Alleud: UCB Institute of Allergy 1997:14–47.

20. Evidence for an increase of atopic disease and possible causes. Clin Exp Allergy 1993; 23:484–492.

21. Wiesch DG, Samet JM. Epidemiology and natural history of asthma. In Middleton E, Reed CE, Ellis EE, Adkinson NF, Yunginger JW, Busse WW (Eds), Allergy. Principles and practice (5th ed.). St. Louis: Mosby 1999, pp. 799–815.

22. Cockroft DW, Murdock KY, Berscheid BA. Relationship between atopy and bronchial hyperresponsiveness to histamine in random population. Ann Allergy 1984; 53:26–29.

23. Burrows B, Martínez FD, Halonen M, Barbee RA, Cline MG. Association of asthma with serum IgE levels and skin-test reactivity to allergens. N Engl J Med 1989; 320:271–277.

24. Burrows B, Sears MR, Flannery EM, Herbison GP, Holdaway MD. Relations of bronchial responsiveness to allergy skin reactivity, lung function, respiratory symptoms, and diagnoses in 13-year-old New Zealand children. J Allergy Clin Immunol 1995; 95:548–556.

25. Sporik R, Holgate ST, Platts-Mills TAE, Cogswell JJ. Exposure to house-dust mite allergen (Der p I) and the development of asthma in childhood. A prospective study. N Engl J Med 1990; 323:502–507.

26. Martínez FD, Wright AL, Taussig LM, Holberg CJ, Halonen M, Morgan WJ. Asthma and wheezing in the first six years of life. N Engl J Med 1995; 332:133–138.

27. Gruber W, Eber E, Steinbrugger B, Modi M, Weinhandl E, Zach MS. Atopy, lung function and bronchial responsiveness in symptom-free pediatric asthma patients. Eur Respir J 1997; 10:1041–1045.

28. Baena-Cagnani CE, Patiño CM, Neffen HE, Cuello MN. Mite allergen sensitisation and exposure in asthmatic patients in Latin America. Allergy Clin Immunol Int 1999 (in press).

29. Pearce N, Pekkanen J, Beasley R. How much asthma is really attributable to atopy? Thorax 1999; 54:268–272.

30. Martínez FD. Role of viral infections in the inception asthma and allergies during childhood: could they be protective? Thorax 1994; 49:1189–1191.

31. Erb KJ. Atopic disorders: A default pathway in the absence of infection? Immunol Today 1999; 20:317–322.

32. Weiland SK, von Muttius E, Hüsing A. Intake of trans fatty acids and prevalence of childhood asthma and allergies in Europe. Lancet 1999; 353:2040–2041.

33. GINA. Global Initiative for Asthma. Global strategy for asthma management and prevention. NHLBI/WHO Workshop report. NIH Publ No. 95–3659.

Etiologic Agents in Occupational Asthma

Cristina Elisabetta Mapp*

Keywords: Occupational asthma, etiology, allergens, chemicals

To date, about 250 agents have been identified as specific causes of occupational asthma with latency in the workplace. Isocyanates are widely used in many industries and are the leading cause of occupational asthma. The prevalence of isocyanate-induced asthma in exposed workers is nearly 10%. In the last decade, protein allergens in natural rubber latex gloves have emerged as an important cause of work-related respiratory allergic and skin disorders, especially in health-care workers. Agents that cause occupational asthma (OA) are classified as either high-molecular-weight (HMW) agents derived from natural plant and animal sources or as low-molecular-weight (LMW) chemicals. Occupational agents can be subdivided into those that are IgE-dependent and those that are IgE-independent. Asthma induced by these two groups of agents differs in clinical presentation, type of asthmatic reaction induced during inhalation challenge, and characteristics of people at risk. Chlorine and ammonia are the most common occupational agents that can induce occupational asthma without latency. The primary treatment of occupational asthma is strict avoidance of exposure to the sensitizing agent.

About 250 agents can cause occupational asthma [1, 2]. Isocyanates are widely used in many industrial processes and are responsible for many cases of occupational asthma. In the last decade, protein allergens in natural rubber latex gloves have emerged as an important cause of work-related respiratory allergic and skin disorders especially in health-care workers [2]. Agents that cause occupational asthma (OA) with latency (OA develops after a period of exposure that may vary from a few weeks to several years) include natural substances derived from natural plant and animal sources, and chemicals [3]. Some examples are shown in Table 1. These occupational agents can be classified into those that are IgE-dependent and those that are IgE-independent. Asthma induced by these two groups of agents differs in clinical presentation, type of asthmatic reaction induced during inhalation tests, and the characteristics of people at risk [1]. Chlo-

Table 1. Common agents that cause occupational asthma with latency.

Occupational agent	Workers at risk
HMW agents	
Cereals	Bakers, millers
Animal-derived allergens	Laboratory animal handlers
Enzymes	Detergent and pharmaceutical users, bakers
Latex	Health professionals
Gums	Carpet makers, pharmaceutical workers
Seafoods	Seafood processors
LMW agents	
Isocyanates	Spray painters, insulation installers, manufacturers of foam, rubber, plastics
Wood dusts	Forest workers, carpenters, cabinetmakers
Anhydrides	Users of plastics, epoxy resins
Fluxes	Electronic workers
Amines	Solderers, shellac and lacquer handlers
Chloramine-T	Janitors, cleaners
Dyes	Textile workers
Persulfate	Hairdressers
Formaldehyde, glutaraldehyde	Hospital staff
Acrylate	Adhesive handlers
Drugs	Pharmaceuticals workers, health professionals
Metals	Solderers, refiners

rine and ammonia are the most common agents that can induce occupational asthma without latency (OA follows exposure to high concentrations of irritant gases, fumes, or chemicals on one or several occasions) [4]. The mechanisms of induction or sensitization by which occupational agents induce asthma are largely unknown, but are believed to be mainly related to immunologic mechanisms. An immunologic mechanism does not necessarily

* Istituto di Medicina del Lavoro, Universita' degli Studi di Padova, Italy

imply an IgE-mediated immunity, but possibly also cell-mediated immunity and mixed reactions.

Asthma is a complex disease in which both genetic and environmental factors are necessary for the expression of the phenotype [5]. HLA associations have been described in isocyanate-induced asthma [6], in acid anhydride-induced asthma [7], in platinum salts-induced asthma (Newman Taylor A, 1998, personal communication), and in red-cedar-induced asthma [8]. These preliminary studies suggest that major histocompatibility complex (MHC) class II proteins may be important determinants of the specificity of the response to occupational agents.

IgE-dependent occupational asthma is a relevant model of allergic asthma. The responsible agents include HMW agents (> 5000 daltons) and some LMW agents as platinum salts and acid anhydrides. HMW agents include flour, animal proteins, and biologic enzymes. Most HMW agents induce asthma by producing specific IgE antibodies. LMW are usually chemicals, some of which occur naturally, i. e., plicatic acid present in the sap of western red cedar, and they often induce asthma through an IgE-independent mechanism. HMW agents act as complete antigens, whereas LMW agents need to react with autologous or heterologous proteins to produce a complete antigen. The critical cells for airway sensitization are the antigen-presenting cells (APC), especially dendritic cells present in the airway epithelium, which through high- and low-affinity receptors for IgE capture allergens, process them, and after migrating to regional lymph nodes, present selected short peptides of the allergens in the groove of their MHC class II antigens to the T cell receptor. Studies in mice have identified at least two types of activated T helper lymphocytes (Th1 and Th2), and there is evidence that these populations exist in humans as well [9]. In genetically susceptible subjects, antigen presentation to naive CD4+ T cells shifts them to a Th2-like T cell with the ability to secrete cytokines encoded on the interleukin 4 (IL-4) gene cluster present in the long arm of chromosome 5. In IgE-dependent OA, inhaled sensitizing agents bind to specific IgE on the surface of mast cells, basophils, and probably also macrophages, eosinophils and platelets. The specific reaction between antigen and IgE causes a cascade of events which give rise to the activation of inflammatory cells. Preformed and newly generated inflammatory mediators are released, and they orchestrate the inflammatory process [10].

Typically, sensitization to natural HMW agents at work may result in allergic contact urticaria, rhi-nitis, conjunctivitis, and/or asthma. The most common agents are flour-dust allergens affecting bakers and animal protein allergens affecting laboratory animal handlers. Latex-glove protein has emerged as a major allergen in health-care facilities. Sensitized workers are at risk for intraoperative anaphylaxis following mucosal exposure to latex glove proteins during surgical or dental procedures and after ingestion of chestnuts, kiwi, avocados, and bananas because these foods share cross-reactive antigens with latex proteins.

The IgE-dependent mechanism does not explain some types of occupational asthma induced by LMW agents (e. g., isocyanates, red cedar) that occur in nonatopic subjects. Specific IgE antibodies have not been found, or have been found in only few subjects sensitized to isocyanates, and they may be markers of exposure rather than cause of disease [11]. However, sensitivity falls with time from last exposure; to maximize sensitivity, serum for testing should be taken during or within 1 month of exposure to isocyanates [12].

IgE-dependent mechanisms may be involved in nonatopic asthma since a relationship between serum IgE concentrations and asthma prevalence regardless of the atopic status has been described [13], and since an increased number of cells expressing the high-affinity IgE receptor has been found in bronchial biopsies obtained from both atopic and nonatopic asthmatic patients [14].

T cells appear to orchestrate the inflammatory process in occupational and nonoccupational asthma [15]. These cells may also be directly involved in the inflammatory process, since proliferation of peripheral-blood lymphocytes has been reported after stimulation with cobalt, nickel [16], and isocyanates [17] in sensitized subjects.

Pathologic airway changes are similar to those observed in nonoccupational asthma. An increased number of activated eosinophils and T lymphocytes has been found in mucosal and submucosal layers, whereas the increase in mast cells was confined to the epithelium [18]. Similar features have been described in bronchial biopsies from subjects with red-cedar-induced asthma [19]. Airway-wall thickness, edema, hypertrophy of smooth muscle, subepithelial fibrosis, and obstruction of the airway lumen by exudate or mucus have also been described. Recent studies have reported that neutrophils are also important in some types of occupational asthma (asthma-like syndromes), i. e., asthma induced by exposure to grain dust [20]. *In vitro* experiments have shown that extracts of grain dust are able to recruit neutrophils by several mechanisms, including endotoxin-induced and nonendotoxin-induced chemotaxis, activation of complement, and release of alveolar macrophage-derived neutrophilic activity [21]. However, eosinophilia and nonspecific airway hyperresponsiveness, the classical features of asthma, are absent in grain-dust-induced asthma.

The mechanisms of occupational asthma without latency (termed "irritant-induced asthma") are largely unknown. Recently, a retrospective investigation of 86 subjects affected by "irritant-induced asthma" was performed by Brooks and coworkers [22]. Sudden-onset type was similar to the reactive airways dysfunction syndrome (RADS), and symptoms began immediately or within a few hours following an accidental, brief, but massive exposure. The non-sudden-onset type appeared after nonmassive and nonbrief exposure to irritants, and asthmatic symptoms took longer to evolve. In this type of occupational asthma without latency, an interaction between environmental and host factors is likely to occur, since preexisting asthma and atopy are considered risk factors [22]. Pathological airway changes include subepithelial fibrosis with a thickness that can reach 30–40 microns, severe damage of epithelium, infiltration of submucosa by mononuclear cells, few T lymphocytes, and occasionally eosinophils.

In conclusion, in recent years, greater recognition has been attained of etiologic agents as well improved diagnostic tools and better knowledge of the mechanisms and natural history of the disease. It is unlikely that occupational asthma will ever disappear, because new chemicals are continually being introduced into the workplaces. Immunochemical assays that can better quantify exposure to workplace occupational sensitizers are necessary to determine ambient exposure limits required to prevent sensitization and asthmatic symptoms at work. Experimental models which define mechanisms and predict allergenic potential of new occupational agents before their introduction and use in the workplace are also required.

Address for correspondence:

Cristina E Mapp, MD
Istituto di Medicina del Lavoro
Via Giustiniani 2
35128 Padova
Italy

Tel. +39 049 821-2562
Fax +39 049 821-2566
E-mail mapp@ux1.unipd.it

References

1. Chan-Yeung M, Malo JL. Occupational asthma. Review article. N Engl J Med 1995; 333(2):107–112.
2. Bernstein DI. Allergic reactions to workplace allergens. JAMA 1997; 278(22):1907–1913.
3. Chan-Yeung M, Malo JL. Etiologic agents in occupational asthma. Eur Respir J 1994; 7:346–371.
4. Bherer L, Cushman R, Courteau JP, et al. A survey of construction workers repeatedly exposed to chlorine over a three to six months period in a pulpmill: Follow-up of affected workers by questionnaire, spirometry, and assessment of bronchial responsiveness 18 to 24 months after exposure ended. Occup Environ Med 1994; 51:225–228.
5. Barnes KC, Marsh DG. The genetic and complexity of allergy and asthma. Immunol Today 1998; 19:325–332.
6. Balboni A, Baricordi OR, Fabbri LM, et al. Association between toluene diisocyanate-induced asthma and DQB1 markers: A possible role for aspartic acid at position 57. Eur Respir J 1996; 9:207–210.
7. Young RP, Barker RD, Pile KD, Cookson OCM, Newman Taylor AJ. The association of HLA-DR3 with specific IgE to inhaled acid anhydrides. Am J Respir Crit Care Med 1995; 151:219–221.
8. Home C, Quintana PJE, Keown PA, Dimitch-Ward H, Chan-Yeung M. Distribution of HLA class II DQB1 and DRB1 alleles in patients with occupational asthma due to western red cedar. Am J Respir Crit Care Med 1997; 155:A135.
9. Romagnani S. Human Th1 and Th2 subsets doubt no more. Immunol Today 1991; 12:256–257.
10. Bochner BS, Undem BJ, Lichtenstein LM. Immunological aspects of allergic asthma. Annu Rev Immunol 1994; 12:295–355.
11. Frew AJ, Chan H, Dryden P, Salari H, Lam S, Chan-Yeung M. Immunologic studies of the mechanisms of occupational asthma caused by western red cedar. J Allergy Clin Immunol 1993; 92:466–478.
12. Tee RD, Cullinan P, Welch J, Burge PS, Newman Taylor AJ. Specific IgE to isocyanates: A useful diagnostic role in occupational asthma. J Allergy Clin Immunol 1998; 101:709–715.
13. Burrows B, Martinez FD, Halonene M, Barbee RA, Cline MG. Association of asthma with serum IgE levels and skin test reactivity to allergens. N Engl J Med 1989; 320:217–227.

14. Humbert M, Grant JA, Taborda-Barata L, et al. High-affinity IgE receptor (FcεRI)-bearing cells in bronchial biopsies from atopic and nonatopic asthma. Am J Respir Crit Care Med 1996; 153:1931–1937.

15. Kay AB. T cells as orchestrators of the asthmatic response. Ciba Found Symp 1997; 206:56–67.

16. Kusaka Y, Nakano Y, Shirakawa T, Morimoto K. Lymphocyte transformation with cobalt in hard metal asthma. Ind Health 1989; 137:1494–1498.

17. Gallagher JS, Tse CST, Brooks SM, Bernstein IL. Diverse profiles of immunoreactivity in toluene diisocyanate (TDI) asthma. J Occup Med 1981; 23:610–616.

18. Bentley AM, Maestrelli P, Saetta M, et al. Activated T-lymphocytes and eosinophils in the bronchial mucosa in isocyanate-induced asthma. J Allergy Clin Immunol 1992; 89:821–828.

19. Frew A, Chan H, Lam S, Chan-Yeung M. Bronchial inflammation in occupational asthma due to western red cedar. Am J Respir Crit Care Med 1995; 151: 340–344.

20. Parks HS, Jung KS, Hwang SC, Nahm DH, Yim HE. Neutrophil infiltration and release of IL-8 in airway mucosa from subjects with grain dust-induced occupational asthma. Clin Exp Allergy 1998; 28:724–730.

21. Von Essen SG, Robbins RA, Thompson AB, et al. Mechanisms of neutrophil recruitment to the lung by grain dust exposure. Am Rev Respir Dis 1998; 138: 921–927.

22. Brooks MS, Hammad Y, Richards I, Giovinco-Barbas J, Jenkins K. The spectrum of irritant-induced asthma. Sudden and not-so-sudden onset and the role of allergy. Chest 1998; 113:42–49.

Bronchial Challenge Tests with Allergens

PM O'Byrne, LJ Wood, GM Gauvreau*

Keywords: Allergens, airway inflammation, eosinophils, mast cells, cysteinyl leukotrienes, early responses, late responses

Allergen inhalation is an important cause of asthma. The inhalation of allergens by sensitized subjects results in an early asthmatic response, which reaches a maximum within 30 min and generally resolves within 1–3 h. In some subjects, the bronchoconstriction recurs after 3–4 h and reaches a maximum over 6–12 h. This is the late asthmatic response. The early asthmatic response is caused by bronchoconstrictor agonists released from airway mast cells through IgE-mediated mechanisms and also, possibly, from airway eosinophils. The mediators responsible are the cysteinyl leukotrienes, histamines, and stimulatory prostaglandins. Evidence is also available to support a role for cysteinyl leukotrienes in the pathogenesis of the late response. Allergen-induced airway hyperresponsiveness and airway inflammation may also be mediated, in part, by cysLTs. The late response is associated with increased numbers of airway eosinophils and metachromatic cells, associated with increases in circulating eosinophil progenitors measured as colony forming units (Eo/B CFU), 24 h after inhaled allergen. After allergen inhalation, signals are sent from the airways to the bone marrow (possibly IL-5), which increases production of Eo/B progenitors, by acting on progenitors more responsive to IL-5, thereby making more cells available to be recruited into the airways. The use of the late asthmatic response as a laboratory model to study the pathogenesis of asthma does have limitations. However, despite these limitations, it is likely that much of the morbidity suffered by allergic asthmatics is a consequence of allergen-induced airway inflammation.

Introduction

The observation that allergen inhalation can cause symptoms of asthma, which can last several days was originally made more than 100 years ago by Blackley [1], who was investigating his own allergy to grass pollen. The first thorough description of the airway responses to inhaled allergen was make by Herxheimer [2] in the early 1950s, who identified two distinct components to the response to inhaled allergen, which he called the immediate and late reactions. The first studies on the pathogenesis of allergen-induced airway responses were undertaken in the late 1960s [3]. Also, about this time Altounyan [4] described another important consequence of the inhalation of allergen, in that exposure to grass pollen during the grass pollen season could increase airway responsiveness to inhaled histamine in sensitized subjects. Subsequently, Cockcroft and coworkers [5] demonstrated that the increase in histamine and methacholine responsiveness that occurs after inhaled allergen, occurs in association with the allergen-induced late asthmatic response.

Allergen-Induced Asthmatic Responses

The inhalation of allergens by sensitized subjects will result in an early asthmatic response, identified as bronchoconstriction developing within 10–15 min of the inhalation, which reaches a maximum within 30 min and generally resolves within 1–3 h (Figure 1). In some subjects, the bronchoconstriction persists and either does not return to baseline values or recurs after 3–4 h and reaches a maximum over 6–12 h. This is the late asthmatic response (Figure 1). The late asthmatic response need not necessarily be preceded by a clinically evident early response. Thus, in a subset of sensitized subjects, the inhaled antigen does not cause an early

* Asthma Research Group, St. Joseph's Hospital and the Department of Medicine, McMaster University, Hamilton, Ontario, Canada

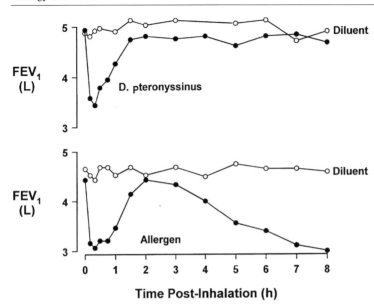

Figure 1. An isolated early asthmatic response following inhalation of house dust mite extract *(D. pteronyssinus)* (upper panel). An early followed by a late asthmatic response following inhalation of house dust mite (lower panel). The control measurements (open circles) are made after inhalation of the diluent alone. The measurements made after allergen inhalation (closed circles) are made at the same time points as the control measurements.

response, but is followed 3 to 8 h later by a late asthmatic response (isolated late response).

The late asthmatic response has been described to occur in approximately 50% of adults [6], and between 70–85% of children [7] who develop an early asthmatic response. The explanation for the apparently higher prevalence in children is not known. Whether the development of a late asthmatic response is dependent on the individual's response to the allergen or also on which allergen is inhaled is unclear.

The Pathogenesis of the Early Asthmatic Response

The early asthmatic response is caused by bronchoconstrictor agonists released from airway inflammatory cells following allergen inhalation. The release of these mediators is from airway mast cells through IgE-mediated mechanisms and also, possibly, from airway eosinophils. The mediators responsible have been clarified over the past 10 years as being the cysteinyl leukotrienes, histamine and stimulatory prostaglandins (PGD_2 and thromboxane).

The cysteinyl leukotrienes are eicosanoids, derived from the cell membrane phospholipid constituent arachidonic acid, which is selectively cleaved by phospholipase A_2 from cell membranes. Arach-

idonic acid is converted sequentially to 5-hydroperoxyeicosatetraenoic acid (5-HPETE) and then to leukotriene (LT)A_4 by a catalytic complex consisting of 5-lipoxygenase (5-LO) and the 5-lipoxygenase activating protein (FLAP). In the presence of leukotriene C_4 synthase, glutathione is adducted at the C6 position of LTA$_4$ to yield the molecule known as LTC$_4$, which is exported from the cytosol to the extracellular microenvironment where the glutamic acid moiety is cleaved by γ-glutamyltranspeptidase to form LTD$_4$. Cleavage of the glycine moiety from LTD$_4$ by a variety of dipeptidases results in the formation of LTE$_4$. LTC$_4$, LTD$_4$, and LTE$_4$ constitute the material formerly known as SRS-A. All three cysteinyl leukotrienes have the same range of biological effects; however, LTE$_4$ is much less potent than its precursor molecules. Among the cells in the lung that possess the enzymatic activities to produce the cysteinyl leukotrienes are mast cells eosinophils and alveolar macrophages.

There is, now, compelling information which implicates the cysteinyl leukotrienes as mediators of the allergen-induced early response. Increased production of the cysteinyl leukotrienes, as measured by increases in urinary excretion of LTE$_4$ has been demonstrated after allergen inhalation [8, 9]. Treatment with drugs which inhibit the synthesis of the cysteinyl leukotrienes or block the Cys LT$_1$ receptor, which mediates the action of the cysteinyl leukotrienes in the airways, markedly attenuates the early response by up to 80% [10, 11] (Figure 2). The residual component of the bronchoconstriction during the early response is caused by histamine [12] released from mast cells and by thromboxane A_2 [13]. An isolated early response is not associated with marked increases in airway eosinophils [14] or prolonged changes in airway hyperresponsiveness [15].

The Pathogenesis of the Late Asthmatic Response

The factors which might predict the development of a late asthmatic response have been examined by several investigators [16–18]. These were mainly indices of high circulating IgE antibody to the inhaled allergen, such as a high IgE RAST with the allergen and a low antigen concentration in the skin eliciting a late cutaneous response. Boulet et al. [17] have also demonstrated that if a late cutaneous response followed a small early cutaneous response (wheal < 5 mm), then a late asthmatic response was more likely to occur after an early response. Thus, an important determinant of whether an individual will develop a late asthmatic response is the level of circulating IgE antibody, which maybe considered the degree of sensitization against the allergen. The other major determinant of the late asthmatic response is the size of the early response [19]. Thus, the greater the degree of airway narrowing during the early response the more likely a late response will develop. As with the early response, the late response appears to be IgE mediated. Several in-

vestigators have demonstrated that the development of a late asthmatic response is related to high levels of allergen specific serum IgE [17, 18]. Also, Kirby et al. [20] have shown that inhaled anti-IgE caused late asthmatic responses.

Inflammatory Cells and the Late Response

The late response is associated with increased numbers of airway eosinophils and metachromatic cells. De Monchy et al. [14] performed BAL during the late asthmatic response 6–7 h after inhaling allergen and showed that numbers of eosinophils were increased in lavage fluid, with no significant change in any other cell type, including neutrophils. Metzger et al. described increases in eosinophils, neutrophils and lymphocytes 48 h after local allergen into the airways [21] A more recent focus has been the examination of the state of activation of the inflammatory cells after allergen inhalation. These studies have identified that eosinophils are activated, as indicated by increased levels of eosinophil cationic protein (ECP) and positive staining for the marker for cleaved ECP (EG2), as early as 3 h and persisted for more than 24 h in BAL after allergen inhalation and this change preceded the increase in total number of eosinophils after allergen inhalation [22].

More recently, a less invasive method than bronchoscopy has been developed, using sputum induced by the inhalation of hypertonic saline, to quantify and characterize inflammatory cells in

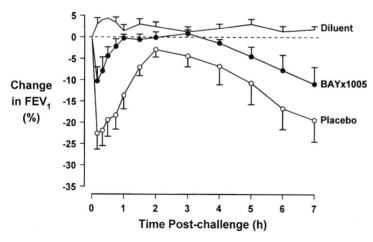

Change in FEV_1 (%)

Time Post-challenge (h)

Figure 2. Mean (± SEM) percent change in FEV_1 from baseline during the early and late asthmatic response to allergen inhalation after treatment with the leukotriene synthesis inhibitor, BAYx1005 (●) and placebo (○) and after inhaled diluent. * $p < 0.05$; ** $p < 0.001$. (Reproduced with permission from [11].)

223

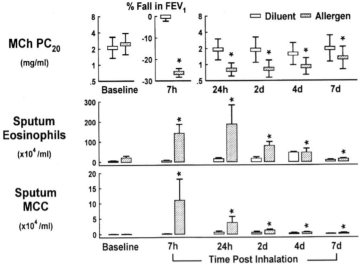

Figure 3. Increases in sputum eosinophils and metachromatic cells followed for 7 days after inhaled allergen in subjects who have developed allergen-induced dual asthmatic responses and methacholine airway hyperresponsiveness. The increases in metachromatic cells were maximal 7 h after inhaled allergen, while the increases in eosinophils were maximal 24 h after allergen. (Reproduced with permission from [23].)

asthmatic airways. Studies using this method have demonstrated that eosinophils increase markedly in sputum samples as early as 7 h after allergen inhalation, and which can persist for up to 7 days after allergen [23] (Figure 3). Also increases in airway metachromatic cells occur after allergen inhalation, which are most marked 7 h after inhalation [23]. The late response is also associated with an increased number of airway eosinophils immunopositive for the eosinophil chemoattractant chemokines eotaxin and RANTES and for interleukin (IL)-5 [23].

These increases in airway eosinophils and metachromatic cells are associated with increases in circulating eosinophil progenitors measured as colony forming units (Eo/B CFU), 24 h after inhaled allergen [24], suggesting the inhaled allergen stimulates bone marrow production of these progenitors. This has recently been confirmed in a study where bone marrow progenitors were directly measured in bone marrow aspirated 24 h after allergen inhalation in mild asthmatic subjects [25]. This study demonstrated an increased responsiveness of the bone marrow to IL-5 after allergen, which was associated with an increased expression of the IL-5 receptor on the progenitors [26]. Taken together, these studies suggest that after allergen inhalation, signals are sent from the airways to the bone marrow (possibly IL-5), which increases production of Eo/B progenitors, by acting on progenitors more responsive to IL-5, thereby making more cells available to be recruited into the airways.

The allergen-induced influx of airway eosinophils and metachromatic cells into the airways can occur independent of late responses. Using a more recently developed method for allergen inhalation in the laboratory, which is repeated low dose challenge over 5 days, marked increases in both eosinophils and metachromatic cells were demonstrated in the airways with a clinically important late response developing [27]. These changes were, however, associated with increases in airway hyperresponsiveness.

Mediators and the Late Response

The bronchoconstrictor mediators mainly responsible for the late responses have been clarified. Considerable evidence is also available to support a role for cysteinyl leukotrienes in the pathogenesis of the late response. Pre-treatment with specific $cysLT_1$ receptor antagonists [10, 28] and LT biosynthesis inhibitors [11] have been shown to partially attenuate the late response by approximately 50% (Figure 2). As with the early response, the residual bronchoconstriction not attenuated by anti-leukotrienes, is likely mediated by histamine release [12].

Allergen-induced airway hyperresponsiveness and airway inflammation may also be mediated, in part, by cysLTs. Pretreatment with the $cysLT_1$

antagonist, Pranlukast, significantly reduced allergen-induced methacholine airway hyperresponsiveness [28]. Also, the $cysLT_1$ antagonist, Zifurlukast, reduced allergen-induced increases in airway inflammatory cells [29].

Taken together, these studies have demonstrated that allergen inhalation by sensitized subjects causes histamine and cysLT release from airway mast cells resulting in the EAR. Also, as a consequence of the EAR, eosinophils and mast cells or basophils, are attracted into the airways and activated. This results in further release of histamine and the cysLTs, causing the LAR. Also, the bone marrow increases its responsiveness to IL-5, which causes increases in eosinophil and basophil production, which propagates the inflammatory response.

Conclusions

It has now been clearly demonstrated that allergic responses in the airways has both an acute and a prolonged component, which, in most instances, is more important clinically and more difficult to treat than the early, relatively short-lived component of these reactions. By focusing on the late responses, in the airways, the importance of airway inflammation in causing both late asthmatic responses and the increases in airway responsiveness after inhaled allergen has become clear. This, in turn, has identified the need to use anti-inflammatory drugs, such as corticosteroids, in treating exacerbations of asthma after exposure to inflammatory stimuli, such as inhaled allergen.

The use of the late asthmatic response as a laboratory model to study the pathogenesis of asthma does have limitations. For example, in many instances airway hyperresponsiveness and asthma are present in subjects who are not allergic to any identifiable allergen. In addition, inhalation of allergen or occupational exposure to a sensitizer can occasionally increase airway responsiveness without a measurable late response occurring. However, despite these limitations, it is likely that much of the morbidity suffered by allergic asthmatics is a consequence of airway inflammation, which is manifest in many subjects as a late asthmatic response. Therefore, continuing studies of the late response is likely to improve our understanding of the pathophysiology of asthma.

Address for correspondence:

PM O'Byrne
Firestone Regional Chest and Allergy Unit
St. Joseph's Hospital
50 Charlton Ave East
Hamilton, Ontario L8N 4A6
Canada
Tel. +1 905 521-6115 ext. 3694
Fax +1 905 521-6125
E-mail obyrnep@fhs.mcmaster.ca

References

1. Blackley CH. On the quantity of pollen found floating in the atmosphere during the prevalence of hay fever and its relationship to the intensity of the symptoms. In Anonymous, Experimental researches on the causes and nature of catarrus aestivus. London: Balliere, Tindell, Cox 1873.

2. Herxheimer H. The late bronchial reaction in induced asthma. Arch Allergy 1952; 3:323–328.

3. Booij-Noord H, Vries Kd, Sluiter HJ, Orie NG. Late bronchial obstructive reaction to experimental inhalation of house dust extract. Clin Allergy 1972; 2:43–61.

4. Altounyan REC. Changes in histamine and atropine responsiveness as a guide to the diagnosis and evaluation of therapy in obstructive airways disease. In J Pepys, AW Frankland (Eds), Disodium cromoglycate in allergic airways disease. London, UK: Butterworth and Co. 1970, pp. 47–53.

5. Cockcroft DW, Murdock KY. Changes in bronchial responsiveness to histamine at intervals after allergen challenge. Thorax 1987; 42:302–308.

6. Robertson DG, Kerigan AT, Hargreave FE, Dolovich J. Late asthmatic responses induced by ragweed pollen allergen. J Allergy Clin Immunol 1974; 54:244–254.

7. Price JF, Hey EN, Soothill JF. Antigen provocation to the skin, nose and lung, in children with asthma; immediate and dual hypersensitivity reactions. Clin Exp Immunol 1991; 143:998–1001.

8. Taylor GW, Black P, Turner N, Taylor I, Maltby NH, Fuller RW, et al. Urinary leukotriene E4 after antigen challenge and in acute asthma and allergic rhinitis. Lancet 1989; i:585–587.

9. Manning PJ, Rokach J, Malo JL, Ethier D, Cartier A, Girard Y, et al. Urinary leukotriene E4 levels during early and late asthmatic responses. J Allergy Clin Immunol 1990; 86:211–220.

10. Taylor IK, O'Shaughnessy KM, Fuller RW, Dollery CT. Effect of a cysteinyl leukotriene receptor antag-

onst, ICI 204–219 on allergen-induced bronchoconstriction and airway hyperactivity in atopic subjects. Lancet 1991; 337:690–694.

11. Hamilton AL, Watson RM, Wyile G, O'Byrne PM. A 5-lipoxygenase activating protein antagonist, Bay 1005, attenuates both early and late phase allergen-induced bronchoconstriction in asthmatic subjects. Thorax 1997; 52:348–354.

12. Roquet A, Dahlen B, Kumlin M, Ihre E, Aanstren G, Binks S, et al. Combined antagonist of leukotrienes and histamine produces predominant inhibition of allergen-induced early and late phase airway obstruction in asthmatics. Am J Respir Crit Care Med 1997; 155:1856–1863.

13. Manning PJ, Stevens WH, Cockcroft DW, O'Byrne PM. The role of thromboxane in allergen-induced asthmatic responses. Eur Respir J 1991; 4:667–672.

14. de Monchy JG, Kauffman HF, Venge P, Koeter GH, Jansen HM, Sluiter HJ, et al. Bronchoalveolar eosinophilia during allergen-induced late asthmatic reactions. Am Rev Respir Dis 1985; 131:373–376.

15. Cartier A, Thomson NC, Frith PA, Roberts R, Hargreave FE. Allergen-induced increase in bronchial responsiveness to histamine: Relationship to the late asthmatic response and change in airway caliber. J Allergy Clin Immunol 1982; 70:170–177.

16. Crimi E, Brusasco V, Losurdo E, Crimi P. Predictive accuracy of late asthmatic reaction to *Dermatophagoides pteronyssinus*. J Allergy Clin Immunol 1986; 78:908–913.

17. Boulet LP, Roberts RS, Dolovich J, Hargreave FE. Prediction of late asthmatic responses to inhaled allergen. Clin Allergy 1984; 14:379–385.

18. Cockcroft DW, Ruffin RE, Frith PA, Cartier A, Juniper EF, Dolovich J, et al. Determinants of allergen-induced asthma: Dose of allergen, circulating IgE antibody concentration, and bronchial responsiveness to inhaled histamine. Am Rev Respir Dis 1979; 120:1053–1058.

19. Hargreave FE, Dolovich J, Robertson DG, Kerigan AT. The late asthmatic response. Can Med Assoc J 1974; 110:415–424.

20. Kirby JG, Robertson DG, Hargreave FE, Dolovich J. Asthmatic responses to inhalation of anti-human IgE. Clin Allergy 1986; 16:191–194.

21. Metzger WJ, Richerson HB, Worden K, Monick M,

Hunninghake GW. Bronchoalveolar lavage of allergic asthmatic patients following allergen bronchoprovocation. Chest 1986; 89:477–483.

22. Aalbers R, Kauffman HF, Smith M, Koeter GH, Timens W, de Monchy JG. Allergen-induced recruitment of inflammatory cells 3 h and 24 h after allergen challenge. Am Rev Respir Dis 1992; 145:A20 Abstract.

23. Gauvreau GM, Watson RM, O'Byrne PM. Kinetics of allergen-induced airway eosinophilic cytokine production and airway inflammation. Am J Respir Crit Care Med 1999; in press.

24. Gibson PG, Manning PJ, O'Byrne PM, Girgis-Gabardo A, Dolovich J, Denburg JA, et al. Allergen-induced asthmatic responses. Relationship between increases in airway responsiveness and increases in circulating eosinophils, basophils, and their progenitors. Am Rev Respir Dis 1991; 143:331–335.

25. Wood LJ, Inman MD, Watson RM, Denburg JA, Foley J, O'Byrne PM. Bone marrow inflammatory progenitor cells after allergen inhalation in asthmatic subjects. Am J Respir Crit Care Med 1998; 157:99–105.

26. Sehmi R, Woods L, Watson RM, Foley R, Hamid Q, O'Byrne PM, et al. Allergen-induced increases in IL-5 a subunit expression on bone marrow derived CD34[+] cells from asthmatic subjects: A novel marker of progenitor cell commitment towards eosinophil differentiation. J Clin Invest 1997; 100:2466–2475.

27. Sulakvelidze I, Inman MD, Rerecich TJ, O'Byrne PM. Increases in airway eosinophils and interleukin-5 with minimal bronchoconstriction during repeated low dose allergen challenge in atopic asthmatics. Eur Resp J 1998; 11:821–827.

28. Hamilton AL, Faiferman I, Stober P, Watson RM, O'Byrne PM. Pranlukast, a leukotriene receptor antagonist, attenuates allergen-induced early and late phase bronchoconstriction and airway hyperresponsiveness in asthmatic subjects. J Allergy Clin Immunol 1998; 102:177–183.

29. Calhoun WJ, Lavins BJ, Minkwitz MC, Evans R, Gleich GJ, Cohn J. Effect of Zafirlukast (Accolate) on cellular mediators of inflammation: Bronchoalveolar lavage fluid findings after segmental allergen challenge. Am J Respir Crit Care Med 1998; 157:1381–1389.

Virus-Induced Asthma

William W Busse*

Keywords: Asthma, respiratory viruses, asthma exacerbations

Viral respiratory infections are the major cause of asthma exacerbatons. Of the respiratory viruses associated with these asthma exacerbations, the common cold virus, rhinovirus, is the most frequent cause. To determine the mechanisms by which rhinoviruses cause an increase in asthma, subjects have been inoculated with live rhinoviruses. From these studies, rhinovirus inoculations have been shown to increase airway inflammation. Thus, respiratory viruses, like rhinovirus, appear to increase asthma severity by enhancing airway inflammation.

Respiratory viruses can have two major effects on airway function and asthma. In children, respiratory infections with respiratory syncytial virus or parainfluenza virus can cause episodes of wheezing. These wheezing episodes are usually associated with the first infection. Although recurrent episodes of wheezing can occur in these children, the frequency with which this occurs and the likelihood that this leads to asthma has yet to be established.

In individuals with existing asthma, respiratory infections are major causes of exacerbations. In this situation, epidemiological studies have indicated that the common cold virus, rhinovirus, is the respiratory infection most commonly associated with these episodes. The discussion that follows will focus on the role of rhinovirus infections and exacerbations of asthma.

Epidemiology

For children or adults with asthma, respiratory viruses are the most frequent cause of asthma exacerbations [1–3]. Initial studies designed to establish the relationship between respiratory infections and asthma used culture of respiratory secretions to identify the causative pathogen. Since these techniques are relatively insensitive, early assessments of the frequency by which respiratory viruses caused asthma were likely an underestimate.

In a seminal study by Johnston and colleagues [2], nasal secretions were obtained from 9-to-11-year-old children over a 13-month period of time. In this cohort of children, the investigators were able to identify respiratory infections in association with asthma exacerbations in approximately 80% to 85% of this school-aged population of children. Using PCR techniques, the most commonly detected virus was rhinovirus. In adults, the frequency with which rhinovirus has been associated with episodes of asthma has been somewhat less but is, nonetheless, still the major cause of acute wheezing [3].

These and other studies have indicated the importance of respiratory infections, particularly rhinovirus, as the major cause of asthma exacerbations. With the use of PCR to identify viruses, a more accurate relationship of viral infections to asthma has been defined and the importance of rhinovirus infections to acute wheezing episodes established.

Mechanisms of Rhinovirus-Induced Asthma

There is considerable evidence that airway inflammation is a major component and factor in the pathogenesis of asthma. Therefore, considerable effort has been directed to understand how rhinovirus infections of the upper airway can cause lower airway dysfunction in patients with asthma. A number of studies have used experimental inoculation with rhinovirus of patients with allergic disease and asthma and evaluated the effects of these infections upon airway dysfunction.

In an initial study, Lemanske and colleagues [4] identified 10 patients with allergic rhinitis, and

*   University of Wisconsin, Madison, WI, USA

inoculated them with rhinovirus. The effects of this experimental illness on airway responsiveness and the airway response to antigen were assessed. These investigators found that rhinovirus upper respiratory tract infection increased airway responsiveness and also the frequency with which late-phase allergic reactions occurred. These observations raised the possibility that the respiratory infection enhanced the likelihood of allergic inflammation and hence the possibility of more severe asthma.

In a subsequent study by Calhoun and colleagues [5], bronchoscopy with segmental antigen challenge was performed prior to and during an experimental rhinovirus infection. In these studies, the investigators found an increase in eosinophil recruitment to the airway following antigen challenge at the time of the respiratory infection. Furthermore, the enhanced recruitment of eosinophils following antigen challenge persisted for 4–6 weeks after the infection. Therefore, the possibility exists that there is an increased recruitment of eosinophils during the respiratory infection, and that this enhanced recruitment may account for the development of the late phase allergic reaction. Moreover, Fraenkel and colleagues [6] evaluated the effect of rhinovirus infection on mucosal inflammation with the use of bronchial biopsy. These investigators found that rhinovirus infection caused an increase in cellular inflammation, principally eosinophils and neutrophils. During the acute infection, the presence of inflammation was noted both in normal and allergic subjects; however, in the allergic subjects, eosinophilic inflammation persisted for a longer period of time.

The above data indicate that rhinovirus infections increase a number of factors that are associated with airway inflammation, principally the development of late-phase, allergic reaction and also the recruitment of inflammatory cells to the airway. Given these observations, it is important to determine how rhinovirus infections can affect events in the lower airway and lead to increased inflammation.

Epithelial cells

The epithelial cell is the principal host cell for rhinovirus infection, and the degree of rhinovirus replication in the epithelial cell strongly influences the severity of symptoms with a cold [7]. Using *in vitro* techniques, a number of investigators have evalu-

ated the effect of inoculating epithelial cells, or epithelial cell lines, with rhinovirus. Rhinovirus inoculation causes the generation of a wide variety of cytokines, including IL-1β, IL-6, IL-8, IL-11, tumor necrosis factor-α, RANTES and GM-CSF [8–13]. If these events were to occur *in vivo*, one would have an adequate explanation for the change in the inflammatory milieu in the lower airway, i. e., an increase in the presence of these proinflammatory mediators would enhance the function of inflammatory cells.

To extend some of these observations to the *in vivo* situation, Einarsson and colleagues [9] measured the effect of respiratory infections on IL-11 levels in nasal secretions. These investigators found higher levels of IL-11 in patients who experienced wheezing with the respiratory infection. This is of particular interest as IL-11 may promote the development of airway hyperresponsiveness.

In addition, Grünberg and colleagues [14] analyzed nasal secretions of volunteers with allergic asthma who were given an experimental infection with rhinovirus 16. These investigators found an increase in IL-8 in nasal secretion of subjects inoculated with the respiratory virus. Furthermore, the quantity of IL-8 generated correlated with the subjects' cold symptoms and asthma symptom scores and changes in airway responsiveness. Thus, from *in vivo* and *in vitro* observations, present data indicate that epithelial cells can be infected with rhinovirus and as a consequence generate a wide variety of proinflammatory mediators, which can promote the inflammatory capacity of cells in the airway.

Macrophages. Airway macrophages are also likely to be involved in the host response to respiratory virus. These cells express ICAM-1 on their cell surface and bind rhinovirus *in vitro* [15, 16]. Furthermore, these cells can secrete a variety of cytokines when macrophages interact with rhinovirus, including IL-1, TNF-α, and interferon-α [15, 16]. Nasal secretions of volunteers infected with respiratory virus have been shown to contain IL-1 [17, 18]. Whether cytokines sicj as IL-1 arise from epithelium or from macrophages is not defined.

T-lymphocytes

Lymphocytes are also a potential source for cytokines during infections. Evidence to suggest that these cells play a role in the acute response to infections is work in progress. However, it is unlikely that these cells contribute significantly to the acute generation of the inflammatory response seen early during the infection. T-cell responses usually require 7–10 days to express themselves following a virus infection. There is usually an acute fall in circulating lymphocytes during a cold, and it is assumed they are recruited to the airway [19]. The role of T lymphocytes in rhinovirus-induced asthma awaits further study [20].

Summary

Respiratory infections are a profound factor in asthma exacerbations. Evidence at the present time suggests that rhinoviruses are the principal respiratory virus associated with asthma exacerbations. To define the mechanisms associated with these responses, evidence has indicated that this virus interacts with epithelial cells as the primary host. Following this, a variety of cytokines are generated which then changes the inflammatory environment in the airway and promotes the likelihood of allergic inflammation. Interestingly, the regulation of this response by current therapeutics has not been as successful as that noted with asthma following allergic driven processes. Therefore, although corticosteroids will provide some benefit in virus-provoked asthma, other modalities may prove to be more effective.

Address for correspondence:

William W Busse
Department of Medicine
Allergy/Clinical Immunology
H6/367 Clinical Science Center
600 Highland Avenue
Madison, WI 53792-3244
USA
Tel. +1 608 263-6183
Fax +1 608 263-3104
E-mail wwb@medicine.wisc.edu

References

1. Busse WW, Gern JE. Viruses in asthma. J Allergy Clin Immunol 1997; 100:147–150.

2. Johnston SL, Pattemore PK, Sanderson G, Smith S, Lampe F, Josephs L, Symington P, O'Toole S, Myint SH, Tyrrell DA, Holgate ST. Community study of role of viral infections in exacerbations of asthma in 9–11 year old children. Br Med J 1995; 310:1225–1229.

3. Nicholson KG, Kent J, Ireland DC. Respiratory viruses and exacerbations of asthma in adults. Br Med J 1993; 307:982–986.

4. Lemanske RF Jr, Dick EC, Swenson CA, Vrtis RF, Busse WW. Rhinovirus upper respiratory infection increases airway hyperreactivity and late asthmatic reactions. J Clin Invest 1989; 83:1–10.

5. Calhoun WJ, Dick EC, Schwartz LB, Busse WW. A common cold virus, rhinovirus 16, potentiates airway inflammation after segmental antigen bronchoprovocation in allergic subjects. J Clin Invest 1994; 94:2200–2208.

6. Fraenkel DJ, Bardin PG, Sanderson G, Lampe F, Johnston SL, Holgate ST. Lower airway inflammation during rhinovirus colds in normal and in asthmatic subjects. Am J Respir Crit Care Med 1995; 151:879–886.

7. Gern JE, Calhoun WJ, Swenson C, Shen G, Busse WW. Rhinovirus infection preferentially increases lower airway responsiveness in allergic subjects. Am J Respir Crit Care Med 1997; 155:1872–1876.

8. Dicosmo BF, Geba GP, Picarella D, Elias JA, Rankin JA, Stripp BR, Whitsett JA, Flavell RA. Airway epithelial cell expression of interleukin-6 in transgenic mice – uncoupling of airway inflammation and bronchial hyperreactivity. J Clin Invest 1994; 94:2028–2035.

9. Einarsson O, Geba GP, Zhu Z, Landry M, Elias JA. Interleukin-11: stimulation *in vivo* and *in vitro* by respiratory viruses and induction of airway hyperresponsiveness. J Clin Invest 1996; 97:915–924.

10. Garofalo R, Mei F, Espejo R, Ye G, Haeberle H, Baron S, Ogra PL, Reyes VE. Respiratory syncytial virus infection of human respiratory epithelial cells up-regulates class I MHC expression through the induction of IFN-β and IL-1 α. J Immunol 1996; 157:2506–2513.

11. Johnston SL, Papi A, Bates PJ, Mastronarde JG, Monick MM, Hunninghake GW. Low grade rhinovirus infection induces a prolonged release of IL-8 in pulmonary epithelium. J Immunol 1998; 160:6172–6181.

12. Stellato C, Beck LA, Gorgone GA, Proud D, Schall TJ, Ono SJ, Lichtenstein LM, Schleimer RP. Expression of the chemokine RANTES by a human bronchial epithelial cell line. J Immunol 1995; 155:410–418.

13. Terajima M, Yamaya M, Sekizawa K, Okinaga S, Suzuki T, Yamada N, Nakayama K, Ohrui T, Oshima T, Numazaki Y, Sasaki H. Rhinovirus infection of primary cultures of human tracheal epithelium: role of ICAM-1 and IL-1β. Am J Physiol 1997; 273:L749-L759.

14. Grünberg K, Timmers MC, Smits HH, De Klerk EPA, Dick EC, Spaan WJM, Hiemstra PS, Sterk PJ. Effect of experimental rhinovirus 16 colds on airway hyperresponsiveness to histamine and interleukin-8 in nasal lavage in asthmatic subjects *in vivo*. Clin Exp Allergy 1997; 27:36–45.

15. Gern JE, Dick EC, Lee WM, Murray S, Meyer K, Handzel ZT, Busse WW. Rhinovirus enters but does not replicate inside monocytes and airway macrophages. J Immunol 1996; 156:621–627.

16. Hayden FG, Albrecht JK, Kaiser DL, Gwaltney JM Jr. Prevention of natural colds by contact prophylaxis with intranasal α_2-interferon. N Engl J Med 1986; 314:71–75.

17. Noah TL, Henderson FW, Wortman IA, Devlin RB, Handy J, Koren HS, Becker S. Nasal cytokine production in viral acute upper respiratory infection of childhood. J Infect Dis 1995; 171:584–592.

18. Proud D, Gwaltney JM Jr, Hendley JO, Dinarello CA, Gillis S, Schleimer RP. Increased levels of interleukin-1 are detected in nasal secretions of volunteers during experimental rhinovirus colds. J Infect Dis 1994; 169:1007–1013.

19. Levandowski RA, Ou DW, Jackson GG. Acute-phase decrease of T lymphocyte subsets in rhinovirus infection. J Infect Dis 1986; 153:743–748.

20. Gern JE, Busse WW. Role of T cells in virus-induced asthma. In Liggett SB, Meyers DA (Eds), The genetics of asthma. New York: Marcel Dekker, 1996, pp. 39–66.

Asthma Mortality in Latin America

HE Neffen*, CE Baena-Cagnani**

Keywords: Asthma mortality, Latin America, LASAI

During the 1980s, the Latin American Society of Allergy and Immunology coordinated a multicenter study to provide reliable data for gaining of knowledge about the present situation in Latin America. The following countries participated in this study: Argentina, Brazil, Chile, Colombia, Costa Rica, Cuba, Ecuador, Mexico, Paraguay, Peru, Uruguay, and Venezuela. Asthma mortality rates were analyzed in accordance with two variables: Age-adjusted rates (5–34) and total death rates through a uniform protocol. The total population studied was 117,624,058 inhabitants. The highest death rate was found in Uruguay and Mexico (5.63), and the lowest in Paraguay (0.8) and Colombia (1.35). Age-adjusted (5–34) rates were higher in Costa Rica (1.38) and lower in Chile (0.28). In the southern Latin American countries such us Chile, Uruguay, Paraguay, and Argentina, which have marked climatic differences, deaths occurred mainly in the winter. It is important to emphasize that in most countries deaths from asthma occurred at home: Chile (60.7%), Argentina (63.4%) and Paraguay (88%). However, in Uruguay, 58.6% occurred during hospitalization. In Argentina during 1990–1997, asthma mortality, both global and age-adjusted, rates showed a gradual decreasing tendency, especially from 1992 onwards, reaching the following values in 1997: 1.76 and 0.20, with mean values in the 1990–1997 period being 2.80 and 0.43, respectively, and thus lower than in the 1980s (3.38 and 0.61). Concomitantly, it is important to analyze the changes in total antiasthmatic drug sales in Argentina that show a 52.2% reduction in xantine, an increase of 25.6% in inhaled β_2 agonists, a reduction of 52.04% in oral β_2 agonists, and an increase of 308.7% in inhaled steroids. This situation may be related to the fourfold increase in the use of inhaled corticosteroid therapy in Argentina. Changes in asthma mortality should be especially sensitive to changes in the quality of management. For this reason, we are disseminating guidelines for asthma management and prevention around the country to implement them at public and private health-care providers in order to consolidate the decreasing tendency in asthma mortality and improve the patient quality of life.

Introduction

Asthma-related deaths continue despite the substantial advances achieved in our knowledge of this disease, and the availability of improved pharmacotherapy for treating it.

Mortality rates will help us to reconsider the importance of asthma, analyze its causes, and implement therapeutic measures to reduce them since bronchial asthma can be fatal at any age. During the last decade there was a progressive increase in asthma-related mortality rates in the United States [1, 2, 3], as well as in Canada, France, Great Britain, Australia, and New Zealand [4, 5]. Such an increase in mortality rates also correlated with increased hospitalizations due to bronchial asthma, which have lead to higher morbidity and mortality of the disease [6, 7].

More recently a gradual decrease of asthma mortality rates has been observed in several other countries such as Australia, Canada, West Germany, England, and Wales [8]. Global rates have been stable in the United States during the 1990s, at a level 50% higher than in 1979, implying that factors involved in the previous rise are still active [9].

There was a lack of data concerning asthma mortality in Latin America until the publication of a multicenter study coordinated by the Latin-American Society of Allergy and Immunology [10]. This work has provided reliable data for gaining of knowledge about our present situation, which is an indispensable prerequisite to changing it.

Latin America in the 1980s

The following countries participated in the above-mentioned multicenter study: Argentina, Brazil, Chile, Colombia, Costa Rica, Cuba, Mexico,

* Head Allergology Unit, "R. Gutiérrez" Children's Hospital, Santa Fe, Argentina
** Head, Division of Allergy, Pulmonology and Immunology, Municipal Infantile Hospital, Córdoba, Argentina

Table 1. Asthma mortality in Latin America. Population studied: 117,624,058.

Country	Rate x	Age-adjusted 5 / 34 x	Town/country	No. surveyed	Period
Argentina	3.38	0.68	Country	32,470,000	1980/1989
Brazil	2.04	0.48	Sao Paulo City	9,466,701	1980/1991
Chile	1.80	0.28	Country	13,473,347	1980/1990
Colombia	1.35	0.33	Atlantico-Bolivar Province	2,902,876	1986/1990
Costa Rica	3.76	1.38	Country	3,087,685	1982/1991
Cuba	4.09	1.8*	Country	10,700,000	1983/1992
Mexico	5.63	N.A.	Monterrey State	3,080,466	1980/1990
Paraguay	0.8	N.A.	Country	3,121,640	1991
Perú	3.7	N.A.	Lima City	5,992,600	1986/1991
Uruguay	5.63	0.59	Country	3,094,214	1984/1990
Venezuela	3.1	0.82	Country	19,773,000	1980/1989
Ecuador	1.8	0.38**	Country	10,501,529	1990/1991
Average	3.09	0.65		117,624,058	

* 5–44, ** 15–44

Paraguay, Peru, Uruguay, and Venezuela (being able at present to include data from Ecuador). A uniform protocol was designed in Santa Fe (Argentina) and supervised by the "Emilio Coni" National Epidemiological Institute. Population data were provided by the National Statistics and Census Institutes of each country. Mortality rates were estimated according to the following requirements:

1. Total population was divided into age groups in accordance with the World Health Organization (WHO) norms for vital statistics and mortality global and age-adjusted (5–34) rates were evaluated.
2. Total deaths from asthma were collected, according to sex and age, and based on death certificates. Deaths certificates also provided information about date and place of death.
3. Rates were calculated based on death registers coded according to the ninth revision of the International Classification of Diseases and Death Causes (ICD-9) that went into effect January 1, 1979. This ninth revision is of a great importance since it classifies asthma separately from other chronic obstructive pulmonary diseases. Code 493 is only assigned to bronchial asthma.

This classification is useful when the patient is alive but not when the cause of death is to be coded since most deaths from asthma occur at home without medical assistance. Furthermore, the professional who completes the death certificate is usually not the specialist who has been treating the disease and does not know its etiological causes.

Table 1 shows mean mortality and age-adjusted

(5–34) rates in the different countries. The total population studied was 117,624,058 inhabitants.

The highest death rates were found in Uruguay and Mexico (5.63) and the lowest in Paraguay (0.8) and Colombia (1.35). Age-adjusted (5–34) rates were higher in Costa Rica (1.38) and lower in Chile (0.28). Data provided by Cuba included an age group from 5 to 44 (1.8) and by Ecuador from 15 to 44 (0.38).

As to sex, the analysis of the information provided by seven countries showed a slight predominance of females (52.21%) over males (48.02%). Male deaths prevailed in the mid-1980s in Peru and Chile, but thereafter a progressive increase in female deaths was observed.

In the southern countries of Latin America such as Chile, Uruguay, Paraguay, and Argentina, which have marked climatic differences, deaths occurred mainly during the winter. In the Santa Fe province (Argentina) [9], the 26% of total deaths occurred in June and July, and were more frequent on Fridays (15.2%) and Saturdays (15.2%) [11].

It is important to emphasize that, in most countries, deaths from asthma occurred at home: Chile (60.7%), Colombia (62.2%), Argentina (63.4%), Ecuador (76%), and Paraguay (88%). However, in Uruguay, 58.6% occurred during hospitalization. In Colombia, deaths at home dropped from 73.6% in 1979 to 44% in 1994, while a simultaneous increase in deaths occurred in hospitals (25.2% up to 50.3%). This could be partially explained by the increase in the accessibility of health care providers [12].

In Argentina, the average rate of deaths from

asthma during the 1980s, based on data provided by the "Emilio Coni" National Epidemiological Institute, was 3.38, showing the lowest value in 1982 (3.03) and the highest in 1987 (3.6).

Death rates in industrialized areas with great economic development and in huge urban conglomerates (3.82 ± 64), where inhabitants are exposed to high pollution levels combined with some poor areas and overcrowded living conditions, prevailed over those in less developed Argentinean provinces (2.09 ± 0.19) [13].

As a confirmation of these data, global death rates from asthma in Santa Fe and Cordoba, two Argentinean provinces with major industrial development, during the 1980s were 4.17 and 5.02, respectively. It is worth noting that during this decade, deaths from asthma were highest in 1985: 135 (rate: 5.0) in Santa Fe and 176 (rate: 6.81) in Córdoba [14].

In Santa Fe in 1987, 23,333 people died from various causes; 1476 from nontraumatic diseases of

the respiratory system (codes from 466 to 529) and 129 from bronchial asthma. Asthma represented 0.55% of total deaths and 8.73% of deaths due to nontraumatic diseases of the respiratory system, which put it in 5th place in this last subgroup. It was also more common in females (Table 2).

Similar results were found in Uruguay, where 7% of total deaths in 1990 were due to nontraumatic diseases of the respiratory system. Bronchial asthma represents 7.6% of these nontraumatic diseases and 0.54% of total deaths [15].

Argentina in the 1990s

Between 1990–1997, asthma mortality global and age-adjusted rates in Argentina showed a gradual decreasing tendency, especially from 1992 onwards, reaching the following values in 1997: 1.76 and 0.20, respectively; mean values in the 1990–1997 period were 2.80 and 0.43, respectively (Figure 1).

This occurs when the prevalence of asthma in Argentina increases, in accordance with data provided by different epidemiological studies carried out in Rosario (1968) and Córdoba (1980) [16], in comparison with more recent works using the ISAAC

Table 2. Number of deaths, Province of Santa Fe 1987.

Inhabitants	2,725,000
Asthma Mortality Rates	4.7 per 100,000

Number of Deaths	
Males	13,104
Females	10,223
Total	23,336

Number of deaths from nontraumatic diseases of the respiratory system (codes 466 to 529)	
Males	889
Females	587
Total	1476

Number of deaths from asthma (code 493)	5–34	all ages
Males	10	62
Females	3	67
Total	13	129
Rate per 100,000	1.01	4.7

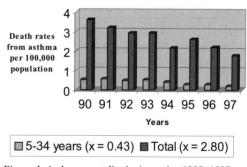

Figure 1. Asthma mortality in Argentina 1990–1997.

Table 3. Prevalence of asthma in children in Argentina.

Period of Study	Population studied	Age (years)	Sample size	Actual (%)	Methodology
1968	Rosario	6–13	3,257	5.6	Questionnaire
1980	Córdoba	6–12	977	2.9	Questionnaire
1996	Bs As / Rosario	6–7	6,012	15.4	ISAAC Questionnaire
1996	Bs As / Rosario	13–14	6,004	11.8	ISAAC Questionnaire
1997	Córdoba	13	3,044	11.2	ISAAC Questionnaire

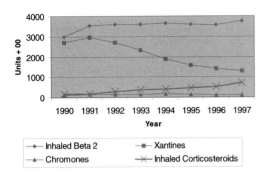

Figure 2. Antiasthmatic drug sales in Argentina from 1990–1997.

questionnaire in Buenos Aires – Rosario (1996) [17] and Córdoba (1997) [18]. Despite the different methodologies employed, there were clear differences that ranged from 2.9% to 5.6% in the former and from 15.4 at 6–7 years of age to 11.2% at 13–14 using the ISAAC protocol (Table 3).

Concomitantly, it is important to analyze the changes in total antiasthmatic drug sales (TADS) in Argentina in 1990 in comparison with 1997 (Figure 2) and their relationship with mortality rates.

In 1990, β_2 agonists represented the 33.79% of TADS, oral β_2 agonists 16.6%, xantines 30.30%, chromones 1.23%, inhaled steroids 1.94%, and systemic steroids 2.28%. In 1997, inhaled β_2 agonists represented 43.25%, oral β_2 agonists 7.28%, xantines 14.85%, chromones 1.32%, inhaled steroids 8.13%, and systemic steroids 1.16%.

The most important changes during these 7 years were a 52.24% reduction in xantine, a 25.06% increase in inhaled β_2 agonists, a 52.04% reduction in oral β_2 agonists, and a 308.73% increase in inhaled steroids.

Another important change is the increase in the use of inhalation route to administer antiasthmatic drugs. Inhaled route represented 43.7% of all drugs administered in 1990 and the 69.73% in 1997. Drugs administered by oral route decreased from 56.94% to 30.27%.

A look at the inhaled β_2 agonists shows that the most prescribed drug in 1990 was salbutamol, followed by fenoterol. The ratio between these two drugs was 1.9 in 1990 and 1.65 in 1997. Total salbutamol sales from 1990 to 1997 increased by 6.7%, while fenoterol sales increased by 33.9%.

Considerations and Future Measures

Our vast continent with its geographical and climatic differences and economic and racial inequalities forms a very heterogeneous population with numerous obstacles to making a global assessment. Our aim of evaluating asthma-related mortality in Latin America during the 1980s based on death certificates presented two main difficulties:

1. In some countries, before implementation of the ICD-9, bronchial asthma was not individually identified as a cause of death. It was included within the codes of other respiratory pathologies such as chronic bronchitis, bronchiectasis, emphysema, unspecified bronchitis, and extrinsic allergic alveolitis (490–496).
2. Death certificates were only occasionally completed by the professional who had been treating the disease. Generally the person who signed the death certificate was not present at the time of the death.

Death rates showed great variations due to environmental, racial, socioeconomic, and medical causes as well as because of the methodology applied to filling out death certificates in the different Latin-American countries.

Medical variables are related to undergraduate and postgraduate education. Physicians should be able to identify asthma properly, both when the patient is alive and when completing a death certificate.

The average number of deaths in the Southern Cone countries (Argentina, Uruguay, Paraguay, and Chile) (x = 2.56) in the 1980s is lower than that in the region called "Bolivariana" (Colombia, Peru, and Venezuela), Central America (Cuba and Costa Rica), and Mexico (x = 3.60). The average number of deaths in all countries studied (x = 3.14) is similar to the values found in Great Britain and Wales; lower than in Australia, New Zealand, West Germany, and Japan; and higher than in the United States and Canada [19].

Countries with marked climatic differences show an increase in the winter when the prevalence of viral and bacterial infections of the airways is high. Such infections can trigger off asthma exacerbations in patients with bronchial hyperreactivity [20, 21].

Deaths occurred more frequently at home. The

most common and important factor associated with this has been the patient's inability to appreciate the severity of the asthmatic attack, leading to an inevitable delay in seeking appropriate medical treatment and assistance.

It is interesting to analyze the decreasing tendency in asthma-related mortality rates in Argentina during the 1990–1997 period, when prevalence was high according to the ISAAC score [17]. This trend in asthma mortality invites comparison with changes in treatment.

In 1997, total rates were lower than 2 per 100,000 inhabitants, which is the first time this has occurred since 1970. It is even more important to note that age-adjusted rates (5–34) decreased to 0.20.

This reduction may be related to changes regarding the greater use of inhaled corticosteroid therapy, which increased fourfold in Argentina in this period. Different studies support the clinical improvements using inhaled steroid therapy and their protective effects against mortality [22, 23].

Recent data from Australia showed similar results, with the 5-fold increase in inhaled corticosteroid use from 1989 to 1993 and the decrease in mortality rates occurring at the same time [24].

The prescription of the inhaled β_2 agonists salbutamol and fenoterol increased from 1990 to 1997. These drugs might be replacing oral β_2 agonists and xantines to some extent. For this reason, the gradual decreasing mortality rate in Argentina should not be attributed to a reduction in inhaled β_2 agonist use.

Changes in asthma mortality should be especially sensitive to changes in quality of management. Most deaths from asthma are probably avoidable, and it is necessary to stress the importance of postgraduate education programs for general practitioners and pediatricians to achieve optimal asthma management and prevention in order to recognize a patient with high mortality risk from asthma.

The dissemination of the Global Initiative for Asthma in Argentina began in 1995. In 1996/1997, 600 specialists and more than 5000 physicians including pediatricians, general practitioners, and family doctors were contacted all around the country. They participated in workshops and symposia where they became aware of the new concept of asthma management and early implementation of antiinflammatory therapeutic strategies in accordance with the Global Strategy for Asthma Management and Prevention (WHO/NHLBI) [19].

During the dissemination of the GINA in Argentina, an interactive computerized questionnaire was answered using keypads before and after the symposia in order to evaluate the impact of the program among health-care providers. Our results showed that the GINA program was found to be an important educational strategy that effectively modified health-care providers' opinion on key concepts of asthma [25].

It is important to recall that one may be successful in changing physician knowledge without changing physician behavior [26]. For this reason, in Argentina we are strongly working to implement guidelines for asthma management and prevention among public and private health-care providers in order to improve asthma management and patient quality of life, reduce morbidity and costs of asthma, and consolidate the decreasing tendency in asthma mortality through different post-graduate education programs.

Asthma is a serious global health problem. People of all ages in Latin American countries are affected by this chronic airway disorder that can be severe and sometimes fatal. Health ministries of all countries do not consider asthma to be a significant issue. Therefore, we should provide them with sound epidemiological studies to make them change their attitude towards this disease and thus be involved in the international crusade against asthma.

Address for correspondence:

Hugo E Neffen, PhD
Irigoyen Freyre 2670
Santa Fe 3000
Argentina
Tel. +54 342 453-7638
Fax +54 342 456-0773
E-mail interasm@neffen.satlink.net

References

1. Sly R. Increases in deaths from asthma. Ann Allergy 1984; 53:20–25.

2. Paulozzi L, Coleman J, Buist A. A recent increase in asthma mortality in the Northwestern United States. Ann Allergy 1986; 56:392–395.

3. Rachelefsky GS, Lewis MA, Lewis CE. An increase in asthma deaths in California. J Allergy Clin Immunol 1987; 79(1).

4. Jackson R, Sears MR, Beaglehole R, Rea HH. International trends in asthma mortality 1970 to 1985. Chest 1988; 94:914–918.

5. Buist A. Asthma mortality: Trends and determinants. Am Rev Resp Dis 1987; 136:1037–1039.

6. Evans, R Recent observations on increases in morbidity and mortality from asthma. N.E.R. Allergy Proc 1986; 7(5).

7. Friday GA, Stillwagon P, Page R, Asman B, Skoner D, Fierman P. Increased hospitalizations from asthma without increased deaths at Pittsburgh Children's Hospital, from 1968–1985. J Allergy Clin Immunol 1987; 79(1).

8. Sly M, O'Donnell R. Stabilization of asthma mortality. Annals Asthma Immunology 1997; 78:347–354.

9. Lang D. Trends in US asthma mortality: Good news and bad news. Annals Allergy Asthma Immunol 1997; 78:333–336.

10. Neffen H, Baena-Cagnani C, Malka S, Solé D, Sepúlveda R, Caraballo L, Caravajal E, Rodriguez Gavaldá R, González Díaz S, Guggiari Chase J, Diez C, Baluga J, Capriles Hulett A. Asthma mortality in Latin America. J Invest Allergol Clin Immunol 1997; 7(4):249–253.

11. Busaniche H, Neffen H, Sanchez Guerra ME. Tasa de muerte por asma en la provincia de Santa· Fe (1980–1987). Arch Arg Inmunol Clin 1991; 22(11):13–20.

12. Vergara C, Caraballo L. Asthma mortality in Colombia. Annals Allergy Asthma Immunol 1998; 80:55–59.

13. Neffen H, Busaniche H, Sanchez Guerra ME. Asthma mortality in Argentine Republic. Proceedings XIV INTERASMA World Congress. Jerusalem 1993.

14. Baena-Cagnani C, Salvucci K, Jalil M, Patiño C, Gurne S, Mareca O. Estudio de la mortalidad por asma en la provincia de Córdoba entre 1980 y 1991. Arch Arg Alerg Inmunol Clín 1994; 26(2):91–99.

15. Baluga JC, Spagna F, Ceni M. Mortalidad por Asma en Uruguay. Período 1984–1994. Rev Med Uruguay 1997; 13:12–22.

16. Carrasco E. Epidemiological aspects of asthma in Latin-America. Chest 1988; 93:S58-S61.

17. ISAAC Steering Committee. Worldwide variations in the prevalence of asthma symptoms: The International Study of Asthma and Allergy in Childhood (ISAAC). Eur Respir J 1998; 12:315–335.

18. Baena-Cagnani CE, Patiño C, Cuello M, Minervini M, Fernández A, Garip E, Salvucci, K, Sancho M, Corelli S, Gómez R. Prevalence and severity of asthma and wheezing in an adolescent population. Int Arch Allergy Immunol 1998; T1–326.

19. Global strategy for asthma management and prevention – NHLBI/WHO workshop report – Chapter II: Epidemiology. Publication No 95-3659, Pag. 13–16 January 1995.

20. Baena-Cagnani C, Patiño C, Tregnaghi M, González S. Infección Viral y Asma: Epidemiología y Mecanismos. Alergia (México) 1990; 37:193.

21. Cypcar D, Stark J, Lemanske R. Impacto de las Infecciones Respiratorias sobre el asma. Clin Ped N Am 1992; 6:1351.

22. Toogood JH, Jennings BH, Baskerville JC, Lefcoe NM. Aerosol corticosteroids. In EB Weis, M Stein (Eds), Bronchial asthma: Mechanisms and therapeutics, 3rd edition. Boston: Little, Brown & Co 1993, pp. 818–841.

23. Ernst P, Spitzer WO, Suissa S, Cockroft D, Habbick B, Horwitz RI, Boivin JF, McNutt M, Buist AS. Risk of fatal and near-fatal asthma in relation to inhaled corticosteroid use. JAMA 1992; 268:3462–3464.

24. Wilson JW, Jenkins C. Asthma mortality: Where is it going? Med J Austr 1996; 164:391–393.

25. Baena-Cagnani CE, Neffen H, Abbate E, Balanzat A, Gene R, Patiño C. Impact of Gina Dissemination Programme among Health Care Providers (HCP). Eur Resp J 1998; 12(suppl 29):62s.

26. Lomas J. Holding back the tide of caesareans: Publishing recommendations is not enough to stop the rise. Br Med J 1998; 297:569–570.

The Natural History of Occupational Asthma

Cristina Elisabetta Mapp*

Keywords: Occupational asthma, outcome, risk factors, natural history

Our understanding of natural history of occupational asthma is improving through the establishment of a more precise definition of occupational asthma. Risk factors for the development of occupational asthma include genetic factors, atopic status, cigarette smoking, and specific occupational environments. Asthma affects 5 to 10% of all persons worldwide. The proportion of newly diagnosed cases of asthma in adults due to occupational exposure is unknown. At present, several hundred occupational agents have been identified, accounting for between 10 and 15% of adult asthma. Asthma resulting from occupational exposure differs little in its clinical or pathologic features from nonoccupational asthma. Airway hyperresponsiveness is present, and it is considered a consequence rather than a predisposing factor in occupational asthma. Atopy is a risk factor for those occupational agents that induce specific IgE antibodies, whereas in occupational asthma related to low molecular weight agents, nonsmokers and nonatopic subjects are at greater risk. A genetic predisposition may be present. The majority of subjects with occupational asthma with latency do not recover and suffer permanent impairment or disability. Early diagnosis and early removal from exposure generally increase the likelihood of recovery. A better knowledge of the natural history of occupational asthma may also improve the understanding of the natural history of nonoccupational asthma.

Our understanding of the natural history of occupational asthma is determined by a few criteria: First, a precise definition of the disease that allows identification of the affected subjects; second, longitudinal data that allow us to monitor the disease from onset to remission or to persistence; and finally, the understanding of the effect of the cessation of exposure to the sensitizing agent and of therapy on the course of disease and its outcome.

Two types of occupational asthma are recognized, depending on whether or not it develops after a latency period. Occupational asthma with latency (developing after a period of exposure that may vary from a few weeks to several years) is the most common type. Occupational asthma without a latency period, termed "irritant-induced asthma," follows exposure to high concentrations of gases, fumes, or chemicals [1]. Asthma-like syndromes have been reported in workers exposed to cotton and grain dust, and these are probably associated with endotoxin inhalation. Similarly, potroom asthma is usually considered to be a separate condition from occupational asthma, the causative agent being unknown. The definition of occupational asthma with latency is precise, whereas the definitions of occupational asthma without latency and of asthma-like syndromes are more difficult and have some limitations. The mechanisms of occupational asthma with latency are more clearly understood [2], and the pathological airway changes are similar to those described in nonoccupational asthma [3–5]. There is an increase in airway wall thickness, edema, hypertrophy of smooth muscle, increased subepithelial fibrosis, epithelial desquamation, and in severe cases, obstruction of the airway lumen by exudate or mucus. T lymphocytes, eosinophils, and mast cells are key cells in the inflammatory process and exhibit signs of activation. The mechanisms of occupational asthma without latency are largely unknown. Cases have been reported after accidental inhalation of ammonia, chlorine, acid, fumes, and sulphur dioxide [6]. Striking fibrosis of the bronchial wall was found in some patients [7]. Neutrophil infiltration and release of interleukin 8 (IL-8) have been described in airway mucosa of subjects with grain dust-induced asthma [8]. However, this syndrome differs from typical occupational asthma in many aspects: It is associated with cross shift change, no eosinophilia, no airway hyperresponsiveness, no previous exposure necessary, no specific IgE, and chronic airflow limitation.

Exposure is the most important determinant of whether occupational asthma develops. In occupational asthma with latency, the higher the degree of

---

* Istituto di Medicina del Lavoro, Universita' degli Studi di Padova, Italy

exposure to the sensitizing agent, the higher the prevalence of asthma [9]. Atopy and cigarette smoking are important determinants for occupational agents that induce asthma through an IgE-dependent mechanism [10]. Cigarette smoking is more important than atopy in predisposing subjects to sensitization to platinum salts [11]. Atopy and smoking are not important determinants for agents that induce asthma through IgE-independent mechanisms [11, 12]. The duration of exposure is not important. About 40% of subjects with occupational asthma develop symptoms within 2 years of exposure, whereas in 20% symptoms develop after 10 years of exposure [13]. A role for a genetic component of asthma has been hypothesized based on the observations that asthma tended to cluster in families. Few studies have investigated the genetic component in occupational asthma, and all reported human leukocyte antigen (HLA) associations [14–17]. Preexisting allergic/atopy and/or preexisting asthma are significant contributors of occupational asthma without latency, in the so-called "not-so-sudden irritant-induced asthma" [18]. It is likely that genetic factors interact with occupational exposure to cause the phenotype of the disease, but we do not know which type of interaction occurs.

Most subjects with occupational asthma still report symptoms of asthma and exhibit nonspecific airway hyperresponsiveness even years after cessation of exposure to the sensitizing agent [19, 20]. Factors than can affect the outcome have not been elucidated. Specific sensitization remains for a long time [21], and pathology partially reverses with time [22–24]. It is established that the persistence of asthma after cessation of exposure is associated with a longer duration of exposure before and after the onset of symptoms and with a more severe asthma as defined by the degree of airway obstruction and nonspecific airway hyperresponsiveness at the time of diagnosis [19, 20]. The improvement is very slow and gradual and continues for many years after removal from exposure. Barker and coworkers [25] reported persistent symptoms and airway hyperresponsiveness in occupational asthma induced by tetrachlorophtalic anhydride (TCPA), despite avoidance of exposure for 12 years and a progressive fall in specific IgE. Recently, it was reported that subjects removed for more than 5 years show better outcome. The duration of the interval from cessation of exposure appears to be a factor determining this finding [26].

There are few follow-up data available on the outcome of "irritant-induced asthma." Bherer and

coworkers reported that 75% of pulpmill workers who developed asthmatic symptoms after acute exposure had nonspecific airway hyperresponsiveness 18–24 months after exposure [27].

Most follow-up studies of subjects with occupational asthma were carried out at a time when inhaled glucocorticoids were not widely used in the treatment of asthma. A recent study showed that inhaled glucocorticoids combined with removal from exposure led to a significant improvement of asthma [28]. Early diagnosis and early removal from exposure increase the likelihood of recovery.

In conclusion, asthma resulting from occupational exposure differs little in its clinical or pathologic features from nonoccupational asthma. Therefore, the occupational model is relevant to studies of outcome, and gives us a view into the possible natural history of both occupational and nonoccupational asthma.

Address for correspondence:

Cristina E Mapp, MD
Istituto di Medicina del Lavoro
Via Giustiniani 2
I-35128 Padova
Italy
Tel. +39 049 821-2562
Fax +39 049 821-2566
E-mail mapp@ux1.unipd.it

References

1. Chan-Yeung M, Malo J-L. Occupational asthma. Review article. N Engl J Med 1995; 333(2):107–112.
2. Mapp CE, Saetta M, Maestrelli P, et al. Mechanisms and pathology of occupational asthma. Eur Respir J 1994; 7:544–554.
3. Saetta M, Di Stefano A, Maestrelli P, et al. Airway mucosal inflammation in occupational asthma induced by toluene diisocyanate. Am Rev Respir Dis 1992; 145:160–168.
4. Frew A, Chan H, Lam S, Chan-Yeung M. Bronchial inflammation in occupational asthma due to western red cedar. Am J Respir Crit Care Med 1995; 151:340–344.
5. Fabbri LM, Danieli D, Crescioli S, et al. Fatal asthma in a subject sensitized to toluene diisocyanate. Am Rev Respir Dis 1988; 137:1494–1498.
6. Brooks SM, Weiss MA, Bernstein IL. Reactive airways dysfunction syndrome (RADS). Persistent

asthma syndrome after high level irritant exposures. Chest 1985; 88(3):376–384.

7. Gautrin D, Boulet LP, Boutet M, et al. Is reactive airways dysfunction syndrome a variant of occupational asthma? J Allergy Clin Immunol 1994; 93:12–22.

8. Parks HS, Jung KS, Hwang SC, Nahm DH, Yim HE. Neutrophil infiltration and release of IL-8 in airway mucosa from subjects with grain dust-induced asthma: comparison with allergic asthma. J Korean Med Sci 1998; 13:21–26.

9. Chan-Yeung M. Occupational asthma. Chest 1990; 98(suppl.):148s–161s.

10. Chan-Yeung M. Assessment of asthma in the workplace. Chest 1995; 108:1084–1117.

11. Venables KM, Dally MB, Nunn AJ, et al. Smoking and occupational allergy in workers in a platinum refinery. Br Med J 1989; 299:939–942.

12. Mapp CE, Boschetto P, Dal Vecchio L, Maestrelli P, Fabbri LM. Occupational asthma due to isocyanates. Eur Respir J 1988; 1:273–279.

13. Malo JL, Ghezzo H, D'Aquino C, L'Archeveque J, Cartier A, Chan-Yeung M. Natural history of occupational asthma: Relevance of type of agent and other factors in the rate of development of symptoms in affected subjects. J Allergy Clin Immunol 1992; 90:937–944.

14. Balboni A, Baricordi OR, Fabbri LM, et al. Association between toluene diisocyanate-induced asthma and DQB1 markers: A possible role for aspartic acid at position 57. Eur Respir J 1996; 9:207–210.

15. Young RP, Barker RD, Pile KD, Cookson OCN, Newman Taylor AJ. The association of HLA-DR3 with specific IgE to inhaled acid anhydrides. Am J Respir Crit Care Med 1995; 151:219–221.

16. Home C, Quintana PJE, Keown PA, Dimitch-Ward H, Chan-Yeung M. Distribution of HLA class II DQB1 and DRB1 alleles in patients with occupational asthma due to western red cedar. Am J Respir Crit Care Med 1997; 155:A135.

17. Soriano JB, Ercilla G, Sunyer J, et al. HLA class II genes in soybean epidemic asthma patients. Am J Respir Crit Care Med 1997; 1156:1394–1398.

18. Brooks MS, Hammad Y, Richards I, Giovinco-Barbas J, Jenkins KI. The spectrum of irritant-induced asthma. Sudden and not-so-sudden onset and the role of allergy. Chest 1998; 113:42–49.

19. Paggiaro PL, Vagaggini B, Bacci E, et al. Prognosis of occupational asthma. Eur Respir J 1994; 7:761–767.

20. Mapp CE, Chiesura Corona P, De Marzo N, et al. Persistent asthma due to isocyanates: A follow-up of subjects with occupational asthma due to toluene diisocyanate. Am Rev Respir Dis 1988; 137:1326–1329.

21. Banks DE, Rando RJU, Barkman HJ. Persistence of toluene diisocyanate-induced asthma despite negligible workplace exposures. Chest 1990; 97:121–125.

22. Chan-Yeung M, LeRiche J, McLean L, Lam S. Comparison of cellular and protein changes in bronchial lavage fluid of symptomatic and asymptomatic patients on follow-up examination. Clin Allergy 1988; 18:359–365.

23. Saetta M, Maestrelli P, Di Stefano A, et al. Effect of cessation of exposure to toluene diisocyanate (TDI) on bronchial mucosa of subjects with TDI-induced asthma. Am Rev Respir Dis 1992; 145:169–174.

24. Saetta M, Maestrelli P, Turato G, et al. Airway wall remodelling after cessation of exposure to isocyanates in sensitized asthmatic subjects. Am J Respir Crit Care Med 1995; 151:489–494.

25. Barker RD, Harris JM, Welch JA, Venables KM, Newman Taylor AJ. Occupational asthma caused by tetrachlorophtalic anhydride: A 12-year follow-up. J Allergy Clin Immunol 1998; 101:717–719.

26. Perfetti L, Cartier A, Ghezzo H, Gautrin D, Malo JL. Follow-up of occupational asthma after removal from or diminution of exposure to the responsible agent. Relevance of the length of the interval from cessation of exposure. Chest 1998; 114:398–403.

27. Bherer L, Cushman R, Courteau JP, et al. Survey of construction workers repeatedly exposed to chlorine over a three to six months period in a pulpmill: Follow-up of affected workers by questionnaire, spirometry, and assessment of bronchial responsiveness 18 to 24 months after exposure ended. Occup Environ Med 1995; 51:225–228.

28. Malo JL, Cartier A, Coté JU, et al. Influence of inhaled steroids on recovery from occupational asthma after cessation of exposure: An 18-month double-blind crossover study. Am J Respir Crit Care Med 1996; 153:953–960.

Clinical Aspects and Diagnosis of Occupational Asthma

Michael G Pearson*

Keywords: Occupational asthma, serial peak flow, sensitization, diagnostic criteria, prognosis

Definitions of occupational asthma are variables which makes a positive diagnosis relatively more difficult and renders international comparisons of incidence and causation difficult. Nevertheless occupational causes are well described and the diagnosis can be made confidently in many subjects. More care than usual is required because the consequences of the diagnosis on both the patients' and sometimes their colleagues' future employment can be severe. The diagnosis rests on proving that the patient does have objective asthma which is related to specific exposures within the workplace. Once this has been established serial peak flow measurement is the single most useful tool for confirming a work relationship but is by no means infallible. Specific challenge tests are the gold standard for diagnosis but are difficult to perform safely. In all cases there is often a medicolegal angle overlying the case which can blur the issues and make it difficult to obtain full information. Confirmation of the history and timing of illness can often be obtained retrospectively from the primary care or occupational health records and these contemporary notes may be the key data to help avoid the need for challenge testing. Prognosis depends upon early diagnosis and removal form the causative agent.

What is Asthma?

The International Consensus Report [1] on the diagnosis and management of asthma defined asthma as:

"a chronic inflammatory disorder of the airways in which many cells play a role, including mast cells and eosinophils. In susceptible individuals this inflammation causes symptoms which are usually associated with widespread but variable airflow obstruction that is often reversible either spontaneously or with treatment, and causes an associated increase in airway responsiveness to a variety of stimuli."

There is no reference to "cause" of the asthma in this definition, and nor is there any reference to the degree of airflow limitation, the variability of the airflow limitation or the level of inflammation that should be present. Documents from other sets of national guidelines are similarly unclear. Thus, it is hardly surprising that the clinical criteria used to define asthma varies significantly both between asthma specialists and particularly within primary care.

It is generally accepted that, in most individuals, the inflammation that characterizes asthma is the result of an abnormal response to an external, usually inhaled, substance. As more causes of asthma come to light so the proportion of cases that can be labelled as intrinsic asthma becomes ever smaller. However, for most asthmatics it is impossible to define a single causative substance and because most are treated with anti-inflammatory drugs, usually inhaled steroids, that block the response regardless of provoking factor, the clinician does not look too hard for the cause.

The most common allergens that lead to asthma vary from country to country. In the damp UK climate the house dust mite *Dermatophagoides pteronnyssimus* causes measurable antibodies in about 70% of asthmatics, but in dry, hot climates or at altitude other antigens predominate. Occupational asthma is therefore a specific subgroup within the overall spectrum of asthma caused by a specific factor at a workplace. Definitions of occupational asthma are even more varied that for the generic condition. However, the consequences of the diagnosis on both the individual patient and

---

* Consultant Physician, Aintree Chest Centre, University Hospital Aintree, Liverpool, UK; Director of the Clinical Effectiveness and Evaluation Unit, Royal College of Physicians, London; Visiting Professor, University of Salford, Salford, UK

sometimes on his/her work colleagues can be considerable and this imposes a burden on the clinician that is often not appreciated.

What is Occupational Asthma?

The variable definitions are outlined by Berstein et al. [2], resulting in a consensus definition between the 4 editors:

"Occupational asthma is a disease characterized by variable airflow limitation and/or airway hyperresponsiveness due to causes and conditions attributable to a particular occupational environment and not to stimuli encountered outside the workplace. Two types of occupational asthma are distinguished by whether they appear after a latency period:

1. With a latency period – encompasses all instances of immunologic asthma for which and immunologica mechanism has been identified and includes most high and some low molecular weight agents. For some agents causing occupational asthma, evidence of and immunological mechanism is still lacking or may not exist.
2. Without a latency period – best illustrated by irritant induced asthma or the reactive airways dysfunction syndrome (RADS).

Under certain conditions both may co-exist."

This definition excludes the situation where a person with preexisting asthma and hyper reactive airways responds to irritants at work that others tolerate with ease.

Epidemiology of Asthma and Occupational Asthma

Asthma is common affecting about 6% of UK adults and 10% of children. The prevalence has approximately doubled in the last 25 years. While the incidence varies between countries with the UK at the higher end of the spectrum, the evidence that asthma is increasing worldwide is strong [3]. The reasons for this increase are much debated and not agreed. Asthma occurs fairly uniformly across the whole of the UK, and affects all social classes. It is of similar prevalence in both cities and rural communities. Asthma most often begins in childhood, but may come on at any age and in adult life is more common in females than males. The proportion of all asthma caused by exposure to substances in the workplace is small. Scandinavian estimates rise to 6% of the workforce, most UK figures are rather smaller at 2% [4]. Thus, the great majority of asthmatic patients presenting to a clinic will not have occupational asthma, even though most adults who develop asthma will be at work.

For specific occupations, however, the rates of asthma are much higher. The incidence rates for spray painters are 50- to 60-fold higher than for woodworkers [5] and bakers, chemical workers, and farmers are also much higher. It follows therefore that workers who develop asthma while in these occupations are relatively more likely to have occupational asthma than asthma due to other factors in daily living. Men are more likely to get occupational asthma than women probably reflecting the differences in occupational exposures.

There are many well documented causes of asthma from the workplace. The commonest and best understood group of agents are the isocyanates.

Table 1. A few examples of the more common causes of occupational asthma sorted according to the nature of the asthmogenic agent.

Provoking factors	Examples of types of occupation
Animal dusts – from excretions, secretions or furs	Laboratory animal workers, food processors, bird breeders, farm workers
Plant materials – plant allergens or from associated storage mites	Grain handlers, bakers/millers, tea workers and food process workers
Wood dusts – especially western red cedar and hardwoods	Woodmill workers, carpenters
Enzymes and drugs	Pharmaceutical and detergent manufacturers
Low molecular weight chemicals – Di-isocyanates, colophony, anhydrides	Spray painters, foam manufacturers, electronics plants, glues
Metals and salts – platinum salts chomates	Metal refining and plating

These small molecular weight substances are widely used in paints, foams and resins and are used with hardening agents. They are gaseous at most ambient temperatures and are given off from the setting resin or drying paint. Particularly high concentrations occur when paints are sprayed as the smaller paint droplets which can be inhaled contain 10-fold higher concentrations due to surface tension effects holding them in the droplet. Early studies from the USA [5] showed that in a manufacturing plant, about 4% of employees became sensitized to isocyanates over a 5-year period. No textbook can now list all the causes of occupational asthma on a single page. Agents can be grouped in a number of ways (Table 1)

For the most common causes of occupational asthma the evidence of a causal effect is overwhelming, with epidemiological, immunological and physiological evidence that has usually included a direct challenge of patients with the suspected agent. However, for many if not most of the causative agents on many of the lists, the evidence for their asthmogenicity depends on case studies or studies of small numbers of workers. The strength of the evidence is therefore variable and often depends upon extrapolation of what is known for the more common causes. The voluntary reporting systems, such as the SWORD scheme [6] in the UK, record details of all cases suspected on clinical grounds by physicians. The scheme justifies its overinclusiveness because it serves to raise suspicion that may at a later stage justify more formal study of a particular industry of plant.

Clinical Patterns of Occupational Asthma

The Bernstein definition at the start of this article refers to two types of occupational asthma with the defining characteristic being latency. This refers to the finite time required to develop an immunological reaction. Thus, an employee might commence in a job and cope well with no respiratory symptoms for a period of weeks, months or years despite being exposed. Then over a short period they develop an immunological reaction to the substance, which leads to inflammation characteristic of asthma and the development of wheeze and the other asthma symptoms. This sensitization is often dramatic in that the person becomes unable to tolerate exposure to minute concentrations many fold less that those they had worked under previously. The sensitization may commence abruptly or may get progressively worse over a period of weeks or sometimes longer. Typically the worker will notice coughing and wheezing after exposure that may start within 15 minutes at the beginning of the day and get worse during the day with improvement over the evening and night only to recur next day when exposed again. At weekends with a longer period of non-exposure the person may return to complete normality. Holiday periods may produce an even greater contrast. The precise pattern will vary with the job – some workers will only handle the offending substance once or twice in the day and can then relate symptoms quite easily to that task. Others with more prolonged or haphazard exposure pattern give a correspondingly less clear story. Most of these "immediate" type reactions are likely to involve IgE mediated responses. It is important to recognize that most cases will also have delayed responses mediated by IgG or cell mediated factors and that if this is the only mechanism present the symptoms may only come on in the evening after work so that the work relationship may easily be overlooked.

This concept of sensitization to minute quantities of agent, differentiates immunologically mediated asthma from the irritant response that is to be expected in a preexisting asthmatic. A person with bronchial hyperreactivity is likely to wheeze when exposed to small concentrations of chlorine (or similar irritant gases) whether the exposure occurs whilst cleaning the kitchen at home or from non-significant (for other workers) exposures at the workplace. This is a feature of their underlying disease rather than of occupationally caused asthma. There is a debate as to whether such low dose irritant exposures are damaging in the long term for asthma patients with strong protagonists on both sides fuelled by the spectre of medicolegal claims against employers. The definition used above does not accept this as occupational asthma.

The factors that cause a person to become sensitized are still unknown. An acute spillage leading to a high dose exposure, a viral infection in an exposed person, or a cumulative dose factor have all been mooted. It is important to note that only a minority of workers in a given exposed occupation will develop asthma meaning that there are significant host factors which must be important. Atopic individuals appear to be more likely to respond to the biological agents than non-atopics, and in some studies smokers are at more risk than non-smokers. The clinician trying to make a diagnosis does not have a easily definable list of questions to sort out the genuine occupational case from the rest and thus the diagnosis continues to be one based on all the available evidence and not only on history.

Making a Diagnosis

There are three parts to making a diagnosis of occupational asthma.
- First, prove that the person really does have asthma
- Second, show that there has been exposure to an agent capable of causing occupational asthma
- Third, demonstrate that asthma is linked to the suspected agent.
  1) a history compatible with exposure
  2) a record of symptoms at the appropriate times, made in the works or other medical records
  3) a serial PEF record at work and at home
  4) specific challenge tests

Demonstrating the Patient Does Have Asthma

In primary care asthma is common and the doctor will often make a clinical diagnosis based on a history of cough, wheeze and nocturnal waking. Drugs will be prescribed and the response monitored. If there is not a dramatic response, then the doctor can reconsider th diagnosis. However, when occupational asthma is suspected this clinical approach is usually inadequate because of the consequences that may emanate from the diagnosis. A worker may become concerned about their safety of their job and be unhappy going to work. If kept off work, the worker will become worried about their livelihood. Other workers or the employer may become involved and the future of the whole process or work area may become uncertain. Once doubts are raised it becomes very difficult to resolve them with certainty. There is also the chance that a worker will seek compensation from the employer through the courts at which stage it is extremely helpful to have objective measurements.

For all these reasons, it is advisable to try and document the asthma with greater care than normal if occupational factors are suspected. Methods of objectively demonstrating asthma include
- observing an obstructive pattern on spirometry

with a marked (> 500 ml) response to bronchodilator;
- observing serial PEF measurements over 2 to 3 weeks and noting diurnal variations of greater than 15 – 20%;
- observing an markedly improved FEV or PEF after introducing asthma therapy;
- performing an asthma exercise test and showing a drop in FEV_1 after exercise;
- showing that there is marked bronchial hyperreactivity to histamine or metacholine;
- noting variable lung function measurements over time.

Over the last 15 years this author has often tried to sort out the diagnosis of patients who have become embroiled in legal claims and in a number of cases it has proved impossible to document any objective evidence of asthma. Sadly, by the time the case has got this far, the individual is often so distrustful as to be beyond reassurance, with the consequence that not only do they not have a claim, but they also have no job.

Showing There Has Been Exposure to an Asthma Causing Agent

If the patient works in a job where there is known exposure to one of the agents with proven potential to cause asthma, it is still necessary to demonstrate that the exposures were of a level and timing to explain the reported symptoms. A detailed history is required of all the jobs the patient has performed, of the work practices in the jobs including details such as how the fumes or dusts were being generated and most important, of the temporal relationships between exposure and symptoms.

Symptoms after exposure to certain processes, or on specific tasks, or marked weekend and/or holiday improvements are strong pointers. In many cases the story is less clearcut and the doctor will be left uncertain. In such cases it is helpful to know what agents are likely to be present at the workplace. For the situation of laboratory animal workers the exposures are easy to enquire about, but for the chemical process worker the "recipe" of ingredients may not be known. In the UK and most European countries there are health and safety regulations that stipulate a data sheet be present at the workplace for every potentially dangerous chemical and be available to each worker. Most workers in the UK can get hold of these data sheets and the results can often be surprising and very informative. Once the exposures are identified the history may need to be taken again focussing on the specific process under suspicion.

If no asthmogenic agent can be identified, the diagnosis must not be immediately dismissed. If further tests such as serial PEF values show an occupationally linked fall in PEF, then either something has been missed in the history or it is possible that a new cause of asthma exists that justifies detailed investigation possibly including a challenge test.

Showing That the Records Support the Diagnosis

If there is any clinical doubt (and always if there is a legal claim), the earlier records of the patient should be obtained and inspected. Contemporary records may confirm the timing and substance of the history and thus add much credibility to the history based diagnosis, but on occasion they can also show either a very different pattern of disease, a total lack of symptoms, or that there was pre-existing asthma. It is particularly useful to have support from the records when an employee has either already left the job or otherwise ceased to be exposed because it is not possible to obtain serial PEF charts at work and home in such cases.

Serial PEF Recording

This has become the main objective diagnostic tool for occupational asthma. PEF is simple to perform and cheap. It is possible to ask a worker to record their PEF as often as 2 hourly (and always more than 4 times daily) and to plot the data as a serial chart (see Figure 1). On this chart the median, maximum and minimum value for each day are plotted with the timing of work exposures added to the chart. It is possible to show in clearcut cases that the median PEF is lower on days of exposure and that the PEF range is greater. Often charts are not as clear as this and to counter this and add a degree of objectivity, computer programs have been developed to help in the interpretation of the changes in PEF. One such system [7, 8] claims considerable success, although it is used routinely by relatively few clinicians and others remain sceptical, preferring to rely on their own visual assessments of charts. In general the objectivity introduced by computerized analysis should be welcomed but with the caveat of whether the data being entered are reliable. Canadian studies have shown that individuals are not reliable when completing their charts and even when aware that the results are being monitored persist in either writing in values for measurements they did not make or of misrecording values by more than 50 l/min for as many as half of all readings [9, 10].

Despite these limitations, most doctors given a suggestive history, documented asthma and a supportive PEF chart would make a firm diagnosis of occupational asthma and advise the patient about further exposures etc. This is a reasonable approach but for the reasons above is not infallible so on occasions it is necessary to look for further confirmation.

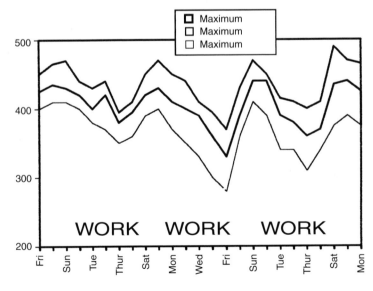

Figure 1. Chart of serial peak flow measurements made every 2 to 4 hours throughout the day and then plotted as the maximum, median, and minimum values for each day to demonstrate the relationship of PEF and work exposures.

More Specific Tests

The gold standard test for occupational asthma remains a challenge test in which the actual exposure conditions are simulated in the laboratory, and shown to be capable of reproducing the patient's asthmatic response. Challenge tests are not easy to perform and are not without danger. The basis of the test is to expose a person to a substance that is expected to induce an immunological reaction that may continue for many hours, leading to inflammation and associated bronchospasm. If the dose is too high the reaction may be too vigorous, and the consequent asthmatic episode difficult to control.

There must be good reason for performing the challenge test such as:
– proving a response to an agent not previously recognized as asthmogenic;
– resolving significant doubt about the diagnosis with a man's employment depending on the outcome.

Simply proving the point for a legal case is usually not sufficient reason.

It is beyond the scope of this paper to discuss the detailed methodology for challenge testing but it is important when interpreting results to ask the following:
– Did the challenge involve concentrations similar to those in the workplace?
– Were comparable placebo challenges performed to indicate what the persons normal daily variability is? Were the challenges open or single blind?
– Did the patient exhibit a response within an appropriate time period and of sufficient size to be both statistically and clinically relevant?

Challenge tests are difficult and time consuming to perform, but there is no doubt that positive tests have been extremely important in establishing which agents are truly asthmogenic and may also offer important opportunities for studying the trigger mechanisms of asthma under controlled circumstances.

What Does the Diagnosis Mean?

Prognosis

If a person becomes sensitized to a substance at work and the link is recognized quickly ie within a few months of symptoms commencing, and further exposure avoided then many if not most cases will resolve spontaneously and may have no more symptoms at all [11]. Some cases, however, develop a persistent asthma becoming sensitized to other common allergens and sensitive to non-specific stimuli such as intercurrent viral infections. If cases are not diagnosed early and the problem becomes firmly established then the likelihood of complete recovery is much less and in one study of isocyanate workers up to 80% were still symptomatic 4 years after diagnosis [12]. The emphasis is therefore on early diagnosis leading to cessation of exposure.

Effects of the Diagnosis on the Worker

Once a firm diagnosis of occupational asthma has been made, the person should if at all possible be removed from further exposure. This may be achieved by altering the working conditions to prevent exposure by either enclosing a process, by installing good exhaust ventilation or changing the agents being used, or if none of these is possible by removing the man from that job. All too often the latter means losing a job and the associated income since especially in small firms it is difficult to find alternative employment which does not entail continued exposure. It is particularly difficult because once sensitized and individual responds to levels many times lower than previously tolerated, which are within permitted exposure limits.

This often leads to the employee seeking redress from his employer through the courts. In many countries there are statutory bodies that dispense a modest level of workers compensation but this rarely matches the wages of the job and thus civil actions are becoming more common. In the UK the experience of these actions is that the levels of compensation are often not high and often insufficient to make up for the loss of a job.

Effects on the Employer and Other Employees

If working conditions are sufficiently poor for an individual to become sensitized and develop asthma, it follows that others in similar jobs are also at risk. The physician should therefore seek to alert

245

appropriate authorities of the likely risk. Employers may be reluctant to spend money modifying their plant or fitting extra ventilation and in the UK there are employment medical advisors and factory inspectors employed by government with powers to order modifications to a premises or process and to close the operation down if the changes are not implemented. Since prevention of asthma is undoubtedly better than cure, this is sensible medicine, but it may not be sensible for the employer or other staff. If the costs of modification are considerable then the business may become uncompetitive with other similar operations especially when they are in countries where no regulation exists. Whether the need to prevent other cases of asthma justifies the economic penalty for employers or other employees is justified is a political judgement. In general the health argument should win out since it is morally unsatisfactory to knowingly put employees at any risk and especially if the risks are avoidable.

The Legal Situation

The physician who makes a diagnosis of occupational asthma must always be aware of the potential for a legal claim to arise from that diagnosis. Good records by the doctor can be important to the chances of success especially as the doctor could be called as a witness in the case. Casual or careless statements may return to haunt the doctor. It is important not to make too precipitate a diagnosis and not to raise expectations too much. Good documentation of the basis for the diagnosis and treatment given is especially important

Conclusion

There is no single clearcut definition of occupational asthma, and no single test differentiates occupational from non-occupationally caused asthma. Because the consequences of the diagnosis may have effects that go far beyond the individual patient being treated, physicians should make an objective diagnosis and spend more time than usual exploring the relationships between putative exposure and the alleged effects. However, a correct diagnosis offers the potential for avoidance and sometimes "cure" as well as the opportunity to pro-

tect other colleagues within the same work environment. Finally, by defining specific causes and chemicals, the diagnosis offers opportunities for understanding the causation of asthma in a way that is not possible for the non-occupational case with a multitude of triggers.

Address for correspondence:

Michael G Pearson
Consultant Physician
Aintree Chest Centre
University Hospital Aintree
Liverpool L31 3DL
UK
Tel. +44 151 529-3857
Fax +44 151 529-2873
E-mail mikepearson@email.msn.com

References

1. International Consensus Report on the Diagnosis and Management of Asthma. Clin Exp Allergy 1992; 22(suppl):1–72.

2. Bernstein IL, Chan-Yeung M, Malo J-L, Bernstein DL. Asthma in the workplace. New York: Marcel Dekker 1993, pp. 1–3.

3. Jarvis D, Burney P. The epidemiology of allergic disease. BMJ 1998; 316:607–609.

4. Meredith S, Nordman H. Occupational asthma: Measures of frequency from four countries. Thorax 1996: 51:431–435.

5. Weill H, Butcher B, Dharmarajan V, Glindmeyer H, Jones R, Carr J, O'Neill C, Salvaggio JE. Respiratory and immunologic evaluation of isocyanate exposure in a new manufacturing plant. NIOSH technical report No. 81–125. US Government Printing Office, Washington 1981.

6. Meredith S. Reported incidence of occupational asthma in the United Kingdom, 1989–1990. J. Epidemiol Community Health 1993; 47:459–463.

7. Gannon PFG, Newton DT, Pantin CFA, Burge PS Effect of the number of peak expiratory flow readings per day on the estimate of diurnal variation. Thorax 1998; 53:790–792.

8. Bright P, Sherwood Burge P. The diagnosis of occupational asthma from serial measurements of lung function at and away from work. Thorax 1996; 51: 857–863.

9. Malo J-L, Trudeau C, Glazzo H, L'Archeveque J, Cartier A. Do subjects investigated for occupational asthma through serial peak flow measurements falsify

their results. J Allergy Clin Immunol 1995; 96:601–607.

10. Verschelden P, Cartier A, L'Archeveque J, Trudeau C, Malo J-L. Compliance with and accuracy of daily self-assessment of peak expiratory flow (PEF) in asthmatic subjects over a 3 month period. Eur Respir J 1996; 9:880–885.

11. Ross DJ, McDonald JC. Health and employment after a diagnosis of occupational asthma. Occup Med 1998; 48:219–225.

12. Losewicz S, Assouffi BK, Hawkins R, Newman-Taylor AJ. Outcome of asthma induced by isocyanates. Brit J Dis Chest 1987; 81:14–22.

Nerve Growth Factor and Asthma

Sergio Bonini*, Alessandro Lambiase**, Francesca Properzi***, Megon Bresciani****,
Guido Sacerdoti****, Stefano Bonini**, Luigi Aloe***

Keywords: Nerve growth factor, asthma, eosinophil, mast cell, lymphocyte

Increasing evidence accumulated from research performed in our own and other laboratories – and briefly reviewed below – indicates that the role of nerve growth factor (NGF) is not confined to the central and peripheral nervous system, but also extends to allergic diseases and asthma. (1) NGF serum levels are increased in patients with allergic diseases and asthma and related to the severity of the inflammatory process and disease. In vernal keratoconjunctivitis, NGF plasma levels correlate with the number of mast cells infiltrating the conjunctiva and with circulating levels of substance P. In a mouse model of allergic airway inflammation and asthma, an increased number of NGF-positive cells was detectable in the inflammatory infiltrate of the lung, and increased levels of NGF were present in serum and bronchoalveolar lavage fluids. In humans, increased mRNA for NGF is found in nasal mucosal scrapings of patients with allergic rhinitis who also show high levels of NGF in serum and nasal fluids, further increasing after specific allergen challenge. (2) NGF is released by several modulatory and effector cells of allergic inflammation and asthma, such as Th2 CD4 positive cells, mast cells, and eosinophils. NGF also increases airway hyperreactivity to histamine in a guinea pig model of asthma. (3) NGF receptors are expressed on epithelial cells of patients with allergic conjunctivitis as well as several inflammatory cells. These are able to respond to NGF with activation and mediator release. NGF administration to the eye in humans has a profound effect on fibroblast activation and reparative processes of corneal ulcers, suggesting a role for NGF also in tissue remodelling processes occurring in asthma. (4) In the mouse, anti-NGF treatment reduces airways hyperreactivity induced by ovalbumin topical challenge of sensitized animals. The above data strongly suggest that NGF is an important mediator in allergic diseases and asthma.

Introduction

Koch's postulates have often been adapted to test the hypothesis that a new molecule adds to the mediators involved in asthma [1]. To answer these postulates, the substance should:
1. be found in the biological fluids of asthmatic patients in physiological concentrations and correlate with disease activity;
2. be produced and released by inflammatory cells implicated in asthma;
3. reproduce the key features of the disease;
4. be antagonized by specific treatment with subsequent improvement of asthma symptoms.

This paper presents recently accumulated evidence that nerve growth factor (NGF), the best characterized member of the neurotrophin family, answers the above postulates and might therefore have a role in inflammatory and remodelling processes of bronchial asthma.

NGF is Increased in Biological Fluids of Asthmatic Patients

In 1996, we first reported that NGF is increased in the serum of patients with allergic diseases and asthma [2]. NGF serum levels were measured in 49 patients with asthma and/or rhinoconjunctivitis and/or urticaria angioedema and related to clinical parameters such as bronchial reactivity, total and specific serum IgE, and circulating levels of eosi-

* Allergology and Clinical Immunology and Department of Internal Medicine, Second University of Naples, Italy
** Department of Ophthalmology, University Tor Vergata, Rome, Italy
*** Institute of Neurobiology, Italian National Research Council, Rome, Italy
**** Department of Internal Medicine, Second University of Naples, Italy

nophils cationic protein (ECP). NGF was significantly increased in the 42 allergic (skin test/RAST positive) subjects compared to the 18 matched controls (49.7 ± 28.8 pg/ml vs 3.8 ± 1.7 pg/ml). Asthma patients had higher NGF serum values (87.6 ± 59.8 pg/ml) than rhinoconjunctivitis and urticaria-angioedema patients, particularly those with a documented sensitization to airborne allergens (132.1 ± 90.8 pg/ml).

NGF serum levels correlated with total IgE serum values ($p = 0.43$; $p < 0.02$), the highest values being found in asthma subjects with a high degree of bronchial reactivity to histamine and high serum values of ECP.

Interestingly enough, in vernal keratoconjunctivitis – a severe allergic inflammatory disease of the eye with mast cells, eosinophils, and CD4-Th2-type lymphocytes – the increased NGF serum value correlates with the increased number of mast cells infiltrating the conjunctiva [3] and with the circulating levels of substance P [4].

The increase of NGF in asthma has been recently confirmed by Braun et al. [5], who reported increased NGF levels in bronchoalveolar lavage during late asthmatic responses to allergen challenge, associated with an increased number of eosinophils and Th2 cytokines.

Accordingly, in allergic rhinitis patients Sanico et al. [6] found that NGF (and mRNA for it) is over-expressed in nasal mucosal scrapings and increased in nasal fluids, particularly after allergen challenge [7].

Therefore, NGF is increased in biological fluids of patients with asthma and allergic disease and correlates with disease activity.

NGF Is Produced and Released by Inflammatory Cells Implicated in Asthma

The first observation that mast cells synthesize, store, and release NGF was published in 1994 by Leon et al. in rats [8]. More recently, also human mast cells have been reported to be a source of NGF [9–10].

CD4+ lymphocytes with a Th2-type cytokine profile are known to play an important role in modulating allergic inflammatory mechanisms in asthma. We have studied NGF levels in culture super-

natants of 5 Th0, 6 Th1, and 5 Th2 clones derived from human circulating mononuclear blood cells [11]. Both Th1 and Th2 clones – but not Th0 clones – secrete NGF in basal conditions. PHA activation induces NGF secretion by Th0 clones and selectively increases the NGF release by Th2 clones.

NGF is also produced and released by human circulating *eosinophils*. In fact, NGF was found in sonicates of blood eosinophils isolated and purified from 7 subjects with mild eosinophilia, in concentrations ranging from 1.5 to 17.8 pg/ml/10 [6] cells [12]. The eosinophil production of NGF was confirmed by the demonstration of mRNA for this neurotrophin by RT-PCR in freshly isolated cells.

NGF Reproduces the Key Features of Asthma

NGF exerts its biological effects by interacting with two specific receptors: a tyrosinkinase high-affinity receptor (TrKA) and a low-affinity receptor belonging to the TNF receptor superfamily [13]. NGF receptors are expressed on several allergic inflammatory cells such as mast cells [9, 10], CD4+ lymphocytes [11], and eosinophils [12]. NGF has a priming effect on anti-IgE histamine release from circulating human basophils [14] and induces a selective release of cytotoxic mediators by peripheral blood eosinophils [12].

Interestingly enough, mast cells, CD4+ lymphocytes, and eosinophils also express NGF receptors. Therefore, we might suggest that an autocrine circuit might be involved in inducing activation and prolonging survival of these cells as has been shown for neuronal cells and B cells (see [13] for a review).

In vivo, NGF topically administered to subjects with corneal ulcers causes intense fibroblast proliferation and tissue healing [15]. All these data support the hypothesis that NGF has a role in inflammatory and remodelling processes in allergic disease and asthma. This hypothesis is more directly supported by experimental studies on the effects of NGF on bronchial hyperreactivity. Intravenously administered NGF potentates, in a dose-dependent way, the histamine-induced bronchoconstriction up to 200% in guinea pigs [16].

Anti-NGF Treatment Reduces Airways Hyperreactivity

The effect of anti-NGF treatment in antagonizing the effects of NGF on allergic inflammation and airways hyperreactivity was studied by Braun et al. [17] in a mouse model of asthma. Nasal application of anti-NGF to ovalbumin-sensitized mice significantly reduces IL-4 and prevents development of airways hyperreactivity induced by specific allergen challenge.

This preliminary observation should prompt further studies on the possibility of modulating allergic inflammation and asthma by reducing the synthesis of NGF or by blocking its activity at specific receptor level.

Concluding Remarks

Since 1990, on the basis of increasing evidence presented by several laboratories, Levi Montalcini, Aloe, and Alleva [18] suggested that the biological effects of NGF are not confined to the nervous system but also extend to the endocrine and immune systems, this molecule possibly representing or link among the integrated adaptive responses of the body to various stimuli. In this paper we have focused on the possible role of NGF in allergic inflammation and asthma.

In fact, NGF is produced by and can act on all major cells involved in the allergic inflammatory events responsible for symptoms in allergic patients. However, it is not clear at present whether NGF has a major causal role in producing allergic inflammation and airway hyperreactivity, or whether it is only an epiphenomenon – and a marker therefore – of it. Certainly, even if we consider NGF a consequence of allergic inflammation, the marked effects of this molecule on peripheral nerves and the autocrine circuits demonstrated for several inflammatory cells should still stay for some additional modulatory effect of this molecule on the complex network of inflammatory cells and mediators operating in allergic inflammation and asthma. But even more convincing are the data obtained *in vivo* about the potent effect of this growth factor on fibroblast proliferation, collagen deposition, and tissue changes during reparative processes following inflammatory events. Studies are in course in our own and other laboratories to evaluate the effects of NGF on human fibroblasts and myofibroblasts and its role in remodelling processes occurring in asthma.

Address for correspondence:

Prof. Sergio Bonini
CNR, Via di Pietralata 190
I-00100 Rome
Italy
Tel. +39 06 3534-6840
Fax +39 06 3540-3017
E-mail se.bonini-CNR@flashnet.it

References

1. Robinson C, Holgate ST. The role of leukotrienes in asthma: Evidence from clinical investigations. Adv Prostaglandin Res 1990; 20:209.

2. Bonini Se, Lambiase A, Bonini St, Angelucci F, Magrini L, Manni L, Aloe L. Circulating nerve growth factor levels are increased in humans with allergic diseases and asthma. Proc Natl Acad Sci USA 1996; 93:10955.

3. Lambiase A, Bonini St, Bonini Se, Micera A, Magrini L, Bracci-Laudiero L, Aloe L. Increased plasma levels of Nerve Growth Factor in Vernal keratoconjunctivitis and relationships to conjunctival mast cells. Invest Ophthalmol Vis Sci 1995; 36:2127.

4. Lambiase A, Bonini St, Micera A, Tirassa P, Magrini L, Bonini Se, Aloe L. Increased plasma levels of substance P in vernal keratoconjunctivitis. Inv Ophthalmol Vis Sci 1997; 38:2161.

5. Braun A, Lommatsch M, Lewin G, Virchow C, Renz H. Neurotrophins: A link between airway inflammation and airway smooth muscle contractility in asthma? Int Arch Allergy Immunol 1999; 118:163–165.

6. Sanico AM, Proud D, Koliatsos V, Stanisz A, Bienenstock J, Togias A. Nerve growth factor in allergic rhinitis. J Allergy Clin Immunol 1999; 103:S172.

7. Sanico AM, Koliatsos VE, Stanisz A, Bienenstock J, Togias A. Neural hyperresponsiveness and nerve growth factor in allergic rhinitis. Int Arch Allergy Immunol 1999; 118:154–158.

8. Leon A, Buriani A, Dal Toso R, Fabris M, Romanello S, Aloe L, Levi-Montalcini R. Mast cells synthesize, store and release nerve growth factor. Proc Natl Acad Sci USA 1994; 91:3739.

9. Nilsson G, Forsberg-Nilsson K, Xiang Z, Hallbook F, Nilsson K, Metcalfe DD. Human mast cell express

functional TrkA and are a source of nerve growth factor. Eur J Immunol 1997; 27:2295.

10. See-Ying T, Tsai M, Yamaguchi M, Yano K, Butterfield JH, Galli SJ. Expression of functional TrkA receptor tyrosine kinase in the HMC-1 human mast cell line in human mast cell. Blood 1997; 90:1807.

11. Lambiase A, Bracci-Laudiero L, Bonini Se, Bonini St, Starace G, D'Elios MM, De Carli M, Aloe L. Human CD4$^+$ T cell clones produce and release nerve growth factor and express high-affinity nerve growth factor receptors. J Allergy Clin Immunol 1997; 100:408–414.

12. Solomon A, Aloe L, Pe'er J, Frucht-Pery J, Bonini St, Bonini Se, Levi-Schaffer F. Nerve Growth Factor is preformed blood eosinophils. J Allergy Clin Immunol 1998; 102:454.

13. Aloe L, Bracci-Laudiero L, Bonini Se, Manni L. The expanding role of nerve growth factor: From neurotrophic activity to immunologic diseases. Allergy 1997; 52:883.

14. Bischoff SC, Dahinden CA. Effect of nerve growth factor on the release of inflammatory mediators by mature human basophils. Blood 1992; 79:2662.

15. Lambiase A, Rama P, Bonini St, Caprioglio G, Aloe L. Topical treatment with Nerve Growth Factor for corneal neurotrophic ulcers. New Engl J Med 1998; 338:1174.

16. De Vries A, Dessing MC, Engels F, Henricks PAJ, Nijkamp FP. Nerve growth factor induces a neurokinin-1 receptor mediated airway hyperresponsiveness. Am J Resp Crit Care Med 1999; 159:A281.

17. Braun A, Appel E, Baruch R, Hera U, Botchkarev V, Paus R, Brodic C, Renz H. Role of nerve growth factor in a mouse model of allergic airway inflammation and asthma. Eur J Immunol 1998; 28:3240.

18. Levi-Montalcini R, Aloe L, Alleva E. A role for nerve growth factor in nervous, endocrine and immune systems. Progr Neuroendocrinimmunol 1990; 1:1.

Measuring the Outcome of Asthma

Michael G Pearson*

Keywords: Asthma outcomes, population measures, clinical views, patient perspectives, clinical governance

The measurement of the outcome of any chronic medical condition is made difficult because it is hard to separate the effects of a treatment intervention from changes due to the continuing presence of diesase. However, it is possible to derive surrogate mesasures – outcome indicators – which, while imprecise, do nevertheless provide a sufficient picture of the care processes to highlight problems that deserve more detailed attention. Indicators such as death rates are relevant for studies of large populations but of little import to individual doctors and not at all to patients. Patient-centred outcomes are hardest to measure, but since the object of medicine is to make patients feel better, they need to be recorded. A recent workshop at the Royal College of Physidans has defined a simple 3-question measure that is useable in every asthma consultation and that can be aggregated to provide a measure of the success or otherwise of individual doctors in controlling their asthma patients. The challenge will be to devise automated methods for collecting and collating such simple measures on a routine basis.

Introduction

The ideal target outcome of medical management is a cure for the patient. However for most chronic medical conditions this is quite unrealistic. The cure has either not yet been discovered the best that can be hoped for is to produce a remission or a slowing of the progression of disease.

In surgery, it is relatively easy to measure whether for example herniorraphy repairs have been successful because there is a clear start point – the presence of the hernia, a clear intervention – surgery, and a clear end point – absence of the hernia. In a chronic medical condition, patients present at varying stages of disease, have different rates of natural progression and moreover there is often no endpoint because the disease progresses slowly over many years. The latter is complicated by the natural ageing process which itself leads to reduced function in most body functions, and also by the presence of other pathology which may mask or make it harder to assess the effect of the first condition.

Asthma is a chronic condition which often starts in childhood but can come on at any age. Childhood asthma may remit completely in early adult life only to recur years later in a proportion or people. Once present, asthma may follow a benign course with treatment controlling most if not all the symptoms, and with no obvious deterioration even over many years. Or it may be a progressive condition that over 20 to 30 years leads to respiratory insufficiency. And of course at any time a small proportion of asthmatics develop an acute attack from which they die. It is therefore a disease with a wide variability between patients and can also be confused with many other chronic medical conditions especially cardiac dysfunction and chronic obstructive pulmonary disease.

Therapy to control the pathologic process of the disease is effective in most patients but there remains no cure. The burden of disease from asthma is substantial with drugs (10% of all drugs prescribed) [1], hospital admissions (3% of all medical admissions) and lost time from productive work costing the UK 500–800 million pounds per year. Thus the incentive to optimize the provision of asthma therapy is considerable. But establishing that treatment is cost-effective implies a need to measure what the outcome of treatment is. Hence the current interest to measure what has previously appeared to be unmeasurable.

* Consultant Physician, Aintree Chest Centre, University Hospital Aintree, Liverpool, UK; Director of the Clinical Effectiveness and Evaluation Unit, Royal College of Physicians, London; Visiting Professor, University of Salford, Salford, UK

What Is an Outcome?

A recent UK report defines a health outcome as

"a change in health, health related status, or risk factors affecting health. A health outcome may be the result of the natural history of the disease or they may be the effect of interventions designed to prevent or treat it." [2]

The report was particularly concerned with the effect of health interventions and recognized that direct outcomes of particular interventions were often not possible but that it might be possible to derive an indicator of outcome from aggregated statistical measures about a group of patients compiled from assessments made on that population. The indicator might not necessarily produce an absolute answer as to whether care is good or bad but it should at least provide a pointer to circumstances that are worthy of further investigation.

Choosing Indicators of Outcome

At different parts of the health system there are different perspective as to what an outcome is. At national level the concern is for the overall picture and national death rates, admission rates are clearly of interest. In contrast, at the level of an individual primary care doctor who may have 1 or 2 patients admitted with asthma each year and may only see an asthma death twice in a career such outcomes are too infrequent to be of any value as indicators of care quality. The different perspectives may therefore relate to

- *the population* – with the aim of the monitoring interventions to reduce deaths, reduce the number of acute attacks and to reduce or avoid risk factors for asthma
- *the clinical picture* – such as the need to detect asthma early, to prevent exacerbations, to return function to normal and to reduce the impact of asthma on general well being
- *the patient* – who is concerned that exacerbations and symptoms are minimized and that asthma should have minimal impact on lifestyle.

The working group that produced the UK Department of Health report considered each of these areas and attempted to recommend indicators for each. For each indicator recommended a detailed

specification was constructed which included a precise definition of both numerator and denominator, the rationale supporting the adoption of a particular measure and comment on the potential uses and of potential confounding factors that could make interpretation difficult. A few of the recommendations are discussed below.

Population Measures

Many countries have collected data on causes of death using standard ICD coding systems to do so. However the accuracy of such data are variable and many studies have shown that 25–30% of deaths attributed to asthma are not in fact due to asthma, although this must be balanced by an unknown number of deaths due to but not coded as asthma. The "signal noise" produced by such "random" errors is considerable but at national level the figures appear to be acceptably robust for monitoring trends in death rates. UK deaths figures from asthma reached a peak in the late 1980s and have been falling from nearly 2000 deaths per year to just over 1300 in 1996 [3]. This is mirrored by a reduction in hospital admissions due to asthma in all age groups from 1994 onwards and since the changes are apparent in all age groups (except the over 85 years group), and are progressive over time, they seem likely to be real [4]. However, while it would be encouraging to believe that the production of national guidelines and of increased medical activity around asthma are responsible, it is not possible to differentiate with any certainty the effect of the health interventions from changes in the natural history of the condition or from other factors such as changes in the environment or even the national diet.

However trends that persist over time are likely to be an indication of the effectiveness or otherwise of the health service and thus are useful for service planning. Data can be expressed in various ways from simple numbers of deaths to examining age specific rates or years of life lost – both of which make allowance of age at death which is clearly a strong potential confounder.

The Clinical View

Doctors are trained to consider asthma as a disease characterized by reversible airflow obstruction in which lung function will vary from normal to ab-

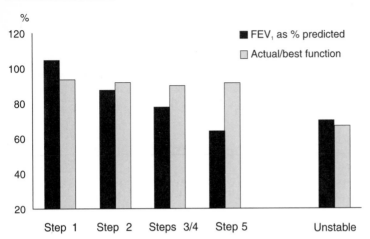

Figure 1. FEV$_1$ and PEF levels.

normal as the disease fluctuates. It therefore makes sense to consider measurements of PEF and FEV$_1$ as markers of asthma control and in addition to add in the number of severe attacks (e.g., bad enough to require admission to hospital). However the variability of the PEF and FEV$_1$ with time in the same patient even within a single day makes it impossible to estimate asthma control from single measurements at one point in time. Serial measurements of PEF are difficult to collect reliably and even more difficult to collect in a standard fashion that can be recorded automatically for analysis by the health service. There are many studies in which PEF recording has been used but the relationship of PEF values to other estimates of asthma control remains variable – likely to be a consequence of the variable standards of data recording by different patients. In occupational asthma studies comparing the values written down by patients with those recorded on a computer chip in the PF meter, as many as 50% of data points were erroneous [5].

A further problem when using change in lung function as an outcome is the need to make allowance for the expected decline due to normal ageing and the huge differences due to gender and different stature. The rate of decline of lung function is potentially of great interest but the challenge of collecting and linking together serial data on many patients during routine practice is daunting. An original way out of these difficulties has been put forward by Connolly et al. [6] who from a serial review of patients attending hospital asthma clinics observed that the actual function recorded at a particular visit could be compared with the best achieved by that individual within the recent past,

e.g., the previous one to two years. This provides a degree of control not only for the variability due to different sizes and gender of patients but also for their disease severity. They divided patients into levels of severity according to the asthma therapy recommended for the five steps of the British asthma guidelines, and found that the actual PEF or FEV$_1$ expressed as percent of predicted fall with increasing disease severity but that the "actual" divided by the "best" (expressed as a percentage) was greater than 85% at each disease level if the patient was well controlled (Figure 1) but reduced when asthma was unstable.

Although the maths and disciplined recording needed to achieve this measure in current routine practice are considerable, the increasing use of computerized records makes it likely that such data based on a series of visits to a surgery or clinic could be collected and could be used to both monitor correct control and also the numbers of patients with progressively declining function. Because it is applicable at all levels of asthma, such a measure would be equally applicable to the hospital clinic and to the primary care centre.

An alternative might be to record the acute episodes of asthma – which represent the failures of disease control. However although hospital admissions are relatively easy to collect from patient admission systems, their value as an indicator is only relevant at a population level because numbers per primary care doctor are too small. With a hospital admission rate in the UK of about 0.8 per 1000 of adult population the indicator only begins to achieve reasonable numbers when populations of small cities are studied. There are many more lesser exacerbations experienced by patients but the problem of defining what constitutes an exacerbation and moreover of finding a way of routinely recording the episodes has so far not been resolved.

Patient Perspectives

Patients have little interest in what the level of lung function is and are little concerned by national death figures that have affected "other people." Their concerns are to do with whether they notice symptoms from their asthma and whether the asthma is interfering with their lifestyle or not. However patient perceptions of asthma vary widely and so too do their attitudes to the impairment it imposes on them. At the extremes, some asthmatics manage to stay at work despite poorly controlled severe asthma with very poor lung function, whilst others become almost housebound despite what appears to the doctor to be mild asthma. Thus the effect of asthma on each individual is variable and accurate measurement is not easy. Detailed measures of lifestyle are possible [7, 8] with questionnaires that examine 4 or more domains of the patients experience and amalgamate the result into a "quality of life score." The utility of these instruments in clinical trials is now well proven and their relationship to other measures of asthma such as lung function, admission rates and responses to treatment are well known. However while it is possible in a research study to ask a patient 32 or 72 questions, the same is not so during a routine consultation.

Various workers have demonstrated that much shorter instruments can obtain data that indicate the same type of information at least when analyzed for groups of patients. Jones [9] developed a 3-question index with very simple yes/no answers and showed that within a single general practice population it was possible to relate the practice score to measures of asthma severity such as admission rates, and to lung function and that over time the measure was also sensitive to changes resulting from an aggressive asthma management plan for those patients with symptoms. Rimington et al. reported a 4-question score [10] and compared the results obtained with that from the Juniper Asthma Quality of Life Questionnaire and found that there was a good group correlation. The Tayside 3-question score has been shown to relate to better care for patients without additional cost to the health service [11]. The potential of these short scores was noted in the asthma outcome indi-

cator report but with the rider that further work should be done to define precisely which form the instrument should take and second how it might be used in routine care.

A workshop was convened by the Clinical Effectiveness and Evaluation unit of the Royal College of Physicians to address this in 1998. It brought together 12 groups from around the UK with experience of working with a short (but different) questionnaire. Each contributed details of their questionnaire and data obtained using their instrument and at the end of a constructive debate there was unanimous agreement that all should work to a single 3-question score based on questions that ought to form part of every asthma consultation at any level of severity. The three questions were:
- In the last week (or month), have you had difficulty sleeping because of your asthma symptoms (including cough).
- In the last week (or month), have you had your usual asthma symptoms during the day (cough, wheeze, chest tightness or breathlessness)?
- In the last week (or month), has your asthma interfered with your usual activities (e. g., housework, work/school, etc.)?

The answers to these questions can be recorded either as yes/no ie the symptom has been present or absent in the past week/month or as a semi quantitative answer along the lines of the Tayside schema, i. e., *None / once or twice per month / once or twice per week / most days/nights.*

Other items were considered for inclusion of which one deserves comment. Many pharmaceutical trials have used a question on the frequency of β_2-agonist use as an indicator of poor control. The group rejected this for two main reasons. First, the information may not be reliable. It is likely to be confounded in those patients who despite the recommendations in the guidelines continue to use their reliever inhaler on a regular qds basis and because the severity trigger for use varies so much between patients. Second, the information can be obtained better from the computerized prescribing records that are held by most general practitioners in the UK which should show exactly how often a patient is receiving repeat prescriptions and moreover this can be collected automatically by programming the computer without need to ask the patient.

The potential for targetting those patients with most symptoms has already been demonstrated by Jones et al. [9]. If the semiquantitative score is used and if a score from 0 to 3 for each question is summed, it is possible to derive an asthma control score (between 0 and 9) for each patient. At the extremes there will be little doubt that a patient with no symptoms (zero score) is well controlled and the patient with lots of symptoms (score of 9) is poorly controlled, but in the individual there are no data to show that the score is sufficiently specific for it to be anything but a general guide for the monitoring of treatment. However if the scores are aggregated over a group of patients attending a single primary care practice, it would be possible to calculate an overall asthma control score for that practice.

If some control were made for the case-mix (social deprivation, age, asthma severity, etc.) of the population, comparisons between the level of symptom control achieved by different practitioners might become possible. Clearly it would be of considerable interest to patients to know that the asthma patients attending their doctor has less symptoms that average for that area, and demonstrating that the average symptom score fell over time as new therapy was introduced or just better application of existing treatment would be useful for the individual doctor and for the authorities charged with monitoring practice standards.

However, this last issue has become highly political in the UK following some high profile failures of medical care. The UK General Medical Council has announced that all doctors must have their standards of clinical practice revalidated at regular intervals and clearly if there are objective measures of outcome then they are likely to be used as part of the assessment.

Many doctors find the concept that their care is to be formally assessed with the results being known to others as professionally threatening. However patients are expecting more of their doctors and it must be better to have some objective measures of the effectiveness of medical care than to rely upon subjective opinion. Good doctors will have nothing to fear – and we should have no brief with those whose care is substandard.

Address for correspondence:

Michael G Pearson
Consultant Physician
Aintree Chest Centre
University Hospital Aintree
Liverpool L31 3DL, UK
Tel. +44 151 529-3857
Fax +44 151 529-2873
E-mail mikepearson@email.msn.com

References

1. Department of Health Asthma. An epidemiological overview. London: HMSO 1994.
2. Pearson M, Goldacre M, Coles J et al. (Eds). Outcome indicators for asthma: Report of a working group to the Department of Health London. Royal College of Physicians Research Unit and Oxford Unit of Health Care Epidemiology, NHSE, London 1999.
3. Campbell MJ, Cog man GR, Holgate ST, Johnston SL. Age specific trends in asthma mortality in England and Wales 1983–5: Results of an observational study. Brit Med J 1997; 314:1439–1440.
4. Decreased admissions data – Burney.
5. Cote J, Cartier A, Malo J-L, Robeau M, Boulet LP. Compliance with PEF monitoring in home management of asthma. Chest 1998; 113:968–972.
6. Connolly CK, Prescott RJ, Alcock SM Gatnash AA. Actual over best function as an outcome measure in asthma. Respir Med 1994; 8:453–459.
7. Jones PW, Quirk FH, Baveystock CM, Littlejohns P. A self complete measure of health status for chronic airflow limitation: The St Georges Respiratory Questionnaire. Am Rev Respir Dis 1992; 145:1321–1327.
8. Juniper E, Guyatt GH, Epstein RS, Ferrie PJ, Jaeschke R, Hiller ER. Evaluation of impairment of health related quality of life in asthma: Development of a questionnaire for use in clinical trials. Thorax 1992; 47:76–83.
9. Jones KP, Charlton I, Middleton M, Preece W, Hill A. Targeting asthma care in general practice using a morbidity index. BMJ 1992; 304:1353–1356.
10. Rimmington L, Aaronovsky L, Mowatt A, Wharburton E, Ryland I, Pearson MG. Use of a simple patient focussed asthma morbidity score. Eur Resp J 1997; 10:194s.
11. Bryce FP, Neville RG, Clark RA, Crombie IK, MacKenzie P. Controlled trial of an audit facilitator in the diagnosis and treatment of childhood asthma in general practice. BMJ 1995;310:838–842.

Intercellular Adhesion Molecules: Clinical Perspectives

Giovanni Passalacqua, Giorgio Ciprandi, Annamaria Riccio, Antonio Scordamaglia, Mercedes Pasquali, Giorgio Walter Canonica*

Keywords: Allergic inflammation, cell adhesion molecules, ICAM-1

Cell adhesion molecules (CAMs) are heavily involved in many biological processes, including tissue architecture maintenance, embryogenesis, and inflammation. Because of their high flexibility, CAMs govern the selective migration and recruitment of inflammatory cells at the site of an allergic reaction. ICAM-1 (CD54) seems to play a central role, and it can be considered a reliable marker of ongoing allergic inflammation. ICAM-1 is promptly expressed on epithelial cells following allergen-specific challenge and, to a lesser extent, during subliminal continuous exposure to allergen. This latter fact represents the so-called minimal persistent inflammation (MPI). Since ICAM-1 is the main receptor for human rhinoviruses, a link between infections of upper airways and asthma attacks can be envisaged. Thus, the pharmacological modulation of CAMs may represent a promising therapeutical target. Several antihistamines, corticosteroids, and specific immunotherapy have been demonstrated as being able to downregulate the expression of CAMs, and this effect parallels the clinical efficacy. Based on these premises, a correct treatment strategy for respiratory allergy should be targeted not only to symptoms, but also to allergic inflammation. In this regard a continuous antihistamine treatment has been proven to be more effective than the "on-demand" one. This fact has been recently substantiated in several *in vivo* studies by means of the nasal and conjunctival models. Finally, the Early Treatment of Allergic Children (ETAC) study confirmed the preventive potential of an early and continuous treatment in children.

Introduction

During the last 10 years, our knowledge of mechanisms sustaining the allergic reaction (namely, allergic inflammation) has developed rapidly, thus producing a complex network of cells and signals. IgE, mast cells, and histamine release still remain the main components involved in the early phases of allergic reaction, but a wide variety of other cells, mediators, and molecules (e. g., T lymphocytes, leukotrienes, cytokines, kinins, and adhesion molecules) contribute to the subsequent events.

The allergic reaction is not only a short-lived phenomenon, but rather a continuous process that leads to an inflammatory infiltration of the target organs (i. e., nose, conjunctiva, and bronchi). An adhesion machinery indeed governs the migration and selective recruitment of inflammatory cells at the site of allergic inflammation [1]. The ICAM-1 molecule is now recognized as a protagonist of cells' migration and a reliable marker of allergic inflammation. Therefore, the knowledge of the kinetics of its expression on epithelia may be regarded as an important topic for both pathophysiology and for new therapeutical strategies [2]. The experimental studies involving adhesion molecules have also led us to discover a possible link between viral infections and asthma in children and promising new therapeutical approaches.

Adhesion Molecules: General Aspects

During the early 1980s, some molecules were described with the apparently unique aim of mediating the cell-to-cell adhesion. These molecules were grouped under the name of cell adhesion molecules (CAMs). CAMs are classified (based on the chemical structure) into four main families: Ig superfamily, integrins, selectins, and cadherins [1, 3]. Adherence processes are involved in many biological

---

* Allergy and Respiratory Diseases, Dept of Internal Medicine, Genoa University, Genoa, Italy

events: inflammation, embryogenesis, wound healing, tissue growth, and tissue structure maintenance. Indeed, immune inflammation, allergic reaction, and autoimmunity are the most extensively investigated fields, as well as the possible pharmacological modulation of CAMs.

The impressive structural etherogeneicity of CAMs is counterbalanced by a common function: the cell-to-cell contact. CAMs are responsible for intercellular adhesion, cell adhesion to epithelia and endothelia, recruitment, selective migration, and homing. The system is highly flexible because of some characteristics: (1) the differential distribution of CAMs (some of them are ubiquitous and others are or cell-type specific); (2) the possible modulation of their expression by inflammatory mediators (inducibility); (3) the existence of soluble forms of CAMs, which may likely act as regulating elements of the system itself; (4) CAMs may also act as activating elements for some cells.

Immunoglobulin Superfamily (Ig-like Structure)

Includes: Igs, TCR, CD3, major histocompatibility complex (MHC) molecules, CD4, and CD8. LFA-2 binds LFA-3, which has wide tissue distribution. ICAM-1 is strongly inducible by inflammatory stimuli and mainly binds the integrin LFA-1, as do ICAM-2 and ICAM-3, but the latter molecules are usually constitutively expressed on endothelial cells and leukocytes. ICAM-1, because of its inducibility, seems to have a pivotal role in allergic inflammation. Finally, the CD28/B7.1-B7.2 system, which seems to be involved in lymphocyte activation process [4].

Integrins (Noncovalent Heterodimers, α and β Chain)

They are further subdivided (based on β chain structure) into β1 integrins or very late antigens (VLA); β2 integrins or leukocyte integrins expressed on leukocytes; β3 integrins or cytoadhesins expressed on endothelial cells and platelets.

Selectins (N-Terminal Lectin Domain) [5]

These are promptly expressed, under inflammatory stimuli, on leukocytes and endothelial cells, and mediate the early phases of adhesion of leukocytes to vessels' endothelium. P-, E-, and L-selectin are the main members of this family.

Cadherins

These have only recently been described. These molecules are different in structure from the others, and usually perform homophilic adhesion.

The selective expression pattern of CAMs and their modulation partly explain the margination and recruitment of inflammatory cells at the site of allergic reaction. This mechanism has been elucidated for eosinophils (and other leukocytes) in asthma [6–8]. The inflammatory mediators release causes vasodilation and bloodstream deceleration; this fact plus the prompt expression of P-sel on endothelial cells induces the "rolling-over" of leukocytes. The next step (firm adhesion) is due to the heterotypic adhesion between leukocyte beta integrins and ICAM-1/ICAM-2. It is of note that ICAM-1 expression on endothelial cells is enhanced by inflammatory stimuli. It is remarkable, too, that eosinophils, but not neutrophils, express VLA-4, which binds VCAM-1, which may explain the selective eosinophil recruitment in allergic inflammation. Members of integrin family operate the binding of leukocytes to extracellular matrix.

The Role of CAMs in Allergic Inflammation

Very recently, the epithelium captured the attention of both basic scientists and allergists. Epithelial cells are no longer considered to be simple bystanders of the allergic reaction; rather, they express to varying degree adhesion molecules, and this expression can be modulated by inflammatory mediators [9]. Both the conjunctival and the nasal challenge represent an ideal model for studying allergic inflammation and CAMs' expression [10]. In fact these procedures apply the stimulus directly to the target organ: They are well tolerated by patients and allow us to use a wide variety of stimuli, including allergen, hyperosmolar solution and histamine. Nasal and conjunctival cells promptly express ICAM-1 upon allergen-specific challenge [11, 12], as well as under natural allergenic exposure, whereas pollenosic patients do not show local inflammatory aspects outside of the pollen season. This is similar to what is observed in the bronchial mucosa of asthmatic subjects [13, 14]. On the other hand, allergic subjects continuously exposed to the offending allergen (i. e., mites) have a mild inflammatory infiltration and a weak expression of ICAM-1 on epithelia, even when they are completely asymptomatic [15]. This phenomenon is called minimal persistent inflammation (MPI). Thus, a continuous allergen exposure may induce a minimal persistent inflammation, without clinical symptoms, and ICAM-1 may be employed as a reliable marker of clinical and subclinical inflammation. It is noteworthy that ICAM-1 has been demonstrated to be a selective receptor for human rhinoviruses [16]. Therefore, the continuous expression of ICAM-1 on epithelial cells in symptom-free allergic subjects should be regarded as a possible triggering event for asthma attacks. In fact, rhinoviral infections are the most frequent event preceding asthma attacks in children.

Clinical Perspectives

Based on the premises above, some interesting therapeutical implications can be derived. In particular, the pharmacological modulation of CAMs and a continuous rather than on-demand drug treatment could be envisaged.

Indeed, some experimental attempts to block ICAM-1 function by means of specific monoclonal antibodies have been made [17–18] with encouraging results, though this approach obviously needs further investigations for its potential role in humans. On the other hand, some of the newer antihistamines have been demonstrated as being able to modulate the expression of ICAM-1 on cultured cell lines (conjunctiva, gut, bronchi) [19–20]. Similar results were obtained with budesonide [21].

Nasal and conjunctival models have been widely used to evaluate the effects of different compounds on ICAM-1 expression. The administration of azelastine to the eye reduced ICAM-1 expression in pollinosic subjects under natural allergenic exposure [22]. Cetirizine reduced the nasal the allergic inflammation under seasonal pollen exposure [23] and the minimal persistent inflammation in perennial rhinitis [24]. Also the glucocorticoid deflazacort was demonstrated as being able of inhibiting the molecular and cellular events of the late-phase reaction after specific ocular challenge, but it did not affect the early-phase reaction [25]. On the contrary, nasal fluticasone reduced both the early- and late-phase events following allergen challenge [26]. Terfenadine (in a 7-day course) reduced

inflammatory infiltration, ICAM-1 expression, and soluble ECP levels in nasal lavage, in symptomatic pollinosic subjects [27]. Finally, loratadine administered orally for 2 weeks, reduced inflammatory phenomena under natural allergen exposure, and its antiallergic effect was superimposable on that of cetirizine [28].

Interestingly, also local immunotherapy appeared able of reducing the inflammatory events (and ICAM-1 expression on epithelia) following specific allergen challenge. This fact has been demonstrated with both local nasal immunotherapy [29] and sublingual/swallow immunotherapy [30]. These effects well correlate with the other inflammatory parameters and the clinical effectiveness.

When the presence of an allergic inflammation underlying clinical features is considered, a continuous treatment is expected to be more effective than an on-demand one. This hypothesis has been substantiated in studies conducted with H1 antagonists [31–32]. In these studies, continuous treatment achieved an effective symptomatological relief and a better control of the inflammatory phenomena.

Finally, continuous treatment (over a 1-year period) with the antihistamine terfenadine was demonstrated as able to reduce the morbidity of upper respiratory infections in children suffering from mite-induced respiratory allergy [33]. The same was demonstrated in a controlled trial of continuous treatment with cetirizine, in which a significant drug-sparing effect was also seen [Ciprandi et al., submitted]. This facts are in agreement with the hypothesis of the involvement of ICAM-1 expression in MPI and viral infections. The preventive potential of antihistamines in atopic children has recently been substantiated by the experimental data of the ETAC study [34].

Conclusions

Adhesion molecules play a relevant role in the processes of allergic inflammation, since they regulate the recruitment of inflammatory cells. In particular, ICAM-1 has been recognized as a hallmark of the allergic inflammation, promptly expressed upon allergen exposure. Nasal and conjunctival challenges represent a reliable and safe experimental tool for studying inflammatory phenomena of allergic reaction. These models allow the study of the antiallergic properties of several compounds, commonly used for the treatment of allergic diseases. Several treatments (new antihistamines, corticosteroids, and immunotherapy) have been demonstrated as being able of reducing both inflammatory infiltration and ICAM-1 expression on nasal and conjunctival epithelial cells, this paralleled by a clinical effect. Moreover, the experimental data obtained so far on the modulation of ICAM-1 and inflammation suggest that the better strategy for upper respiratory allergy treatment is the continuous rather than the on-demand one. In other words, a treatment over the whole period of exposure allows one to achieve both an optimal clinical effect and a control of the allergic inflammation. Finally, the possible preventive action of antihistamine in atopic children is a promising perspective.

Address for correspondence:

Giorgio Walter Canonica
Allergy and Respiratory Diseases – DIMI
L.go R.Benzi 10
I-16132 Genoa
Italy
Tel. +39 010 353-8931
Fax + 39 010 353-8904

References

1. Springer T. Adhesion receptors of the immune system. Nature 1990; 346:425–433.

2. Canonica GW, Ciprandi G, Pesce GP, Buscaglia S, Paolieri F, Bagnasco M. ICAM-1 on epithelial cells in allergic subjects: A hallmark of allergic inflammation. Int Arch Allergy Clin Immunol 1995; 107:99–104.

3. Dustin ML, Springer T. Role of lymphocyte adhesion receptors in transient interactions and cell locomotion. Annu Rev Immunol 1991; 9:27–32.

4. Linsley P, Brady W, Grosmaire L, Aruffo A, Damle NK, Ledbetter JA. Binding of the b cell activation antigen B7 to CD28 costimulates T cell proliferation and IL2 mRNA accumulation. J Exp Med 1991; 173:721–722.

5. Bevilacqua M, Butcher E, Furie B. Selectins: A family of adhesion receptors. Cell 1991; 67:233.

6. Calderon E, Lockey RF. A possible role for adhesion molecules in asthma. J Allergy Clin Immunology 1992; 90:852–865.

7. Smith CH, Barker JW, Lee TH. Adhesion molecules

8. Hansel TT, Walker C. The migration of eosinophils into the sputum of asthmatics: The role of adhesion molecules. Clin Exp Allergy 1992; 22:345–350.

9. Paolieri F, Battifora M, Pesce G, Riccio AM, Canonica GW, Bagnasco M. Intercellular adhesion molecule 1 on cultured human cell lines: Influence of proinflammatory cytokines. Allergy 1998; 53:1178–1181.

10. Ciprandi G, Passalacqua G, Azzarone B, Bagnasco M, Canonica GW. Molecular events in allergic inflammation: Expression of adhesion molecules and their modulation. In G Marone (Eds), Asthma and allergic diseases. London: Academic Press 1998, pp. 309–315.

11. Ciprandi G, Buscaglia S, Pesce GP, Villaggio B, Bagnasco M, Canonica GW. Allergic subjects express intercellular adhesion molecule 1 on epithelial cells of conjunctiva after specific allergenic challenge. J Allergy Clin Immunol 1993; 91:783–792.

12. Ciprandi G, Pronzato C, Ricca V, Passalacqua G, Bagnasco M, Canonica GW. Allergen specific challenge induces ICAM1 expression on nasal epithelial cells in allergic subjects: Relationships with early and late phase events. Am Rev Resp Crit Care Med 1994; 150:1653–1659.

13. Vignola AM, Campbell A, Chanez P, Bousquet J, Lacost P, Michel FB, Godard P. HLA DR and ICAM1 expression on bronchial epithelial cells in asthma and chronic bronchitis. Am Rev Resp Dis 1993; 148:689–694.

14. Djukanovic R, Roche WR, Wilson JW. Mucosal inflammation in asthma. Am Rev Resp Dis 1990; 142: 434–439.

15. Ciprandi G, Buscaglia S, Pesce GP, Pronzato C, Ricca V, Parmiani S, Bagnasco M, Canonica GW. Minimal persistent inflammation is present at mucosal level in asymptomatic rhinitic patients with allergy due to mites. J Allergy Clin Immunol 1995; 96:971–979.

16. Greve M, Davis G, Meyer AM, Forte CP, Yost SC, Marlor CW, Kamark EM, McClelland AM. The major human rhinoviruses receptor is ICAM-1. Cell 1989; 56:839–842.

17. Wegner CD, Gundel RH, Reilly P, Haynes N, Letts G, Rothlein R. Intercellular adhesion molecule 1 in the pathogenesis of asthma. Science 1990; 247:456–460.

18. Kavanaguch AF, Nichols LA, Lipski PE. Treatment of refractory rheumathoid arthritis with anti CD54 monoclonal antibodies. Arthritis Rheum 1992; 35(s): 40.

19. Buscaglia S, Catrullo A, Ciprandi G, Pesce GP, Fiorino N, Paolieri F, Bagnasco M, Canonica GW. Levocabastine eye drops reduces ICAM-1 expression both

in allergic inflammation. Am Rev Resp Dis 1993; 148:s75.

in vitro and *in vivo*. XV European Congress of Allergology and Clin Immunol. Allergy 1995; 26(50):79.

20. Paolieri F, Riccio AM, Battifora M, Ciprandi G, Bagnasco M, Canonica GW. MDL16455A and terfenadine in vitro activity on human continuous cell lines. XV European Congress of Allergology and Clin Immunol. Allergy 1995; 26(50):77.

21. Scordamaglia A, Paolieri F, Battifora M, Milanese M, Riccio AM, Bagnasco M, Canonica GW. Budesonide in vitro action on a human continuous bronchial cell line: ICAM-1 expression. XV European Congress of Allergology and Clin Immunol. Allergy 1995; 26(50): 266.

22. Ciprandi G, Pronzato C, Passalacqua G et al. Topical azelastine reduces eosinophil activation and ICAM-1 expression on nasal epithelial cells: An antiallergic activity. J Allergy Clin Immunol 1997; 98:1088–1096.

23. Ciprandi G, Buscaglia S, Pesce GP, Passalacqua G, Rihoux JP, Bagnasco M, Canonica GW. Cetirizine reduces inflammatory cell recruitment and ICAM1 expression on conjunctival epithelium both in early and late phase reaction after specific allergenic challenge. J Allergy Clin Immunol 1995, 95:612–621.

24. Fasce L, Ciprandi G, Pronzato C, Cozzani S, Tosca MA, Grimaldi I, Canonica GW. Cetirizine reduces ICAM-1 expression on epithelial cells during nasal minimal persistent inflammation in asymptomatic children with mite allergic asthma. Int Arch Allergy Immunol 1996 109:272–276.

25. Ciprandi G, Buscaglia S, Pesce GP, Iudice A, Bagnasco M, Canonica GW. Deflazacort protects against late phase but not early phase reactions induced by allergen specific conjunctival provocation test. Allergy 1993; 48:421–425.

26. Ciprandi G, Ricca V, Passalacqua G, Fasolo A, Canonica GW. Intranasal fluticasone propionate reduces ICAM-1 on nasal epithelium both during early and late phase after allergen challenge. Clin Exp Allergy 1998; 28:293–299.

27. Ciprandi G, Pronzato C, Ricca V, Varese P, Del Giacco GS, Canonica GW. Terfenadine exerts antiallergic activity reducing ICAM-1 expression on nasal epithelial cells in patients with pollen allergy. Clin Exp Allergy 1995; 25:871–878.

28. Ciprandi G, Pronzato C, Ricca V, Passalacqua G, Danzig M, Canonica GW. Loratadine treatment of rhinitis due to pollen allergy reduces epithelial ICAM-1 expression. Clin Exp Allergy 1997; 27: 1175–1179.

29. Passalacqua G, Albano M, Ruffoni S, Pronzato C, Riccio AM, DiBerardino L, Scordamaglia A, Canonica GW. Local nasal immunotherapy to parietaria: Evidence of reduction of allergic inflammation. Am J Resp Crit Care Med 1995; 152:461–466.

30. Passalacqua G, Albano M, Fregonese L, Riccio AM, Pronzato C, Mela GS, Canonica GW. Long-term allergoid treatment with allergoid dust mite immunotherapy in mite induced rhinoconjunctivitis. Lancet 1998; 351:629–632.

31. Ciprandi G, Passalacqua G, Mincarini M, Ricca V, Canonica GW. Continuous versus on demand treatment with cetirizine for allergic rhinitis. Ann Allergy Asthma Immunol 1997; 79:505–507.

32. Ciprandi G, Ricca V, Passalacqua G, et al. Seasonal rhinitis and azelastine: Long- or short-term treatment? J Allergy Clin Immunol 1997; 99:301–307.

33. Ciprandi G, Ricca V, Passalacqua G, Tosca MA, Landi M, Canonica GW. Continuous antihistamine treatment controls allergic inflammation and reduces respiratory morbidity in children with mite allergy. Allergy 1999 (in press).

34. The ETAC Study Group. Pediatr Allergy Immunol 1998; 3:116.

Experimental Studies on Inhaled Corticosteroids Effects

PM O'Byrne*

Keywords: Asthma, inhaled corticosteroids, early intervention

Inhaled corticosteroids have evolved into the most useful and effective drugs currently available to treat asthma. The inhaled route is preferable to minimize unwanted effects. Inhaled corticosteroids improve the physiological abnormalities of variable airflow obstruction and airway hyperresponsiveness, that characterized asthma, as well as reducing the decline in lung function over time that occurs in asthmatics. Inhaled corticosteroids are also cost-beneficial when compared to other treatments, even in patients with milder asthma, treated in primary care. For these reasons, inhaled corticosteroids are now being considered the first line therapy for patients with regular, daily asthma symptoms, and should be started early after a diagnosis is made, rather than delaying until all other treatment options have been tried and not provided optimal control of asthma. There are, however, several issues about the early intervention with inhaled corticosteroids that have not yet been resolved. One such issue is whether inhaled corticosteroids should be used in asthmatic patients who have very mild and infrequent symptoms, or who develop symptoms only after being exposed to an inciting stimulus, such as exercise or cold air, and who have normal airway caliber most of the time. These asthmatics do have evidence of airway inflammation and structural changes in airway biopsies; however, we do not yet know whether they lose lung function more rapidly than nonasthmatics, or whether the morbidity of having very mild asthma warrants the use of regular treatment.

ly Gelfand [2] demonstrated clinical benefit from inhaled cortisone in a small group of patients with both allergic or nonallergic asthma. Subsequently, a multi-center trial run by the Medical Research Council in the United Kingdom demonstrated improvement in acute severe asthma in a placebo-controlled trial [3], and reports at that time described benefit in chronic asthma [4], demonstrating the unequivocal benefit of corticosteroids in asthma. Subsequently, both oral and inhaled corticosteroids have evolved into the most important and useful drugs currently available to treat asthma.

At the time of their introduction to clinical practice in the early 1970s, and for many years after this, the use of inhaled corticosteroids was mainly limited to patients who had persisting symptoms despite aggressive oral or inhaled bronchodilator use. The increased appreciation, in the mid 1980s, of the central role of airway inflammation in the pathogenesis of all asthma [5, 6, 7], provided a rationale for the earlier introduction of inhaled corticosteroids, particularly as the ability of inhaled corticosteroids to reduce airway inflammation [8] and improve some of the airway structural abnormalities associated with asthma was being identified. This has led to a reappraisal of how best inhaled corticosteroids may be used currently and in the future management of asthma.

Introduction

Corticosteroids have been used to treat a variety of airway diseases since the early 1950s. This was following an initial study of Carryer et al. [1], who reported the benefits of oral cortisone on ragweed pollen-induced hay fever and asthma. Subsequent-

Reasons for Earlier Intervention with Inhaled Corticosteroids

Early intervention with inhaled corticosteroids in asthma means beginning this treatment as the first

* Asthma Research Group, St. Joseph's Hospital and Department of Medicine, McMaster University, Hamilton, Ontario, Canada

regular treatment used after a diagnosis is established. An argument for early intervention with inhaled corticosteroids could be made if one or more of the following conditions were met:

1. Inhaled corticosteroids were *more effective* than other regular treatment to achieve optimal asthma control and meet the other treatment objectives.
2. Inhaled corticosteroids prevented the decline in lung function over time that occurs in asthmatics.
3. Inhaled corticosteroids were safer than an *equally effective* treatment modality.
4. Inhaled corticosteroids were cost beneficial as an initial treatment of asthma, as measured by a benefit to the patient and/or to society by reducing the morbidity of asthma, which was not available by using any other medication.

There is little debate in the literature that corticosteroids are the most effective treatment for asthma [9,10], and that the inhaled route is preferable to minimize unwanted effects. There is, however, considerable debate over the early use of inhaled corticosteroids in asthmatic patient considered to have mild asthma [11]. These patient are usually treated with regular inhaled β_2-agonists, or with drugs considered to be less clinically effective than inhaled corticosteroids, such as cromoglycate or nedocromil sodium. In a study of newly diagnosed asthmatics seen in specialty clinics, early intervention with

the inhaled corticosteroid, budesonide, was shown to be an effective first-line treatment, when compared with an inhaled β_2-agonist, as indicated by reduced symptoms, improvements in lung function, and improvements in methacholine airway hyperresponsiveness [12]. However, many patients considered to have mild asthma are not seen in specialty clinics but are managed in primary care practices. It is possible that these patients are, in fact, ideally controlled without the use of inhaled corticosteroids. To address this issue, one study has examined the efficacy and cost-benefit of inhaled corticosteroids, supplemented with bronchodilators as needed, compared to bronchodilators alone, as first line treatment of asthma in primary care practice [13]. This double blind study compared budesonide 400 µg/day, budesonide 800 µg/day, and placebo in patients considered by their primary care physician to have such mild asthma that they would not derive any clinical benefit from inhaled corticosteroids. The study demonstrated that low doses of an inhaled corticosteroid provided better asthma control (Figure 1), and is cost-beneficial, when compared to bronchodilators alone in the management of these patients with mild asthma and supports the early intervention with inhaled corticosteroids for adult patients with regular daily symptoms of asthma. In addition, the study reinforced the need to strive for optimal control of asthma, and once control is achieved, to identify the minimum amounts of medication needed to maintain control.

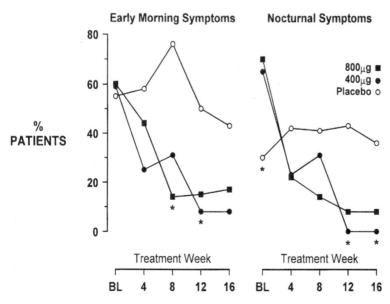

Figure 1. Proportion of patients considered by their family physician as having mild asthma, experiencing early morning symptoms or nocturnal symptoms in the month prior to evaluation at baseline and after treatment with inhaled budesonide at treatment weeks 4 to 16 for patients on placebo (O), budesonide 400 µg/day (●) and 800 µg/day (■). * $p < 0.05$, ** $p < 0.01$, *** $p < 0.001$. (Reproduced with permission from [13].)

Effects of Inhaled Corticosteroids on Lung Function over Time

Asthmatics lose lung function more rapidly than nonasthmatics [14], although less rapidly than cigarette smokers. In occasional asthmatics, this leads to severe, permanent, fixed airflow obstruction, with all of the attendant disability and handicap associated with this condition. A number of recent studies in both adults and children have demonstrated that inhaled steroids provide a protective effect against the deterioration in lung function seen with prolonged regular use of inhaled bronchodilator therapy alone. In one study [15], the investigators had evaluated subjects in whom they had previously reported that the treatment of newly diagnosed asthmatics with inhaled budesonide 1200 µg/day for 2 years improved asthma control as indicated by reduced symptoms, improvements in lung function, and improvements in methacholine airway hyperresponsiveness, when compared to inhaled β_2-agonists [12]. The subjects receiving budesonide were subsequently randomly allocated to continuing for a third year on a lower dose of inhaled budesonide (400 µg/day) or placebo. The improvements in all parameters were maintained on the lower dose of budesonide, but were lost on placebo. The subjects who had previously been treated with inhaled β_2-agonists only were treated with the higher dose of inhaled budesonide for the third year, and while they improved in all parame-

ters when compared to the first 2 years of treatment, the improvement in lung function or methacholine airway hyperresponsiveness was significantly less than that achieved by the subjects treated for the first year of the study with inhaled budesonide. This suggests that these asthmatics had lost lung function which might have been preserved with the early use of inhaled corticosteroids (Figure 2).

A study in asthmatic children has been reported by Agertoft and Pedersen [16], who have studied two cohorts for up to 7 years. One cohort had been treated with inhaled corticosteroids shortly after diagnosis, while the other had received a variety of other anti-asthma medications, including cromones, theophylline and regular inhaled β_2-agonists, but not inhaled corticosteroids. Some children in the second cohort were converted to inhaled corticosteroids, but on average 5 years after an initial diagnosis. These children in whom treatment with inhaled corticosteroids was started later did not achieve the level of lung function of the children treated early, even after 3 years of treatment with inhaled corticosteroids. The study also measured growth velocity in these children and concluded that doses of inhaled budesonide up to 400 µg/day was not associated with a reduction in growth velocity. A subsequent study in adult asthmatics, has confirmed these observations [17].

These studies, taken together, suggest that inhaled corticosteroids can diminish the decline in lung function that occurs in asthmatics, and that early intervention with inhaled corticosteroids can optimize lung function in asthmatics. Each of these studies, however, has limitations, mainly in that

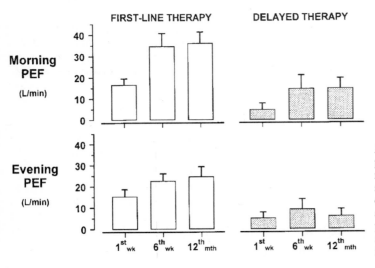

Figure 2. Comparison of the improvements in peak expired flow rates in patients treated with budesonide as first line therapy within one year of diagnosis of asthma and patients treated more than two years after diagnosis. (Redrawn and reproduced with permission from [15].)

none were explicitly designed to address this issue in a prospective fashion. Therefore, while the results are consistent between the studies, the results are not conclusive. This has lead to the development of a very large, multinational, prospective, randomized and placebo-controlled study of the effects of early intervention with inhaled corticosteroids in both childhood and adult asthma. This study, known as the START (Steroid Therapy As Regular Treatment) trial, will evaluate the potential beneficial effects of inhaled corticosteroids treatment started within the first two years of the development of asthma, in patients with very mild disease.

Future Trends in Inhaled Corticosteroid Use

These studies taken together suggest that low doses of inhaled corticosteroids will be used earlier in the onset of asthma and in patients with milder disease. The impact of earlier treatment on the progression of the disease is a critical issue, which needs to be evaluated in future studies. It is plausible that, by preventing the airway structural abnormalities associated with asthma, the development of fixed airflow obstruction and more severe disease can be prevented. Also, it is clear from the studies which have evaluated this, that the severity of asthma is often underappreciated by both patients and physicians. This leads to under-treatment, less than ideal asthma control, and the attendant effects on patients quality of life and increased costs to society. The only way to ensure that this does not happen, is to offer optimal treatment to all patients with established asthma, and this would most often be a therapeutic trial of inhaled corticosteroids.

Conclusions

Inhaled corticosteroids are the most effective medications currently available to treat symptomatic asthma, and are, fortunately, free of clinically relevant unwanted effects, when used in the doses needed to provide optimal control in most asthmatics. Inhaled corticosteroids also improve the physiological abnormalities of variable airflow obstruction and airway hyperresponsiveness, that charac-

terized asthma, as well as reducing the decline in lung function over time that occurs in asthmatics. Inhaled corticosteroids are also cost-beneficial when compared to other treatments, even in patients with milder asthma, treated in primary care. For these reasons, inhaled corticosteroids are now being considered the first line therapy for patients with regular, daily asthma symptoms, and should be started early after a diagnosis is made, rather than delaying until all other treatment options have been tried and not provided optimal control of asthma.

There are, however, several issues about the early intervention with inhaled corticosteroids that have not yet been resolved. One such issue is whether inhaled corticosteroids should be used in asthmatic patients who have very mild and infrequent symptoms, or who develop symptoms only after being exposed to an inciting stimulus, such as exercise or cold air, and who have normal airway calibre most of the time. The current consensus statements do not recommend regular treatment in such patients, and this recommendation should be adhered to until more information is available about the natural history of asthma in such patients. These asthmatics do have evidence of airway inflammation and structural changes in airway biopsies; however, we do not yet know whether they lose lung function more rapidly than nonasthmatics, or whether the morbidity of having very mild asthma warrants the use of regular treatment. This information may be available when the results of the START trial are available. Also, not enough is yet known about the long term effects of even low doses of inhaled corticosteroids. Although the studies of Agertoft and Pedersen [16] has provided details of up to 7 years of treatment on some of the potential unwanted effects in children, these studies may need to be more prolonged before the concerns and fears of using inhaled corticosteroids very early in asthma will be allayed.

Address for correspondence:

PM O'Byrne
Firestone Regional Chest and Allergy Unit
St. Joseph's Hospital
50 Charlton Ave East
Hamilton, Ontario L8N 4A6
Canada
Tel. +1 905 521-6115 ext. 3694
Fax +1 905 521-6125
E-mail obyrnep@fhs.mcmaster.ca

References

1. Carryer HM, Koelshe GA, Prickman LE, et al. The effect of cortisone on bronchial asthma and hay fever occurring in subjects sensitive to ragweed pollen. J Allergy 1950; 21:282–287.

2. Gelfand ML. Administration of cortisone by the aerosol method in the treatment of bronchial asthma. N Engl J Med 1951; 245:293–294.

3. Medical Research Council. Controlled trial of effects of cortisone acetate in status asthmaticus. Lancet 1956; 2:803–806.

4. Foulds GS, Greaves DP, Herxheimer H, Kingdom LG. Hydrocortisone in treatment of allergic conjunctivitis, allergic rhinitis, and bronchial asthma. Lancet 1955; 1:234–235.

5. O'Byrne PM. Airway inflammation and airway hyperresponsiveness [Review]. Chest 1986; 90:575–577.

6. Kirby JG, Hargreave FE, Gleich GJ, O'Byrne PM. Bronchoalveolar cell profiles of asthmatic and non-asthmatic subjects. Am Rev Respir Dis 1987; 136:379–383.

7. Beasley R, Roche WR, Roberts JA, Holgate ST. Cellular events in the bronchi in mild asthma and after bronchial provocation. Am Rev Respir Dis 1989; 139:806–817.

8. Jeffery PK, Godfrey RW, Adelroth E, Nelson F, Rogers A, Johansson SA. Effects of treatment on airway inflammation and thickening of basement membrane reticular collagen in asthma. A quantitative light and electron microscopic study. Am Rev Respir Dis 1992; 145:890–899.

9. Barnes PJ, Pedersen S. Efficacy and safety of inhaled corticosteroids in asthma. Am Rev Respir Dis 1993; 148:S1–S26.

10. Pedersen S, O'Byrne PM. A comparison of the efficacy and safety of inhaled corticosteroids in asthma. Allergy 1997; 52:1–34.

11. Drazen J, Israel E. Treating mild asthma, when are inhaled steroids indicated? N Engl J Med 1994; 331:737–738.

12. Haahtela T, Jarvinen M, Tuomo K, Kiviranta K, Koskinen S, Lehtonen K, et al. Comparison of a β2-antagonist, terbutaline, with an inhaled corticosteroid, budesonide, in newly detected asthma. N Engl J Med 1991; 325:388–392.

13. O'Byrne PM, Cuddy L, Taylor DW, Birch S, Morris J, Syrotiuk J. The clinical efficacy and cost benefit of inhaled corticosteroids as therapy in patients with mild asthma in primary care practice. Can Resp J 1996; 3:169–175.

14. Lange P, Parner J, Vestbo J, Schnohr P, Jensen G. A 15-year follow-up study of ventilatory function in adults with asthma. N Engl J Med 1998; 339:1194–1200.

15. Haahtela T, Jarvinen M, Kava T, et al. Effects of reducing or discontinuing inhaled budesonide in patients with mild asthma. N Engl J Med 1994; 331:700–705.

16. Agertoft L, Pedersen S. Effects of long-term treatment with an inhaled corticosteroid on growth and pulmonary function in asthmatic children. Respir Med 1994; 88:373–381.

17. Selroos O, Pietinalho A, Lofroos AB, Riska H. Effect of early vs late intervention with inhaled corticosteroids in asthma. Chest 1995; 108:1228–1234.

Index of Keywords*

---

* This index was prepared on the basis of the keywords supplied by the authors. The page numbers refer to the first page of the chapter referring to the subject.

Index of Authors